11/2/75

AMERICAN MEDICAL AVARICE

AMERICAN MEDICAL AVARICE

by Ruth Mulvey Harmer

ABELARD-SCHUMAN   New York

Designed by Jack Meserole

Manufactured in the United States of America

Library of Congress Cataloging in Publication Data

Harmer, Ruth Mulvey.
   American medical avarice.
   Includes bibliographical references and index.
   1. Medical fees—United States. 2. Physicians—
United States. 3. Medical economics—United States.
I. Title.
R728.5.H37   1975   338.4'7'36210973   74-9370
ISBN 0-200-04025-1

10 9 8 7 6 5 4 3 2 1

1382036

In another year, I promised that
this book would be for dearest Lowell and Lisa.
It is for them still—with all love.

Contents

Foreword

Here is a book for which the people of America have waited long and all too patiently.

We have known that "something" was radically wrong with the way in which we receive—or do not receive—the medical care we need. But we have not known what that "something" was.

We have known that the cost of doctors' care and especially of hospital care has risen faster than any other element in the sky-rocketing cost of living.

But we have not known why.

We have known that there weren't enough doctors and that those there were concentrated in high income areas, leaving vast rural areas and core cities with hardly any physicians at all.

But we have understood only vaguely why this was so.

Many of us, those fortunate enough to *have* a family doctor, have loved and respected him, and then have wondered why the American Medical Association, to which he in all probability belonged, acted so very differently from the image we had of that family doctor.

We have not understood this.

We have found out that the drug industry is the second most profitable industry—next to oil—in the entire economy. And we have wondered why necessary drugs and medicines cost so much. And why our druggist could not sell us generic drugs at half the price of the branded ones. We have wanted our doctors to be well paid but we have been surprised to find that the medical profession, which is supposed to be devoted to service to people, should have been willing to push the incomes of its members to such heights that physicians as a class make the highest incomes of any occupational group except corporation executives.

It has astonished us to find the American Medical Association opposing almost every proposal for social progress or the relief of human need.

But we have not understood why this was so.

We have wondered why twice as many surgical operations of the same kind take place in the United States as in many other countries.

We have wondered why medical practice has concentrated so much on "wonder drugs" and neglected such basic roads to health as adequate nutrition, free and widespread immunizations, a clean environment and decent housing for the poor.

Especially has it seemed strange to us that the medical-care system—if such it can be called—was geared almost exclusively to episodic curing of disease after it has become serious, instead of to prevention of illness before it occurs in severe form. Stranger still, we have been spending billions for sickness insurance and have found so few ways to provide ourselves with health assurance.

We have wondered about all this but we have not had adequate answers to why these things were so.

Not until Ruth Harmer wrote the book which follows.

But now at last we can begin to understand why all these strange things have been happening to us. Thanks to monumental and meticulously careful research this author has laid out the facts for everyone to see.

She tells us why.

She does far more than that. She suggests a number of things that can be done about the matter—group health prepayment plans for example whose business it is to keep their members well, to control costs, to prescribe expensive drugs and even more expensive operations only when truly necessary, to prevent disease and keep people out of hospitals.

Dr. Harmer's book contains plenty of warnings—warnings about dangerous drugs and why there has been no more protection by government agencies against their use than has been the case. Warnings too that the state of health of the American people as a whole is deteriorating not improving. And warnings about the dangers in nursing homes that are in violation of standards supposed to be prescribed for them.

But in each chapter there are suggested remedies. Out of each gloomy, disheartening story of what has been and is, there shines a ray of light, of hope; if only we the people will rouse ourselves and begin to act in our own defense.

This is a book that almost wasn't. In its original form, different only in its dating, the book was to have been published three years ago. The then prospective publisher had even prepared advertising copy for promotion of the book.

And then it happened. No. The publisher had decided not to publish after all. Why? Well for various reasons—none clearly stated and none very convincing. They just weren't going to do it.

Maybe when the reader has finished absorbing the array of hard facts about the record of the AMA which this book contains —when he sees how fearless the author has been, once her research was complete—then he will begin to understand why he has had to wait three years for the answers to his many disturbing questions.

Maybe too the book will inspire the conscientious doctors of the nation, of whom there are, of course, thousands, to revolt against AMA policies and perform a miracle of change therein.

American Medical Avarice is a timely book if ever there was one.

For there is no doubt that this nation faces its hour of decision in respect to health and medical care. The present solo-practice, fee-for-service system—if such it can be called—is simply no longer able to protect the health of American families at a cost which any but the richest of them can afford.

In 1940 there were 83 general practitioners for every 100,000 persons. By 1967 there were only 32. The traditional family doctor–patient relationship is becoming rare; fewer and fewer families know what doctor to go to for what ailment; and all too often they go not at all until illness has become acute.

Core cities and rural areas are becoming medical care "deserts," with fewer and fewer physicians being willing to practice there. They go to the more affluent suburbs instead and for understandable economic reasons.

The episodic, emergency type of service to which solo, fee-for-service practice leads is wasteful of both health and resources. Lack of rational organization leads to overinvestment—and needless duplication of investment—in the kind of very expensive equipment and facilities which medical technology now requires. There are too many unnecessary operations performed—twice the number per capita that take place in England and Wales, for example. Nor does solo practice make possible the full development of the services of nurse–practitioners or Medex, thus enabling the fully trained physician to increase his efficiency. Only in a group practice setting is such development safe and practical. There are too few ambulatory and extended care facilities, perhaps a few too many acute care hospitals.

Even were no other factors involved, the astronomical increases in the cost of medical care under the present system necessitate change and reform. A year's hospitalization at current charges will cost a family some $40,000. The cost of health care has risen 66 percent per capita over the past five years. Ten years ago the average cost of a hospital day was $45. Today it is more than $100. Although 80 percent of the people have some form of health insurance, claims pay only about 40 percent of the total cost—the rest comes out of the family pocket book, or the taxpayers'. Overemphasis on *hospital* insurance to the exclusion of primary care protection has, it is estimated, caused one hospital bed in four to be occupied by someone who need not be there.

On the other hand group practice prepayment direct service plans have as their main objective to keep people ambulatory and out of the hospital. They are in the business of health maintenance first and foremost. The health maintenance organization (HMO) at its best represents the only attempt in this country to date to rationalize the health care of people, and they do sharply reduce the overall cost. They begin with primary, ambulatory care and they share with their members, at all times, the risks of keeping them healthy. And they are controlled by or in the interest of consumers.

The record of the genuine nonprofit prepayment group health plans is such as to suggest that in a broad proliferation of such plans might be found not only the antidote to the excesses of the AMA of which Dr. Harmer's book speaks but also a better answer to the nation's health-care problem than can be found in any other approach.

Group practice by a balanced team of general practioners and specialists makes possible efficient use by all of them of laboratory, operational, and other expensive equipment which modern medicine requires. Group practice also makes possible ready—and costless—referral of patients by the family doctor to the appropriate specialist. Again, group practice in a direct service comprehensive care plan makes it possible for doctors to be available 24 hours a day every day of the year to care for patients' needs, but also enables members of the team to have undisturbed time off duty, periods of vacation, and opportunity for study.

Most important of all perhaps, group practice in the setting of a prepayment direct service plan enables physicians to practice medical care as it should be practiced. For two principal reasons. First they no longer have to concern themselves with the economic details of solo practice. Their income is assured, and they can spend all their time and energy on the task of keeping the subscribers to their plan in the best possible health. The better job they do, the fewer serious sicknesses that take place, the fewer operations that have to be performed, the less will be their burdens. But their compensation will remain at the same or an even higher level. Second, because the subscribers to the genuine health maintenance organization have already paid for comprehensive care, they are inclined to give the doctor a chance to practice preventive medicine. Instead of waiting, because of fear of exorbitant cost, until sickness has already become serious members of group health plans will usually take advantage of their prepayment by seeing the doctor in the early stages of illness. They will report for periodic check-ups. They will submit to tests, immunizations, and screenings. In fact, the subscribers to a demo-cratically controlled plan are in a position to demand the best of care. For they have paid for it.

The record of such plans speaks for itself. Subscribers to such plans as Group Health Cooperative of Puget Sound or the Kaiser Plans spend year after year less then half the number of days in the hospital, per capita, as do people covered by commercial in-surance or even by Blue Cross. Such subscribers are operated upon less often. In 1966 group health plans averaged only 31 operations per 1000 persons enrolled, compared to 73 per 1000 in Blue Shield Plans.

Since hospital costs and the expenses of operations are the main factors in the escalating cost of medical care, this is why the genuine HMO offers the best hope of checking those rising costs.

The objective and the motivation is, as has been said, to keep people healthy. Everyone associated with such plans has not only a humanitarian but an *economic* reason for pursuing that objec-tive. To that end there are peer reviews of the quality of care, frequent staff consultations, unified complete medical records, ready referrals, and one-stop centers where all kinds of care are available.

When, under these circumstances, a public welfare agency con-tracts to pay a group health plan for the care of a prescribed num-ber of people, and to do so on a capitation basis, the quality of care received by these people is certain to be raised. For all the advantages of the plan's members are available also to the clients of the public agency. And where the information is available—as in Seattle (GHC of PS) and Portland (Kaiser)—we find that the low-income people are receiving high quality comprehensive care at less cost to the public agency paying the capitation than it formerly cost that agency to pay for hit-and-miss episodic care on a fee-for-service basis.

The 176,000 members of Group Health Cooperative of Puget Sound averaged less than half as much as the general population per capita for total cost of drugs in 1972. This plan operates its own pharmacy and drug formulary. Further the hospital costs averaged only $47 per member, compared to a national average of $135.

In general, well-conducted community-based prepayment group-practice plans can save their family members some 25 to 50 percent of what comparable indemnity insurance would cost them.

For decades the movement for this rational method of organizing the delivery of health care and making it available to large numbers of people faced a bitter struggle for existence. For years the AMA opposed such plans and at times attempted to deny physicians associated with them membership in medical societies.

Today all is different. The HMO is suddenly popular. Congress has passed landmark legislation to encourage their development.

And therein lies a lethal danger. It is the danger of prostitution of the concept of group practice, prepayment, direct service, and comprehensive care to private profit. It is the danger of inexperienced people setting up such plans without concern for the welfare of the subscribers to them.

Already the charlatans have moved in. The Auditor General of California has reported that out of $56 million paid by the State Department of Health to supposed health maintenance organizations, 52 percent of that amount was spent for "administration" and only 48 percent for health-care services.

This is what will happen as long as almost anyone is permitted to set up an HMO. That opportunity should be restricted—above all any governmental aid should be restricted—to persons and organizations such as the Group Health Association of America, who can demonstrate both adequate experience and a commitment to the service motive.

The motivation is the all-important matter.

If a farm or labor organization, a city government, an organization of consumers, Blue Cross, a dedicated group of physicians, or even a far-sighted insurance company initiates a plan for the sole purpose of meeting the health needs of people and controlling the cost of medical and hospital care, the motivation will be one of preventing illness, keeping subscribers as well as possible, providing such services as are necessary to accomplish this. The very essence of the effort of such plans will be to so care for the health of subscribers that they will remain ambulatory and not need hospitalization. But if the motivation is private profit for some third party—not providers of service or consumers thereof— then that third party's motivation will tend to be—perhaps inevitably will be—to keep services at a minimum and to compensate the staff at as low a rate as possible.

At present only about six million people in the United States have the advantage of comprehensive and continuous health care in a genuine cooperative group health prepayment plan.

That number could grow significantly in the years to come. It could grow if more employers would emulate Henry Kaiser. It could grow if more mayors would do what Fiorello La Guardia did when he established Health Insurance Plan of Greater New York. It could grow if more labor unions would do what a Teamsters local did in St. Louis when The Labor Health Institute was established there. It could grow if groups of ordinary citizens pooled their time, effort, and money as some of them did in establishing Group Health Cooperative of Puget Sound.

Federal financial help will be needed and on a scale such as Senator Kennedy originally proposed, not on the scale recently provided by the Congress.

But if thirty million people instead of six million were enrolled in good nonprofit health-maintenance plans and if public agencies contracted with them for care of those in greatest need, then their competition in the health care field could do wonders in transforming the delivery of good medical care to the American people as a whole.

And Ruth Harmer's book would not have been in vain.

Ruth Harmer is no "Johnny-come-lately" author. She is an experienced defender of the public good, a careful, seasoned expositor of wrongs and dangers in our society. Her *High Cost of Dying* exposed the abuses of the funeral business, and her *Unfit For Human Consumption* warned of the adulteration of soils and food with pesticides.

She should be listened to.

JERRY VOORHIS

Introduction:
Problems and Paradoxes

My introduction to the profoundly paradoxical nature of American medicine occurred on a sweltering afternoon one August 12 years ago when my husband, who had set off for the library a few minutes earlier, ran down the steps calling, "Phone for an ambulance. Mrs. Blanco has been hurt—badly, I think. She's beside the road, near her house."

I called the city's emergency service, asked that an ambulance be sent, and followed him down the street to wait with Mrs. Blanco. She was sitting on the grass, poised as a Buddha, with her gray, all-season coat bundled about her. One leg stuck out awkwardly before her, the heavy cotton stocking ripped and blood-stained from her fall. Halfway between knee and ankle, a thin sliver of bone protruded through flesh and stocking.

"Don't trouble yourselves," she reassured us calmly, in the rich Boston accent that 40 years in California had not altered. "It's nothing. I'll be all right." I winced, feeling again the nerve-torturing pain of a broken bone. But we played the be-cheerful-it's-nothing game: Mrs. Blanco, my husband, the woman who had been walking up the hill with her when she fell, and I.

The emergency ambulance arrived in less than half an hour. The driver and attendant got a stretcher and, with surprising gentleness, had her settled in a few minutes. Her friend elected to accompany her; and I said, just before the ambulance doors were shut, "If you need anything, call." It was then four-thirty.

A few minutes after seven that evening, the phone rang. "I don't know what to do," Mrs. Blanco's friend wailed. "You've got to help. The ambulance took us to White Memorial Hospital, and we've been here since. But nobody has done anything."

We got into the Microbus and drove the few miles to the hospital, which has one of the finest reputations in Los Angeles. Mrs. Blanco's companion met us at the door and led us into a corridor beyond the lobby; there we found Mrs. Blanco lying on a high, wheeled stretcher-bed. The lines in her face had deepened, but she managed a smile.

My husband and I went to the admitting desk to find out why she was lying there untreated. The woman in charge was remarkably calm. No one had done anything, she agreed. No one "could" do anything until the relative whose name Mrs. Blanco had given on her arrival had been located. Treatment had to be authorized, she said. She did not make it clear why Mrs. Blanco's authorization was not enough. "The bill must be guaranteed." When we objected further, she shrugged: "You could try another hospital."

When we went back to the corridor to consult with Mrs. Blanco, she asked us to do just that. An orderly helped us to wheel her out to the Volkswagen Microbus and settle her on the floor in the back since the center seat had been removed. Mrs. Blanco's friend and I sat beside her to keep her leg from moving.

We drove a short distance to the French Hospital, another reputable and sizable institution in Los Angeles. A young attendant brought out a wheelchair and helped us to get Mrs. Blanco inside. It was then about eight-thirty—four hours since she had been driven off in the ambulance.

The uniformed woman on duty in the front office said that she could do nothing for us. A doctor would have to admit Mrs. Blanco, and "unfortunately" no staff doctor was available. "Maybe you can find a doctor to sign her in. There's a telephone booth down the hall."

We pooled dimes, and I started to work my way down the list of physicians in the yellow pages of the telephone directory, emerging from time to time from the stifling booth with "no luck" bulletins. I decided to make another appeal to the woman at the desk. "It's too bad," she said politely. When I asked her about some doctor in the hospital checking on Mrs. Blanco, she pointed to a man walking down the hallway: "You can try him, but he's off duty."

The off-duty doctor heard us out, looked at Mrs. Blanco with mild interest, and said that there was nothing he could do. "I'm a cancer specialist," he added, as if that explained everything.

My husband suggested that I call the city's receiving hospital nearby to say that we were taking Mrs. Blanco there. People there would have to do something. By that time, I was beginning to feel that unless some magic word were found the nightmare would continue. I dialed the receiving hospital and told the man who answered that we were on our way. "If you refuse to help," I said, "we are going to call the newspapers, our councilman, the mayor. . . ." I think I got as far as the governor.

"Don't get excited, lady," the man soothed. "Our guys would have brought her here this afternoon, but regulations are that pickups have to be taken to the nearest private hospital unless they ask specifically to be taken here for treatment."

The black attendant who had helped us in was the only person we had met who exhibited any real compassion or concern. He got Mrs. Blanco settled in the Microbus, and we then took her to the city receiving hospital. There an orderly and a young doctor lifted her onto a stretcher and carried her into the examining room. The doctor was reassuring. He and his assistant worked quickly, cleansing the wound, applying a splint. All the while, he complimented Mrs. Blanco on her courage. "That's a nasty fracture," he patted her shoulder, "but you'll be all right." For the first time, I saw tears in her eyes.

"There's nothing else for you to do," he dismissed the rest of us. "We'll get her to County Hospital right away." It was then a little after eleven, seven and a half hours since we had made the first call for help.

When Mrs. Blanco was ready to be discharged from the hospital, where her leg had been set and she had been treated for a week, she refused to go to a nursing home. "I couldn't stand any more of this kind of thing," she said, gesturing around the ward where I had gone to visit her.

I appreciated her feeling. The crowded ward gave the impression of something conceived by Jonathan Swift in one of his more savage moods. Some of the elderly women in the beds that lined the place seemed less human than vegetable. They were lying in stupor, fed by solutions dripped into their veins from bottles on racks beside their beds. In one corner, a near skeleton with closed eyes sang hymns in a monotone; another woman moaned steadily; another, beside Mrs. Blanco, carried on a furious and continuing argument with herself.

Mrs. Blanco elected to go home, even though she knew that it would be some time before she could walk unaided. She wanted privacy and was concerned about finances, for the bill for hospital and medical treatment had been almost $500. Also, she felt that she could manage with the aid of her friend, who volunteered to help with the cooking and cleaning. Mrs. Blanco decided that she could prepare some of her food on a hot plate set near her bed. For some time, all was well; but two days after Christmas, a blanket touching the electrical wires caught fire. Mrs. Blanco was dead by the time the firemen arrived.

It was, the local paper noted in the report, "an unfortunate accident."

But accident seemed too easy a word to use about her ordeal and death. Surely there was something wrong with a health-care system that allowed such things to happen. Something was and something is.

Great changes have occurred in American medicine since Mrs. Blanco died—scientific advances, the establishment of social programs like Medicare and Medicaid. But what has not changed is that we have allowed a horse-and-buggy system of medical economics to be used to carry to the American people the space age developments in medical science. And despite changes, things remain the same.

For the past decade and more, newspapers, magazines, radio and television stations, books, and talks have heralded the gains made to heal the sick and prolong life. Physicists, biologists, chemists, and technicians have created ingenious devices to alter damaged functions and replace disabled parts. Laboratories and factories turn out the stuff with which to *rebuild* man: Dacron veins, arteries, and blood vessels; ceramic and metal bones, stainless-steel and plastic joints, silicone tracheas and intestinal walls. Artificial heart valves are now commonly inserted; and natural bones, arteries, substitutes for corneas, kidneys, and even hearts are being transplanted. Surgical instruments of remarkable delicacy allow access to every part of the body; laser beams of intensified light and streams of liquid nitrogen are replacing the scalpel. Telemetric monitoring systems developed in space flight research are being used to detect heart and brain disturbances, skin response, blood pressure. Thermographs record internal processes in terms of infra-red heat emissions. Tiny Geiger counters implanted with hypodermic needles in inoperable tumors allow physicians to predict in hours the value of prescribed drug therapy. Electronic devices prod ailing bladders and allow tortured sufferers from cancer and other ills to "tune in" on respite from pain. Light is being used to kill cancer, and light-dark cycles to influence and regulate hormonal and biochemical processes.

Antibiotics, vitamins, hormones, and other "wonder" drugs are used to avert, arrest, and reverse the course of physical and mental decay. They defend man from the plagues and epidemics that have tormented the race from the beginning of time. Able to penetrate the system's most secret places to kill invading infections and regulate failing processes, they have opened up the mysterious recesses of the mind, breaking down emotional barriers, flooding darkness with light.

Historically, whenever science has achieved a great leap forward, cultural lag—that gap between new knowledge and traditional thought—has hindered its wide application. That was true of earlier revolutions in medical science that occurred in Egypt, when priest-physicians translated into living terms the anatomical knowledge of the *Book of the Dead*; in Greece, when Hippocrates established the foundations of medical science; in seventeenth-century England, when William Harvey transformed physiology with his discoveries about the circulation of the blood; in nineteenth-century Europe, when the Industrial Revolution helped to telescope centuries of medical history into a few decades. Gains made then were regarded as the property of the privileged few.

But when modern medicine began its breakthroughs a generation ago, scientific advances were paralleled by a change in social thinking. The gains, it was universally agreed, were to be placed in the service of humanity. Americans formally pledged themselves to that concept after World War II, when they helped to set up the World Health Organization, which holds that: "The enjoyment of the highest attainable standard of health is one of the fundamental rights of every human being." That pledge seemed near fulfillment during the 1960s, when President Lyndon Johnson signed into law the Medicare and Medicaid programs—guaranteeing medical care to millions of older Americans and the seriously deprived.

Americans willingly contributed to foreign-aid programs so that others might have health care. In even more open-handed manner they have been investing in it for themselves and their families. In 1950, the nation's health expenditures were $12,027,000,000; by 1973, they had risen to $94,070,000,000;[1] by 1974 they had reached more than the $100,000,000,000 mark. And they have continued to soar since.

What were they getting for that money?

They have been assured constantly that they are receiving the best medical care in the world: that since the turn of the century the death rate has been halved; that killer diseases like tuberculosis, pneumonia, influenza, diphtheria, and whooping cough have become minor illness. But that has happened all around the world, in countries where people spend far less money for health care. And many of those countries had made far more striking gains. America has fallen far behind in the longevity race. According to the *United Nations Demographic Yearbook, 1973*, life expectancy for American males was less than for men in such medically advanced countries as Sweden, Norway, Denmark, Israel, England, the Netherlands, Belgium, Iceland, France, Switzerland, Australia, New Zealand, the German Democratic Republic, and even such countries as Bulgaria, Greece, Italy, Puerto Rico, and Ireland.[2] Infant mortality, which some medical experts consider "the most sensitive barometer of the health of a nation," is cause for even greater concern, when the record of the United States is compared with those of other nations. In 1964, this country ranked eleventh; within a decade it had dropped to below twentieth place. Organized medicine insists that the U.S. is on the same plateau with countries like Sweden, Norway, Japan, and other advanced countries; but the 1972 U.S. rate of 18.5 deaths per every 1000 live births is not on the level with 10.8 in Sweden, 12.8 in Norway, and 12.4 in Japan—to say nothing of a country like Iceland, where it is only 12.9.[3] Organized medicine has also sought to dismiss differences by saying that other factors are involved. However, the comprehensive and significant study of all births in New York City in 1968 made recently under the direction of the National Academy of Sciences showed clearly that if all pregnant women had received adequate medical care, the infant death rate in the city would have been only 14.7 instead of the 21.9 per 1000 live births recorded that year.[4]

The high incidence of acute and chronic diseases indicates a serious lack of preventive medical care and even the "crisis" care organized medicine favors. In asking the Senate to override the President's veto of the Emergency Medical Services Act of 1973, Senator Alan Cranston pointed out that 175,000 persons die needlessly each year because they are unable to get adequate medical assistance in an emergency involving an accident, a heart attack, or a stroke.[5] Sometimes, an example of that makes headlines, as in 1974 when a Chicago physician admitted that he failed to respond to an emergency call because the patient's daughter was unable to produce his $30 fee in cash. The patient, a fifty-nine-year-old woman, died of shock eight hours later.[6] More often, however, it is a matter of silent suffering. And what of the chronic diseases that afflict millions of Americans—blindness, deafness, respiratory ills, diabetes, mental and nervous disorders, heart conditions, crippling ailments—that afflict millions, even children, and that could have been averted by adequate medical care?[7] Recent studies have shown that between 20 and 40 percent of children in low income areas suffer from one or more chronic diseases; fewer than half are under treatment. What of the millions of senior citizens whose health care had been insured by Medicare in 1966, but who have given up going to the doctor because they simply do not have the money to pay for the huge increases in premiums?[8] Why should middle class families live with the constant fear of what would happen to them if someone was injured or became ill and the insurance ran out?

This book attempts to answer the question of why we are a sick nation. The answer is complex since it deals with many aspects of our inefficient, inequitable, and often ineffective system. But any consideration of the subject must begin and end with the role of the American Medical Association, whose practices and policies reflect the triumph of nineteenth-century medical economics over twentieth-century medical science.

1 Monopolizing Medicine

The dual nature of the American Medical Association was revealingly portrayed on a cover of its *Journal* in 1972, an issue commemorating the 125th anniversary of its founding. With a primitive's eye for detail, the artist vividly recreated that May afternoon in 1847 in the hall of the Academy of Natural Sciences in Philadelphia: the crowded room, the earnest faces of the frock-coated delegates, and the determined handclasp given the first president by a temporary chairman. With a scientist's concern for accuracy, the artist drew in the forefront, its skull and tusks arched over the gathering, the towering skeleton of a mastodon, an ancient symbol of things to come.[1]

The AMA's contradictory qualities are mirrored in the contrast between its scientific and economic policies, its public pronouncements about national well-being, and its private struggles for profit and power.

At the first annual meeting in 1848, President Nathaniel Chapman had glowed proudly: "This assemblage presents a spectacle of moral grandeur delightful to contemplate." A century later, President Harry S. Truman called it disdainfully "just another mean trust."

Some outsiders have agreed with President Truman, characterizing it even more savagely. Others hold it to be the country's most prestigious scientific organization. And within the profession, that dualistic attitude also prevails. Many doctors insist that it is responsible for America's "medical greatness." But a growing number have been indicating that it has nothing to say to or for

9

them. Among the latter is a physician on the faculty of a major medical school, author of *The Healers,* who wrote recently:

> If anything could accurately mirror the disgusting result of practicing medicine almost solely for profit and only secondarily as a healing science and art, it would have to be the American Medical Association.
>
> Deliberately, consciously and very openly, the A.M.A. has patterned its philosophy and its course of action to achieve the goals deemed most important by a majority of its membership. The A.M.A. *is* today's typical entrenched doctor, with all his cupidity and fraud writ large indeed.[2]

No hint was given at that first meeting that the AMA would follow any but the highest path. The 232 delegates were bent on reforming the dismal state of American medicine. Quacks and charlatans and cultists were bilking and murdering people freely under the guise of providing health care. Many of the medical schools were peddling diplomas for a modest sum; in most states it was possible to practice without even the formality of a mail-order diploma.

The AMA proposed to change all that, spelling out as its purpose that it would upgrade medical education, establish standards for medical practice, promote "the usefulness, honor, and interests" of the medical profession, educate public opinion, advance medical knowledge, encourage concerted action by physicians. It held that its existence was "solely for improvement and helpfulness in everything related to the prosperity and well-being not only of every member of the profession as a whole, but of every citizen."[3]

For long that seemed to be the case. The AMA demanded that governments enact health laws and that "government agencies be run for the protection of the people and not for commercial interests." Under the leadership of men like Dr. William C. Gorgas, Dr. Alexander Lambert, Dr. Isaac M. Rubinow, and others, it sought out and challenged diploma mills, charlatans, political machines, and big businessmen, taking on along the way homeopaths, Christian Scientists, antivivisectionists, and "the Lord knows what else," as the editor of the *Journal of the American Medical Association* railed in 1911.[4] When governments dragged their feet, the AMA prodded them into action or hauled them along in its wake.

To give dignity and safety to American medical care, no risk seemed too great. The powerful drug industry was a particular target. In 1916, when the AMA was brought to the edge of financial ruin by a jury verdict in favor of the makers of "Wine of Cardui," a high-proof alcoholic "remedy" for female ills, the organization nevertheless hailed victory in defeat: "Technically guilty; morally justified."[5] The Council on Pharmacy and Chemistry attacked drug makers for other products; it attempted to end the Bayer aspirin monopoly and other patent practices.

Within a quarter of a century, however, former foes had become leading allies. Instead of inspiring governments to act, the AMA was building roadblocks to hold back every effort to extend medical care; far from fighting court battles with drug makers, the AMA was accepting millions from them. The AMA had made medical care a superbusiness and turned scalpels into swords to defend it from those who envisioned it as something more.

As is frequently the case with institutions and organizations, the decline was built into the rise—the fall made possible only by the highest aspirations.

Medical historians generally agree that the turning point, the Great Attitudinal Shift, came at the annual meeting in New Orleans in 1920, during a confrontation between the socially concerned doctors and the medical entrepreneurs over the issue of a comprehensive national health-insurance program. Actually, however, American medicine's rise to scientific distinction and its descent to flagrant profiteering began in 1904, when the AMA created a Council on Medical Education to encourage the country's medical schools to raise standards. During the last half of the nineteenth century, medical education became such a get-rich-quick business that the number of schools had multiplied wildly, from 52 in 1850 to 160 by 1900. Investigation by the Council revealed only about half the number to be "acceptable": the other half were either "doubtful" or frankly "unsatisfactory."[6]

Concerned that the report might be considered partisan, the Council on Medical Education helped to persuade the Carnegie Foundation to study the schools. The findings were thoroughly detailed in 1910 in Abraham Flexner's report on *Medical Education in the United States and Canada.* People were shocked by the findings; most schools accepted students with only a grammar-school education, if that. A number of them were simply offices from which degrees were mailed to "students" who sent in the required fees.[7]

The AMA proposed itself as the organization to bring about an improvement, and Americans were so shocked by the widely publicized findings that it was given free rein. The AMA acted swiftly, effectively, drastically. By 1915, the number of medical schools had been cut to 104; by 1920, to 88; by 1925, to 80; by 1930, to 76.[8] Good new schools were not encouraged to replace the bad old ones. Instead, the AMA began to openly advocate a policy of "professional birth control" that some doctors had been urging since 1904.[9] Medical schools were not-so-delicately threatened about admitting more students. The weapon used was the continuing survey of schools by the AMA's Council on Medical Education and Hospitals. The AMA president in 1934 said:

> it will require real courage and tenacity to bend the educational processes to the urgent social and economic needs of the changing order. *A fine piece of educational work could be well done if we were to use only half of the seventy-odd medical schools in the United States.* (Italics added.)[10]

The medical schools got the message, as the Council was able to reassure the AMA three years later. They reduced enrollment significantly and continued to do that for almost twenty years.

The AMA was understandably elated about the effects of the reduced enrollment policy on the "welfare" of the future practitioner. It succeeded in blocking measure after measure to expand medical schools. Finally, in 1960, President Kennedy acted on reports that, just to *maintain* the ratio of physicians to the population, 20 new medical schools were needed in a decade. Only then did the AMA acknowledge there was some cause for concern about the number of doctors being graduated. Nevertheless, it has continued opposition.

Until very recently, deans of the medical schools have gone along with the AMA. After all, their institutions were in on the very good thing. As Dr. John H. Knowles, former director of the Massachusetts General Hospital, pointed out to a Senate subcommittee a couple of years ago, the Association of American Medical Colleges has been "as conservative and backward as the AMA." He added: "the two major political forces of American medicine . . . have stuck their heads in the sand and put their backside to the socio-economic problem of medicine."[11]

As a result, all the while the AMA denied that the "birth control" policy would have any effect on medical care, the shortage of doctors was becoming so acute that this country was raiding have-little nations like India, Turkey, Iran, Korea, Spain, and Brazil. By 1972, one half of the net addition to the ranks of physicians in the United States were foreign graduates. Additionally, what the *New England Journal of Medicine* in 1974 called a "medical underground" was flourishing; without certification, without license, as many as 9000 were believed to be working in hospitals and clinics—the majority of them responsible for direct patient care.[12]

The shortage has been exacerbated by the trend toward specialization, as is noted in a later chapter, and by the AMA's determination to eliminate competition, labeling any effort to extend medical care and to provide solutions other than allopathic as "cultist." Since the AMA controls state licensing boards and has, for the most part, drafted state laws, it has been able to carry the day every day. For example, it has waged pitched battles to outlaw osteopaths, chiropractors, optometrists.

Osteopathy is a uniquely American contribution to medical practice, dating back to the post-Civil War period when a Missouri doctor became convinced that the human body is self-healing (not a new discovery), depending on the proper functioning of all systems. Dr. Andrew Taylor Still held that osteopathic lesions were chiefly responsible for health problems; these lesions include

13

abnormalities in the joints of the musculoskeletal system, particularly in the spinal column. Manipulation to realign the abnormalities would correct interference of the nerve and blood supply and allow the body to heal itself. Over the years, however, osteopaths took a more comprehensive approach to medical care, placing only somewhat less emphasis on drugs than traditional medicine. The six osteopathic colleges in the United States provide a high level of training; requirements for admission are similar to those of medical schools. Actually, as Elton Rayack has pointed out, the distinction between a DO (Doctor of Osteopathy) and a medical doctor is "closer to a myth than a reality."[13]

The AMA has recognized only the myth, branding osteopaths as enemies of medical practice. Medical doctors have been prohibited from associating with them in medical societies, in hospitals, in schools. In 1962, California MDs successfully lobbied through a law prohibiting the licensing of new osteopathic physicians and surgeons; however, twelve years later the California Supreme Court declared that unconstitutional, thus making graduates of osteopathic colleges in the country eligible for licensing.[14]

Like osteopathy, chiropractic is based on the theory that scientific manipulation, particularly of the spinal column, can remove the interference with the nerve control of the body's systems that impairs their function and thus induces dysfunction or disease. Also up-graded from their predecessors' beginnings in the United States in the late nineteenth century, many modern chiropractors are well trained, averaging 5021 hours in anatomy, physiology, biochemistry, pathology, microbiology, and other essentials of a medical education, as compared with the average training a medical doctor receives of 5702 hours.[15]

Public acceptance of that form of therapy has been considerable; practically every state in the union recognizes chiropractors; more than 500 insurance companies acknowledge claims for chiropractic treatment; workmen's compensation laws in most states and the Social Security Act provide for payments for chiropractic care. An AMA study some years ago revealed that 70 percent of high school seniors believed a chiropractor to be the best source of help for a painful back injury.[16]

Significantly, a good many medical men also consider that chiropractic has something of value to contribute to American medical care. As one medical doctor pointed out recently in *Medical Economics*, since the musculoskeletal system includes about 60 percent of the body's organ system and since less than 1 percent of the clinical training time of doctors is devoted to that, "we can learn from chiropractors."[17] Dr. Louis Lasagna of Johns Hopkins said that "it is quite possible that organized medicine has overplayed its hand in denouncing them [osteopathy and chiropractic] as cults." He added: "thousands of patients utilize their services, many being completely satisfied with the results; for certain musculo-skeletal disorders, osteopaths and chiropractors have as much, and perhaps more, to offer, than most doctors. . . ."[18]

What is unfortunate is that because the AMA has drawn the lines of battle so decisively, manipulative therapy has become an either-or matter. Patients seek out chiropractors not merely for mechanical dysfunction of the joints, but for all ailments. And unscrupulous chiropractors use that type of therapy for all disorders.

Similarly, optometrists have been branded as "cultists." They are not permitted to utilize their skill and training for maximum public benefit because the opthalmologists, who are medical doctors, are afraid that they will provide economic competition. The AMA has ruled that while it is ethical for the latter to accept referrals from optometrists, it is unethical to consult with them.[19]

Nurses, who have important functions in the medical care of many other advanced countries, are here relegated to inferior roles, despite their skills and their long training. The AMA and its allies have consistently fought against their recognition. In California in 1973, medical school deans were warned by the State Board of Medical Examiners to halt all programs to train nurse–practitioners because the nurses may be "practicing medicine illegally."[20] Consequently, although nurses *do,* they may not *be.* For example, school nurses are prohibited from giving even an aspirin tablet to a feverish child. Yet a nurse I know delivered two babies in the last year in a hospital delivery room for a doctor who was playing golf while his patients labored. Needless to say, the doctor sent the bill for services rendered in full.

Programs launched in recent years to further train and utilize the skills of military medical corpsmen and of such trained paramedics as firemen have also been systematically sabotaged. That has been done despite the many lives they have saved.

Although it boasts of its fight against quackery, the AMA has done much to encourage it by its attitude toward health education, nutrition, and some kinds of unorthodox medicine that have demonstrated their usefulness.

Millions of Americans saw for themselves the remarkable possibilities of acupuncture during the telecasts of President Nixon's trip to China. And the opinions of some distinguished medical sophisticates confirmed what the lay public had witnessed with their own eyes. Dr. Paul Dudley White, Dr. Samuel Rosen, Dr. Victor Sidel, and the President's personal physician said they were very impressed with it after having witnessed the removal of a cataract, a thyroid tumor, an ovarian cyst, a diseased lung— all with acupuncture anesthesia. Indeed, Dr. Rosen summed up the view of his colleagues quite simply: "I have seen the past and it works."[21] Nevertheless, the AMA has been battling furiously and successfully to ban or to rigidly limit that technique from being employed in this country.

Although as much as half of the illness in the country and perhaps more is functional rather than organically induced, the medical establishment continues to attempt to discredit many proven mind-body techniques that have been developed. "Psychological anesthesia" is being used successfully in place of drugs to help patients conquer pain; transcendental meditation to steady heart rhythms, lower blood pressure, relieve the condition of prolonged stress that has been blamed for an assortment of modern ailments ranging from cardiovascular diseases to asthma and ulcerative colitis. According to a recent article in one medical journal, biofeedback, a technique that enables the mind to gain control over a wide range of bodily functions once considered automatic, has enabled stroke and accident victims to regain the movement of paralyzed limbs. An experiment at the New York

University Medical Center was made on mind-body techniques with 36 patients suffering varying degrees of paralysis. All showed gains after practicing the techniques, ranging to full recovery for 34. Among them was a young electrician, paralyzed from the neck down. After several months of training, he regained the use of his hands and arms to such an extent that he could feed himself, shave himself, and even develop a new skill in leatherwork.[22] (An excellent account of that and other mind-body techniques is contained in Marilyn Ferguson's *The Brain Revolution*.)

Anything that interferes with "crisis medicine" is also considered suspect, if not downright "cultist." The medical profession has consistently ignored the vital role of nutrition in maintaining health; only 12 medical schools in the country have departments of nutrition, and most doctors presently practicing have had no training in it at all. Yet according to an expert in the *Journal of the American Medical Association* (*JAMA*), the role of nutrition in maintaining health is *not* secondary to antibiotics, new surgical techniques, tissue transplants, and other commonly cited remedies for illness. Indeed, the extraordinary gains in longevity in Europe and the United States during the nineteenth and twentieth centuries are due largely to improved diet.[23]

Dramatic evidence of this was provided by a recent study in Guatemala. Children in one village were given food supplements; children in another, comprehensive medical care; those in a control group, no assistance. Over a five-year period, the nutrition program was as effective as the comprehensive medical program *in reducing the death rate*. While the medical program reduced the fatality rates of the cases, the nutrition program reduced the incidence of disease.

Health education has been ignored as another important means of preventing disease. According to a survey reported by a presidential panel in 1974, health education in this country is so poorly supported that less than one-fourth of 1 percent of federal health funds go into it. Schools often exclude health education; state laws sometimes prevent it.[24]

Other notable successes that the AMA has scored against preventive medicine have been to defeat the establishment of free cancer detection clinics; it helped to stave off for years orders proposed by the Federal Trade Commission that the tobacco industry issue warnings against cigarette smoking in advertisements as well as on packages. The AMA inhibited the growth of pre-paid, group-practice plans, which operate on the theory that doctors should be rewarded for keeping people well in addition to healing them when they are ill; and a score of maternal and child-welfare programs—despite need—on the grounds that they are "unsound in policy, wasteful and extravagant . . . tending to promote communism."[25]

With no less success, the AMA has defeated almost every other significant measure that has been proposed to lower costs, improve quality, and extend the benefits of modern medical science to everyone in the country.

At the 1920 annual meeting in New Orleans, when the entre-preneurs seized power, the delegates were asked to approve a comprehensive health-insurance program. The program had been proposed by the American Association for Labor Legislation, which was a group of prominent economists, lawyers, political scientists, historians, and some of the most outstanding men of medicine, including AMA president Dr. Alexander Lambert. The proponents had little doubt that they would carry the day for the compulsory health-insurance program. But they did not reckon with the minority that was determined to maintain the fee-for-service system that would, particularly when the supply of doctors was curtailed, insure them of a "rewarding" future.

Even by the time of the New Orleans meeting, it had become clear to some of the practical leaders in Chicago that the AMA could be "a big thing." Membership had increased from 8400 in 1900 to 83,000 by 1920, and the structure made it possible for an organized few to impose its will on a disorganized majority, as Oliver Garceau has noted in *The Political History of the American Medical Association.*

Recently, there have been defections in the ranks; but for long, membership in the AMA was an imperative for all doctors since if they did not join one of the nearly 2000 county and district societies the doors of hospitals would be barred to them. When joining the local society, doctors were also required to become members of the state societies and the AMA as part of the package. The state societies select the members of the policy-making House of Delegates. That has been made up largely of the organization men in the state societies. The real power is vested in the super organization men, the 15-man Board of Trustees. Although technically responsible to the House, the board functions with practically no supervision except for the few days when the House of Delegates is in session. Performing what Garceau and others have called "the typical role of corporate directors," the trustees have absolute control over the AMA's funds and the authority to spend those funds not only for scientific investigations and continuing AMA publications, but "for any other purpose approved by the Board of Trustees." Not the least of their power is the appointment of the editor of the *JAMA* (*Journal of the American Medical Association*), which shapes the opinions of the members of the nearly 2000 local groups. One of the chief benefits of membership, as Professor Garceau has pointed out dryly, is that the doctor "is saved the awkward predicament of having to think."[26]

By the time of the New Orleans meeting, the tightly organized minority in power had also found that it would be profitable to make common cause with outsiders who were also bent on realizing maximum profits by maintaining the status quo in medicine: the insurance companies, which were almost unanimously opposed to comprehensive health insurance. Also the drug industry saw that if it advanced AMA interests, the nation's doctors might act as their salesmen and promoters. Even the aid of the healing cults was enlisted. As a result, the program was voted down and the minority succeeded in having adopted a policy resolution that has continued ever since as the organization's position:

> The American Medical Association declares its opposition to the institution of any plan embodying the system of compulsory contributory insurance against illness or any other plan of compulsory insurance which provides for medical service to be rendered contributors or their de-

pendents, provided, controlled, or regulated by any state or Federal government.[27]

So skillful had been the maneuvering, so swift the rupture, so sudden the decision to get the government out of the business of medicine that many loyal AMA members were astonished to find themselves being denounced as heretics. Not a few scrambled to reverse themselves with bewildered agility.

The man who had the vision to appreciate how the economic policies of the AMA could be sold to doctors and the American people as "good medicine" was a short, frenetic doctor who demonstrated his power at the New Orleans session, when Dr. Lambert and other socially concerned medical men went down to defeat. A physician with the face of a rather jolly owl, the verbal facility of a medicine showman, the ruthlessness of a shark, and a genius for managing people, Dr. Morris Fishbein had arrived at the AMA headquarters a year after his graduation from Rush Medical College in 1912 to serve as assistant editor of the *JAMA*.

The triumphant minority at the AMA convention, the men of the worlds of business and finance and political influence, who appreciated talent for manipulating a meeting and swinging a vote, gave Dr. Fishbein their accolade, appointing him editor of the *JAMA* in 1924. For Dr. Fishbein, it was the path to fame and fortune. For the AMA it was even more so. Dr. Fishbein gave organized medicine its "voice"; he opened up to it the real sources of power, money, legislative action, and public assent. Astonishingly, he managed to hold back the twentieth century for 50 years for the benefit of organized medicine.[28]

It was not hard to persuade most doctors to accept the AMA's policy: they benefited hugely from being able to set their own fees, and they enjoyed the freedom from quality controls. The conservative leadership in state and county societies could be counted on to bring "erring" thinkers into line. Hospital privileges could be and were withdrawn; other local doctors could be counted on to boycott referrals, to preside over "kangaroo courts."[29] For those who continued to express social concerns and to act upon them, the state licensing boards—also made up largely of AMA stalwarts—could be counted on to set them straight or ship them out.

How to get the consent of the public was another matter, for they were the chief victims of the uncontrolled costs, uncontrolled quality of the care that the fee-for-service, self-regulating, and self-policing policy involves. Fortunately for organized medicine, Dr. Fishbein was a salesman rather than a scientist by talent. Words were his stock in trade: words, words, words. Where a scientist would say "the evidence suggests," Fishbein uttered Q.E.D. pronouncements. Fiats rather than hypotheses were his line. Conflicting evidence? New facts? Forget them. Editorials and articles in the *JAMA* did just that. Dr. Fishbein wooed and won laymen through books, articles, and features in periodicals; through his newspaper columns of medical advice, which readers were advised to clip and file so that they would be sure of having a doctor in the house, a rather ingenious method of coping with the shortage and of providing care for those too poor to afford the real thing.

The confusion he generated was so total that even those who were the principal beneficiaries of what there was of "socialized medicine" in the country were campaigning against it. For example, President Dwight D. Eisenhower in 1952 accepted the organized doctors' support and their mandate to resist any support for socialized medicine. "Any move toward socialized medicine is sure to have one result," he declaimed; "instead of the patient getting more and better medical care for less, he will get less and poorer medical care for more."[30]

What was remarkable about his declamation was that neither before nor after he became president did General Eisenhower give any indication that he or his wife or their son and his wife or their grandchildren had any intention of foregoing the delivery-room-to-grave socialized medical care they, like all army people, have received through the courtesy of the American public. So, too, congressmen and senators have considered it good sense to utilize privately what they publicly brand a clear and present danger to the moral fiber of the nation. Former President Richard M. Nixon followed the example in 1974. Only one day after he left Walter Reed Hospital, he was denouncing "socialized medicine."

During the 1930s and 1940s, the chief thrust of the public-relations campaign was to discredit everyone who proposed comprehensive health insurance. Dr. Fishbein and other leaders in Chicago took full advantage of the resolution passed in 1931 declaring that "All opinions made to the public on general, social, legislative, and economic relationships of medical practice should be made only through approved channels of the American Medical Association." That meant the forces of reaction in the AMA.

Dramatic evidence of that was provided in the mid-thirties when the reactionary forces in the AMA managed to have set aside the majority report prepared by the prestigious Committee on the Costs of Medical Care. The report, which advocated extension of health services and which had been prepared by such men as Dr. Ray Lyman Wilbur, former AMA president, was branded by Dr. Fishbein as "incitement to revolution."[31] When 700 of the country's top doctors issued a statement supporting the proposals of the majority, it was suggested that the medical educators among them had been motivated by the possibility of getting government money for clinics and dispensaries.

Outsiders, particularly Democratic politicians who followed the New and the Fair Deal, were attacked even more vigorously. The AMA began to spend huge sums to defeat them.

President Truman's request for health insurance created such consternation at the AMA headquarters that it was decided that Dr. Fishbein and the committee working with him needed help. Public relations and political activity were increased when the AMA engaged the California firm of Whitaker and Baxter. The man-and-wife public relations company had achieved national recognition as one of the most effective in the business. This was the company that helped to shape the political rise of President Richard M. Nixon and that had defeated Governor Earl Warren's proposal for a state compulsory insurance law.

During 1949, the Whitaker and Baxter campaign utilized press, radio, television, magazines, billboards, and posters to convey to the American people the message that national health insurance

was bad medicine. Fifty-five million pamphlets bearing the senti-
mental picture by Sir Luke Fildes of a doctor bending over the
bed of a sick child were distributed with the message "Keep
Politics Out of This Picture." The Communist Party was held to
be the chief promoter of national health insurance.[32] The next
year, the campaign was intensified and more than $1,000,000 was
spent in a single month before the fall election. Money flowed in
from the doctors, who were subjected to a "voluntary" assessment.
Other sources were equally generous; the retail druggists, for example, contributed $2,000,000 "to play public opinion and make
it light up like a pinball machine."[33] In 1949 and 1950, the AMA
achieved the dubious distinction of being the biggest spender
among Washington lobbies. It provided almost double the budget
of the second largest lobby and far more than the National Association of Manufacturers, the AFL-CIO, and some of the veterans
associations.[34]

There has been no let-up of either public relations or politicking since. In the mid-1960s, the AMA spent an estimated $7,000,-
000 to defeat the Medicare bill proposed by President Lyndon B.
Johnson and others. In the 1970s, the principal targets have been
Senator Edward M. Kennedy and Congresswoman Martha Griffiths, whose comprehensive national health-insurance bill is regarded as anathema since it would not only introduce cost controls,
but quality controls as well. State and local societies are also active
in politicking; they, too, play both sides of the aisles, but support
chiefly conservatives and ultra-rightists. Ronald Reagan, onetime
western film star, made it to the governor's mansion in California
with great assistance from organized medicine in that state. Indiana congressman Earl F. Landgrebe, who distinguished himself
during the Watergate affair by his all-out support of Richard
Nixon—"My mind is closed on this issue; don't confuse me with
the facts"—has long been a favorite candidate of the organized
doctors in his state despite some of his rather extravagant views
about health care. He was, for example, the only congressman to
vote in 1974 against a bill providing money for cancer research
on the grounds that such research "will only change the way
you go."[35]

Both the cost and quality of medical services are in dire need of controls. Thanks to doctors' ability to charge what the traffic will bear and to determine how most of the health dollars in the United States are spent, the price Americans pay for medical services is ruinous to many individuals and is breaking the back of the social security system. Thanks to doctors' ability to be sole determiners of quality, the level of much of the service is incredibly low. Although both matters will be considered in detail in later chapters, an example of the kind of peril to which some Americans are being exposed by "the best medical system in the world" came to light in December 1973 in a 196-page decision handed down by a California judge. He awarded a former grocery clerk $3,700,000 for damages resulting from an unnecessary back operation performed six years earlier and which prevented successful treatment of a cancer that was killing him "slowly." The surgeon, who had lost two other malpractice actions, acknowledged he had performed the unnecessary operation badly, that his incompetence resulted from his dependence on "uppers and downers."

In his opinion, the judge said that the surgeon had "for nine years made a practice of performing unnecessary surgery incompetently simply to line his pockets." He said that for the five months of the trial his court had been "a Grand Guignol of medical horrors." And he called the state licensing board "derelict" for not having acted against him despite earlier evidence. He did not comment on the loyal colleagues who had testified at the trial that the doctor had a *fine* reputation.[36]

While the trial for the botched, unnecessary operation was going on in one part of the state, it was found in another that hundreds of school children in one prosperous county had not been given follow-up treatment for positive tuberculosis tests because there were not enough health workers to provide it.[37] According to the Public Health Service, one of every 12 persons with a positive skin test develops active TB within a year. Among other AMA triumphs has been the defeat of meaningful school health programs with its "let-them-see-a-private-doctor" argument.

An increasing number of doctors have been deserting the ranks of the AMA. Others have been expressing strong criticism. Among them is Dr. John Adriani, whose struggle to minimize the drug industry's influence is described in a later chapter. Not long ago, Dr. Adriani told me:

> The biggest problem with the American Medical Association is that it has a self-perpetuating body of trustees, who have an exalted opinion of themselves and think they know all there is to know about the health care needs of the country. They have a paid "bureaucracy" at 535 North Dearborn Street, Chicago, that advises them. Only about half of the doctors in the United States belong, and unless those of us who are members do something to "shake them up" and reorganize the superstructure, the Association is going to deteriorate completely.[38]

In such a case, there might be promise in the advertisements for members that the AMA is now running: "Join us. We can do much more together."[39] What and how much are questions to be answered.

2 Medical Affluence

Young men in college, despite popular mythology, cherish great expectations of the rich full life that will be theirs after graduation. Medical students, however, are among the few who possess absolute certainty that their dreams of wealth, if not fame, will be realized. So positive is the belief than an MD degree is the open sesame to the treasure house that in 1965 when a Stanford University student was flunked out of medical school, he promptly filed suit for $1,500,000, or the amount he would lose if he were not allowed to become a doctor.[1] Today, a similar compensatory demand would have to be for twice that amount.

Doctors have climbed far up the money tree in a very short time, reaching the top 1 percent of the income distribution list, with lifetime earnings far ahead of those of teachers, journalists, lawyers, social workers, clergymen, and other education specialists. In 1933, the reported average net income of physicians in private practice was only $3969. By 1951, when all wage earners were averaging $3384, the average net income of doctors in private practice was $13,482. By 1961, it had risen to $25,000.[2] Since the advent of the Medicare and Medicaid programs in 1966, it has soared. Knowledgeable persons estimate the "average" today is three to four times that figure.

Averages are not always helpful in determining the real nature of medical affluence. Doctors have a greater tendency than most, as the Internal Revenue Service has noted, to consistently underestimate their income. And, they are in a better position than most to whittle down their net income by allowable deductions since their "indispensable aides" frequently include tax lawyers and business managers.

However, a Senate Finance Committee made some interesting discoveries about the incomes of doctors in 1968 during an investigation of Medicare and Medicaid payments. In that year, when thousands of doctors were still boycotting the government programs as socialistic evils, many of their colleagues were taking advantage of what has turned out to be a very good thing for the medical profession. At least 10,000 of them received more than $25,000 from government programs alone, in addition to whatever they were making from private practice. Even in relatively poor states doctors were striking it rich. Practitioner #107082B in Georgia, for example, was paid $83,083; a Kentucky colleague, #3372502AS, made $130,759. Physicians in wealthier states were faring no less well. In New York, Dr. 000048772 drew $130,319, Dr. 000070083, $144,497; in California, Dr. 020A18930 received $126,522, and Dr. 00A109070 was paid $145,708 for treating Medicare and Medicaid patients.[3] And so on through the other states.

Physicians who were working as a team often did much better. In Texas, for example, a couple of doctors working together received $1,409,787. And not quite satisfied with the legal bonanza, some medical men began to figure out ways of making sure that none of the money was taken away in taxes. Some Chicago doctors formed a tax-exempt foundation into which they funneled the $1,600,000 they earned in Medicare fees. Those fees, incidentally, had been for services *never* performed.[4]

Some doctors had the grace to be ashamed, but only after their financial returns were made public. Dr. Sanford Polansky of Benton Harbor, Michigan, returned $169,000 in Medicaid payments he had received in 1968 to the state Blue Shield organization, saying that after the "distorted unfair newspaper publicity," he felt that the money, "though earned and deserved, is simply not worth the retaining."[5]

The American Medical Association was outraged that the revelations were made public and accused the Senate Committee and Internal Revenue Service of having indulged in "political exploitation." It also condemned what it called the "few avaricious physicians" who overcharged patients, and laid loftily of them:

> The medical profession is making a great effort to identify and weed out dishonest doctors who betray their oath as professional men serving the public. We have been successful in this search, but a few physicians remain who still are not identified. We shall search them out and expose them, for the good of the entire profession.[6]

The results of that search and the exposure are still unknown.

Nor have the insuring agencies done anything about the gouging that has been going on. For example, a friend showed me copies of the following three bills submitted in 1972 by a Chicago doctor to her employer. One, for treating a man for a cut thumb, was broken down thus:

½ hr. (Dr.'s time at 125/hr.) exam and treatment	62.50
½ hr. use of emergency treatment room (@ 50/hr.)	25.00
Dressings	3.50
Dispensed medication	8.50
TOTAL	$99.50

Another, for treating a man who had been exposed to "poison oak-ivy" while working, was broken down:

10/7/72	
½ hr. exam and treatment (Dr.'s services 125/hr)	62.50
½ hr. use of emergency treatment room	25.00
medications dispensed, injections, etc.	10.00
10/11/72	
office visit	25.00
injection	5.00
10/19/72	
office visit	25.00
injection	5.00
TOTAL	$157.50

Another, for a man who fell and injured his wrist slightly, was broken down:

10/17/72

½ hr. (Dr.'s time at 125/hr.) exam and treatment	62.50
½ hr. use of treatment and emergency room @ 50/hr.	25.00
Bandages and dispensed materials	7.00
TOTAL	$94.50

Those were the fees submitted and paid at a time when fees for office calls to general practitioners in Chicago were supposed to be $15 to $30; and when the price of a tonsillectomy and adenoidectomy in that city was set at $100 to $125.[7] This kind of overcharging was going on in the very city where the AMA was presumably centering its search.

The search and exposure by the Senate Finance Committee and by investigative reporters did produce results, however. The results were momentarily embarrassing to some physicians, perhaps, but not calculated to have any appreciable effects on their prices or their practices. That was the case with a number of the "Poor People's Doctors" named publicly as a result of the Medicaid probe. All of them had received more than $100,000 in 1971 from the program. In an interview with several of them in 1973, reporter Rudy Maxa met some interesting responses. A northeast Washington, D.C., gynecologist, who received $120,000 in 1971, told the reporter that it had taken him six months to get over the "entire fuss." But, he added, "every patient rallied around me. They'd say, 'if there's anything we can do—go down and protest, talk to the mayor. . . .' " What made him finally able to put all the comments about overcharges behind him, however, was that the publicity resulted in his receiving eight to ten new patients a day.[8] Apparently, these patients had not heard about the affluent medico before. And the feeling is in the Washington, D.C., ghetto, as everywhere else in the country, if a man makes all that money, he must be pretty smart.

The poor and the aged, despite public programs, are still victims of high costs. Two episodes that occurred within weeks of each other in 1975 give some clue as to that. One involved a 23-year-old South Carolina woman whose child was delivered by an ambulance attendant after he had driven her for seven hours from one doctor and hospital to another. Her own doctor had refused to deliver the baby or authorize hospital admission because the family owed him $350 for previous treatment. "If I started taking labor cases for free, I'd have five hundred in a month," was his explanation. None of the 20 other doctors whose aid was sought would discuss the matter. Shortly before that at the other side of the country, a California man offered to sell one of his eyes for $35,000 to pay for a costly operation for his wife. The man, unwilling to accept welfare and without medical insurance because of a heart attack he had suffered, explained his having advertised his eye for sale in a newspaper: "I'm desperate. You just try to get your wife in a hospital with no insurance and no money—it's impossible."[9]

The rich can afford anything, although some of them also smart bitterly. But what about the middle- and lower middle-income families who are not protected by the blanket insurance programs sponsored by the government? The despair often inflicted upon them is devastating, as newspaper headlines and Congressional investigations in recent years have revealed.

Consider a few of the stories.

James Rieger was forced into bankruptcy because of medical bills. He testified recently before Senator Edward Kennedy's subcommittee on health that he thought that the hospitalization insurance he had through his employer would cover the bills for the birth of the child the Riegers were expecting. How wrong he was. The infant, who arrived two months prematurely, was kept in the infant intensive-care unit at Cleveland Metropolitan Hospital for two months. His wife, who had suffered a cardiac arrest while giving birth, was also hospitalized there in the intensive-care unit for two months. Total bills came to about $20,000, of which the insurance paid only $350. With a take-home pay of $120 a week, Mr. Rieger filed a bankruptcy petition. At that point, everything the family had been buying on credit, even their stove and refrigerator, was taken away.[10]

Medical bills are forcing many middle-income people to go on welfare. A UCLA graduate student only two months away from taking his oral exams for a Ph.D. in English found himself in 1971 "as perennially pauperized." Costs of treatment for a kidney disease from which he suffers became so great that he had no alternative but to go on welfare. That was the only alternative given in 1972 to a Pennsylvania family which had exhausted all of its savings for the treatment of a twelve-year-old hemophiliac son. With treatments costing between $900 and $1000 a month and with their savings exhausted, the family appealed to the state director of human services for aid. They were told that in order to qualify as "medically needy," the father would have to quit his $7800-a-year job or persuade the company to give him one at a much lower salary. "It just isn't fair," the mother said. "We want to carry our load. But if that is the game they play, then I guess we will just have to play it."[11]

In 1973, papers all over the world carried the story of Howard Thomas, a Florida steelworker who was suing his wife for a divorce so that she could gain the welfare benefits that would allow her to remain in a nursing home. "I love my wife, but I'm at the end of my rope," he explained. The man's ordeal had begun several months earlier, when the Division of Family Services, which administers the Medicaid program in Florida, cut off the $117 he had been receiving toward the expenses of keeping his wife in a nursing home. His monthly salary was $550; the nursing home bill was $500. "I can't help but feel guilty about it," Thomas said, "but there was nothing else I could do. I just thank God she won't have to know about it. She's nothing but a vegetable anymore. She can't talk and she cannot understand. She's just dwindling away."[12]

For many families, the high price of medical care has results far less dramatic. Often the expenses cause no more than a brief, cruel crunch that throws the budget out of kilter and plays havoc temporarily with plans. An illustration of that was provided when, in Los Angeles a couple of years ago, the father of a small child became so outraged by a $420 bill for surgery that he asked reporters to investigate. They, too, found it hard to believe the story. The four-year-old had apparently stuffed a piece of popcorn in her ear, which the mother discovered shortly after when she was washing her. Rather than risk hurting her by trying to extract it themselves, they took the child to a doctor. Dr. One tried to wash the piece of popcorn out; unsuccessful, he charged the father $11 and sent the family to an ear specialist. The specialist clapped the child into a hospital, where she spent two days, including the few minutes necessary for the "operation." The specialist's bill was $100: $20 for the office call, $80 for the surgery. The hospital bill was $258.90, and the anesthesiologist who put the child to sleep for the operation charged $51. Medical and insurance experts told reporters that they considered the bill entirely appropriate; it "illustrates only the high cost of medical care today."[13]

Organized medicine is generally unconcerned about that. It defends doctors' incomes as eminently reasonable; after all, they invest a lot of time and money in education; the costs of practicing medicine are very high; they work long hours; and "Anyhow, plumbers make more." The economics are less impressive.

It is true that a medical education takes a long time and is expensive. (Students have been carefully screened for their ability to make it without having to take on outside jobs to support themselves. As a consequence, until very recently only 15 percent of medical students were from the 36 percent of the population in the lowest income brackets.[14]) What the doctors also neglect to mention is that their medical education has been largely financed by taxpayers. Tuition and fees paid by students cover only about 5 percent or less of the cost of their training; federal, state, and local governments ante up the rest.[15] The cries of "socialism" are muted when physicians refer to their own socialized medical education.

Doctors also say that they are kept out of the job market for years longer than other wage earners. They spend four years in medical school, an additional year or more as interns, an even longer period for those who take residencies in a specialty. However, economists say that doctors more than compensate for the loss of earnings in their younger years by high incomes during the middle years; that they realize a higher return on their educational investment than any other male college graduates, from artists to zoologists and corporation presidents as well. During the past decade, the image of the impoverished intern has given way to another more prosperous picture. Interns are now earning highly respectable salaries, far more than Ph.D.s in most other categories. In New York hospitals, their income rose by 1650 percent in the sixties.

When they finish, there are jobs waiting in abundance, as there certainly are not for physicists, lawyers, and other degree holders, many of whom have spent equal amounts of time in training. Here are a few of the offerings from the "Physicians wanted" columns in one of the 1973 issues of the *JAMA*:

- General Practitioners in a Mississippi health center; starting salary $25,000 to $26,000, with a 12 percent fringe benefit package.

- Psychiatrist, Pennsylvania; $32,000 to $40,000, with "good" benefit package and opportunities to make more in private practice.

- Internist in Iowa, first year $30,000 plus benefits; partnership promised in 12 months, along with "liberal" vacation and meeting time.

- Emergency Room Physician in Tennessee; $30,000 salary, with paid vacation, hospitalization, and all the conveniences of suburban living—fishing, boating, golf, and assorted lures.

- Pediatrician in California; $30,150, with "liberal" fringe benefits, including sick leave, vacation, holidays, health insurance at nominal costs, and such additional bonuses as a retirement plan and social security payments.

- Residencies are highly promising, with stipends of $14,000, $15,000 and more, with a wide range of benefits.[16]

Those, mind you, are only the salaried positions—often held in contempt by physicians because of the ceilings. Such limitations are misleading since a good many full-time salaried doctors do a brisk business in moonlighting. That has been going on to such extent in California, for instance, that in 1973 Los Angeles County Supervisor Kenneth Hahn ordered a survey to find out how doctors ostensibly working for the county were able to earn substantial salaries as teachers at the same time. According to Supervisor Hahn, a doctor employed at Harbor General Hospital was drawing an annual paycheck for $35,435. At the same time, he was on salary at the University of California Medical School for $20,116. Other doctors at the same institution were also on double salaries from county and state. Reluctant to question the size of the teaching fees paid by a public school, Supervisor Hahn insisted on doctors on county salaries "giving patients the eight-hour day they agreed to give them when they accepted employment."[17]

Other lucrative opportunities wait. An advertisement in the *Los Angeles Times* in 1973 urged doctors in private industry and with existing practices to get into the kind of doctor business that overeating by Americans has made possible. Rewards promised? "As little office time as a single afternoon or evening a week can generate income of $50,000 and more."[18]

With "full-time" jobs often treated as part-time assignments by doctors, "part-time" jobs are even more lightly regarded. Also in 1973 in California, the San Diego Bar Association protested the activities of a doctor hired by the county on a part-time basis to attend jail inmates. Although he was earning a salary of $20,000, he was spending just two hours a day at the jail and seeing patients for an average of two minutes, the organization's report said. "He regards all inmates as malingerers and takes a negative approach to treating them, which precludes effective medical treatment."[19]

High overhead is also cited as a reason for extravagant fees. It costs a doctor plenty just to operate his office. Apparently it does, although that is largely the fault of the solo-practice, fee-for-service manner of operating. Instead of sharing equipment and personnel, each physician has to assume the costs of salaries, drugs and medical supplies, office space, insurance, and similar items The American Medical Association sets those figures very high in computing

34

average earnings. Thus, in 1970, the expenses of a general practitioner were held to be $25,719; surgeons' expenses were set at $28,558. Obstetrics-gynecology specialists paid expenses of $29,-388; lowest estimated expenses were those of psychiatrists and anesthesiologists, $13,032 and $11,132.[20]

However accurate the estimates are, all of those expenses, whether necessary or unnecessary, are passed along to the patients, who are also subsidizing doctors in other ways. Doctors furiously protest what they consider to be their "exploitation" in hospital fund-raising drives. Of course, patients pay that. And they pay enormously for the hospital "workshops" doctors use. The patients often invest as much as $150,000 for each doctor using the facilities. Some doctors carry the "private workshop" idea further than others. Not long ago, a doctor reported of a colleague:

> . . . a millionaire g.p. here who caters to a very exclusive clientele, yet he operates out of a tiny office with just one examining room. When I asked him to let me in on his secret, the guy said: "I don't like to see my patients at the office. It's worth more seeing them at the hospital. I use a place in one of the wealthiest parts of town, so no one feels bad about going there. Generally I'll keep at least 20 patients in at a time and hit them $25 apiece for my daily visit. That's $500 a day just for making my morning rounds. Throw in some surgery, give 'em a few shots, do some lab work and it really adds up."[21]

Patients also subsidize physicians' charity, about which so much has been said in public relations brochures and press releases. A good bit of that charity is kept exclusively at home and comes under the heading of "professional courtesy." That is the euphemism for services rendered without charge to other doctors and their families. According to a *Medical Economics* survey in 1973, surgeons and obstetricians were providing more than their colleagues both in the way of charity and professional courtesy: $2000 and $3000 a year.[22] Considering their incomes, that is not very much. Some of the charity is questionably motivated. Undoubtedly some of the doctors who participated in the "Project Vietnam" were prompted by reports of suffering. But that AMA-sponsored activity was also being widely publicized in medical journals with such titles as "Vacation in Vietnam?"[23] Dangers were held minimal; the mission also enabled participants to enjoy tax-deductible vacations in Australia, Europe, and other places either coming or going.

Although some doctors are dedicated, selfless men, the arguments about medical generosity are not very convincing. Much of the volunteer work goes to other doctors, who are well able to afford it. Much of it is a necessary preliminary to gaining staff privileges at a hospital. Much of it is simply a practical matter. As the Mayo brothers' financial expert pointed out long ago, tearing up a bill (which can be done publicly to great effect) may not only save hard feelings, it saves bookkeeping expenses.

Moreover, a good many of the emotionally moving stories about physicians' generosity raise uncomfortable questions. According to a reasonably typical one recently, professional generosity had made life brighter for a man and his wife who had lost two of their children within several years. The doctors decided to reduce their bills from $5281.20 to $296.61. Just how the family could have survived without that reduction was not made clear since the salary of the bereaved father was $300 a month; the mother did not work; the couple had no insurance.

Doctors also defend their exorbitant incomes on the grounds that they work longer hours than most professionals. The way some of the $100,000-plus physicians have it, they are working seven days a week, 12 or 15 hours a day. Perhaps some of them are seeing as many as 100 patients a day, although that may be of modest comfort to the patients.

Some fields have been more lucrative than others. For example, an Illinois doctor who specializes in weight control told a Senate investigating committee that he and his seven assistants handled 85,000 patient visits in a single year with a gross of about $1,000,000, including commissions of $1200 a month he was paid by a drug company. Another specialist in weight control acknowledged that he handled 11,727 office visits in a single year. His gross income for that was about $220,000.[24]

Psychiatry is also a big money-maker now that group psychiatric sessions are in vogue. One of the doctors who received more than $106,000 in Medicaid payments in 1971 was an India-born practitioner who works in a low-income area in the nation's capital. (In fairness, it should be pointed out that he is one of only 11 who practice in the populous southeast and southwest sections of the city; by contrast, there are about 500 psychiatrists catering to the more affluent northwest section.) Even the District of Columbia Medical Society stirred itself long enough to comment about him. In a report of its investigation about the top money-makers from Medicaid, it was noted that: "Charging the maximum allowable rates, [the doctor] would have had to see Medicaid patients at least 13 working hours, 365 days a year, to account for the $106,835 he collected."[25]

But even general practitioners, who are considered to make the least income of all doctors, are raking it in now that Medicare and Medicaid have opened new markets. A California physician who received $152,458 in a single year from the government program for low-income health care (his private practice gains were not revealed) insisted that he made it all by seeing 60 to 70 patients a day, five or six days a week. Another California physician working in the northern California area received government payments of $121,922 on 8988 claims. He insisted that he was motivated only by his belief in "quality" pediatric care. "The county medical society," he said, "investigated us last year, and, God knows, if there was anything wrong, we would have been nabbed."[26] His reason for that belief is a mystery to anyone who has looked into the actions of organized medicine in regard to ethics and exploitation.

Although those doctors piously insist that without their ministrations persons in low-income areas would be without medical care of any kind, the truth is that the care they are giving is often of an inferior quality and the prices they charge have imperiled the programs. In the mid-1960s that first became apparent when Sargent Shriver, director of the war on poverty, ordered an investigation of the raids being made on the Head Start program by money-hungry doctors and dentists. In Mississippi, the men in white who were being paid a fee for each child they examined were rushing black tots through at such a clip that they were able to collect almost a thousand dollars a day. As Jack Anderson reported: "Some dentists didn't even take time to prepare dental charts on the children." In the Southwest, "doctors were also found processing the Mexican-American children *en masse.*"[27]

Far more than costly education, high overhead, hard work, and assorted other reasons, medicine is a bonanza for practitioners because of organized medicine's policies: the deliberately created shortage of doctors, the fee-for-service, solo type of practice, and the encouragement of price fixing.

The direct relationship between physicians' earnings and what has been called the AMA's "venerable trading stratagem" of restricting the supply of doctors relative to the demand for health care has been commented on by many observers. One of the most perceptive, Seymour E. Harris, says in *The Economics of American Medicine*: "*I know of no more relevant index of shortage of doctors than the great rise of income of physicians.*"[28] Instead of seeking to remedy that, the control on the number of doctors being made available was tightened. In 1950, there were 149 doctors in the country for every 100,000 residents; by 1970, 171 for every 100,000. That could have indicated that there was an improvement if the demand had not been intensified. Before Medicare, Medicaid, and extensive buying of private health-insurance policies, most people did not seek treatment of any kind. Indeed, as an MD wrote some years ago in the *New York State Journal of Medicine*: "What keeps the great majority of people well is the fact that they can't afford to be ill." Conceding that the dictum might cause a "certain number" of curable ills to go undetected, he added: "Is it not better that a few such should perish rather than that the majority of the population should be encouraged on every occasion to run sniveling to the doctor?"[29]

Now that people have the financial encouragement and ability to "run sniveling," the doctors are not there.

The interest in specialization has intensified the "Not In To Patients" attitude among doctors. The family doctor who delivered babies, removed tonsils, treated skin disorders, and offered homespun advice to schizoid adolescents and emotionally disturbed parents is a vanishing species, thanks equally to the higher monetary rewards and the complexity of modern medical science. Medical schools and hospitals concerned with quality care have accentuated the trend. Military services, which grant higher rank, more money, and choicer assignments to specialists enhanced it; so did insurance companies, by paying specialists much higher prices for the same services.

The decrease in the number of general practitioners has become worse since the 1950s. In 1965, 22 percent of the country's physicians were in general practice; by 1970, only 15 percent.

Specialization can be a very good thing in a group-practice setting, where the patient is first seen by a generalist and then directed to the appropriate specialist or specialists if necessary. But in fee-for-service, solo practice, it can be disastrous. For one thing, as Dr. Edward R. Pinckney has pointed out, it encourages self-diagnosis. That is a dangerous practice. For example, a person in a state of depression may elect to visit a psychiatrist. If his disorder has psychological origins, well and good; however, if it is caused by physiological malfunctioning, the services of the specialist are of little use since psychiatrists do not make detailed physical examinations.[30]

Specialization has also encouraged hypochondriacs to further strain medical resources by doctor "shopping." A woman I know who was ill pooh-poohed the idea of a generalist. "They don't really know anything," she insisted and pursued a course from one specialist to another. One day she called to tell me she had found a "wonderful" man. He told her the pain she was suffering was probably due to her watching television from a chair that was "too high." She moved to a lower one and was convinced for a few weeks that her problem was solved. Some months later she died of cancer of the liver, which might have been detected by the battery of tests that a generalist gives and been aided by proper treatment by a specialist.

However bad for the patient, this has been good for the specialists. Although an AMA study indicated that general practitioners were grossing $59,578 by 1970, their expenses were higher and many of them were working longer hours. Gross incomes for specialists in internal medicine in the same year were $66,498; for surgeons, $79,258; obstetricians, $76,482; pediatricians, $59,456. Anesthesiologists, whose business costs are paid largely by hospitals, were taking in $50,564.[31] And those estimates, it should be emphasized again, are very low. A California lawyer-physician told me in 1975 that the state average for specialists was at least $150,000.

In basic terms, in 1972 the first visit to a general practitioner cost $8; to an internist, $15; a general surgeon, $10; an obstetrician–gynecologist, $16; and to a pediatrician, $10.[32] (Some pediatricians, incidentally, worried about the leveling off of a population growth, have recently decided to switch to other specialties.)

An interesting study of how the trend toward specialization has intensified the problem of the shortage of doctors and the high cost of treatment was provided some years ago. In 1952 at Cape Canaveral, 16 doctors, only three of whom were specialists, served a population of 40,000. By 1964, there were 117 doctors representing most of the specialties, and they were having tremendous difficulty in serving a population of 170,000. Although the ratio of physicians to the population had increased by more than 40 percent, the income of doctors had skyrocketed for providing fewer services.[33]

Another economic penalty that has grown out of specialization is fee splitting. This involves an agreement between doctors to give payoffs for referrals, which is unethical. Although both the American College of Surgeons and the AMA have protested the ugly custom, it continues to flourish. A few years ago, a doctor described in detail his introduction to that practice. Well trained as an obstetrician–gynecologist, with five years of hospital work behind him, he was having trouble attracting patients. His rescue was effected by an older man, a general practitioner who had graduated from his medical school and out of a feeling of loyalty to a fellow alumnus had decided to set him straight.

Taking precautions to warn him that if his colleague reported him, he would sue, the doctor said that it was customary for gynecologists to share fees: "If they hit the patient for, say, three hundred dollars, they find a way to get me my consultant's or assistant's fee of one hundred dollars—in cash." Not only would he get the older man's cases under those conditions, but cases from other general practitioners in town when they learned that the new specialist was playing the game.

Needless to say, he did.[34]

In this area, too, group practice involving doctors working together on salary works against such conspiracies to fleece the sick. Organized medicine has fought bitterly against every attempt to encourage group practices. While it has spoken publicly against fee splitting, its policies and practices have provided incentive for that.

Actually, the first indication of the AMA's hands-off policy concerning fee splitting came to public attention in 1900, when two members of the Chicago Medical Society decided to expose the racket in that area. They sent to leading surgeons a letter purportedly written by a country doctor who wanted to know precisely what share of the surgeons' fees would be given for referrals. The two doctors took the answers they received to several newspapers in the city hoping that publicity would halt what professional self-policing had not. The papers, of course, were delighted to publish the letters in full, with the names of the correspondents. The Chicago Medical Society, apparently without objection from the AMA headquartered nearby, set the pattern. It ignored the grossly unethical practices of the fee splitters. Instead, it disciplined the two members who had exposed the racket.[35]

Price fixing is illegal in this country, but the medical profession, which has fought its bitterest battles on the grounds of outsiders setting fees, has found a way around that, too. The way, of course, is to establish price floors. So far as the ceiling goes, the sky has been the limit or, in more mundane terms, whatever the traffic would bear. Doctors in an area could charge less than the agreed-upon floor for special charity cases, but charity is pretty much a thing of the past.

After World War II, when private health insurance became an essential item on most budgets, there was a movement to establish a schedule of fees for particular services rendered. The medical profession sabotaged that effort by insisting on "usual and customary, or reasonable charges." The insurance industry bowed. So did the government. What this policy amounts to is that particular doctors in the same specialty in the same area have agreed to charge a minimum payment for a particular service. The doctors know what the minimums are; the insurers have an idea. The patient is totally in the dark, so that it is almost impossible for him to know that he has been overcharged. However, these days a good many senior citizens are realizing to their sorrow that substantial portions of their doctor bills will not be paid on the grounds that they are unreasonable. Since the patient has already paid the doctor himself or will have to do it, the burden falls on him.

Patients are, of course, invited to discuss the matter with the doctor. They are even informed that they can protest about gross overcharging to the county medical association. This is of relatively little help since doctors are reluctant to interfere with the economic practices of other doctors even when they recognize exploitation.

In a moving speech to the American Medical Association several years before he died, Rabbi Abraham J. Heschel, the distinguished theologian, suggested to delegates as "a therapy for the virus of commercialism" that they make *a personal decision to establish a maximum level of income.*" He reminded his audience:

> The nightmare of medical bills, the high arrogance and callousness of the technicians, splitting fees, vested interests in promoting pharmaceutical products, suspicion that the physician is suggesting more surgery than absolutely necessary—all converge to malign the medical profession.

And reviving the ancient myth, he asked: "The goal is to protect or restore the patient's health. But is it not a Sisyphus act if we cure him physically and destroy him economically?"[36] One would have to read far in most professional journals to hear echoes of that genuinely noble counsel.

The attitude of many leaders of organized medicine was expressed a few months after Rabbi Heschel's speech for a Portland psychiatrist. Analyzing the subconscious reasons for some physi-

42

cians' charging too little, Dr. Robert Mighell laid bare the desires for popularity, the guilt complexes, the self-doubts, and "the selflessness syndrome." His own "philosophy," he wrote, had been formed before he became a specialist. He noted that in the sickrooms of his patients bottles holding expensive antibiotics were usually empty, while those holding inexpensive medicines were nearly always full. His remarkable conclusion was that patients should be handed bills high enough to convince them that the doctor's services were as good as expensive medicine.[37]

Whether or not American men of medicine can navigate with their own sextant the gulf that separates Dr. Mighell's counsel from Dr. Heschel's hope is the issue facing us all.

3 Fees for What Kind of Service?

The quality of medical care throughout history has been cause for concern. The few great men who have risen above the hordes of quacks and incompetents have traditionally received rough treatment for their efforts to elevate standards and introduce proper therapy. Scientifically as well as economically, original thinking has not been greatly esteemed in medical circles.

Balavignus, the great fourteenth-century Jewish physician, was permitted to leave the confines of the ghetto because of his financial acumen, not his medical skill. He was branded a "charlatan" by the College of Physicians in Paris when he attempted to employ sanitation measures to minimize the Black Death that had stalked Europe for more than a century, periodically decimating the population. The filth that was the breeding grounds for rats and their plague-bearing parasites had nothing to do with the terrible killer, the physicians pontificated solemnly. Their advice was that "fat people should not sit in the sunshine."[1]

When the Swiss genius Theophrastus Bombastus von Hohenheim, immortalized as Paracelsus, denounced ideas of witchcraft as the origin of disease and scoffed at other sixteenth-century medical absurdities, he was driven by doctors and religious fanatics from his native country and later from France, Germany, and Italy. They persecuted him unmercifully. Finally, it is believed, they murdered him. Yet it was Paracelsus, through his teachings and writings, who ultimately freed medicine from the rusted ideas

44

of Galen, whose doctrines had been held as gospel truth since the second century. A reformer of surgical practice, Paracelsus also laid the foundations for the science of drugs, although it was not until the nineteenth century that a renewed interest in some of his chemical compounds stimulated the great discoveries.[2]

Opprobrium was heaped upon Edward Jenner for insisting that vaccination with cowpox virus was a better prophylactic against smallpox than bloodletting and plasters. He was threatened with expulsion from his medical society during the eighteenth century for that "dangerous" notion. More than a hundred years later, Ignaz Semmelweis was driven mad by the persecution of his colleagues after demonstrating that merely by washing his hands in chloride of lime he had been able to reduce the high rate of deaths from "childbed fever." In the Vienna General Hospital's maternity ward, his simple expedient cut the toll by 800 percent. The European medical profession fell upon him: "Doctors wash their hands? Preposterous."[3]

Just as attempts to upgrade the quality of medical practice from within the profession were markedly resisted, so were the occasional outside efforts. Perhaps the most dramatic of these occurred in Babylonia in about 1950 BC, when man's oldest code of laws, The Judgments of Righteousness, was promulgated by King Hammurabi. A collection and codification of decrees, some new and some dating back to the days of ancient Sumer, the code set forth in precise terms the rights and duties of all individuals in the society, including the several categories of physicians and their patients.

The Code of Hammurabi rigidly regulated the fees charged by the physician-priests, who were attached to the courts of the king and his high officials and who also served those people who could afford to pay. People, as still continues to be the widespread custom, were required to pay according to their means. The quality of the care doctors provided was guaranteed by terrifying regulations. If an operation ended unsuccessfully in the loss of an eye or the patient's life, the physician's hands were cut off. If a slave died during the course of an operation, the physician had to give the owner a substitute slave. Obviously, such draconian measures would have eliminated all but the most daring of physician-priests if they had been strictly invoked. Dr. Henry S. Sigerist, the great medical historian, is of the reasonable opinion they were not; however: "they represent a first attempt of society to protect itself by way of legislation against misuse of a physician's power, a power granted to him by society and without which the physician cannot function."[4]

Subsequent civilizations have done little to protect society or to encourage high-quality performance among men of medicine. Some time before the French Revolution, Voltaire wrote: "Doctors are men who prescribe medicines of which they know little, to cure diseases of which they know less, in human beings of whom they know nothing."

That epigram admirably summed up the centuries of medical progress to that point. And 150 years after Voltaire had rendered his sardonic comment, Dr. Lawrence J. Henderson of Harvard's Medical School said that a random patient in America in the early part of the twentieth century with a random disease who consulted a doctor at random had no more than a 50-50 chance of benefiting from the encounter.[5]

Times have changed? Not very much, experts agree. Although medical science has come such a long way in the last few decades that to talk about the possibility of "risk" in an encounter with a doctor seems as anachronistic as wearing an asafetida bag to ward off colds, risk is all too often the case. Just a few years ago, Dr. Edward R. Pinckney, former editor of the *JAMA*, said that *patients in the United States today have a less than 50-50 chance of having diseases correctly diagnosed.*[6] The kind and quality of care they receive following that is also a risky matter. After a health-survey team made public its findings in the 1960s, New Yorkers were made aware that: "You have just a little better than a 50-50 chance of getting optimal care from a doctor in a hospital in New York City." Since some control is exercised over the performance of doctors in hospitals and since New York has probably more institutions and medical men of distinguished reputation than any other place in the country, the prospects for most patients are not good.

Fees for What Kind of Service?

It is true that a number of medical centers and doctors in the United States have gained such international fame that many prominent foreigners have come here for treatment. (Although the rich of America, it should be noted, and some not-so-rich frequently travel to Europe for treatment.) Whatever their gratitude, some have been genuinely startled by the cost. British comedian Peter Sellers was delighted with the care he received in the United States when he had a heart attack some years ago. When he saw the bill, he spoofs, he told the doctor: "My heart stopped eight times over." That was reported to be $85,000.

Undoubtedly, he did receive fine care. But the repeated assertions that Americans generally are receiving the finest medical care in the world are meaningless unless they can be related to specific constituents of quality care; they are false if they are contradicted by specific evidence.

What criteria can be used? Dr. W. Palmer Dearing, former executive director of the Group Health Association of America, indicated some of the most important recently: "Medical care is of good quality to the degree that it is available, acceptable, continuous, documented, and that the treatment is based on accurate diagnosis rather than symptomology."[7] The fee-for-service approach has played havoc with all of those standards. It has also encouraged doctors to exploit and endanger patients further by submitting them to unnecessary surgery and other forms of treatment.

Although Medicare and Medicaid have extended the *possibility* of treatment to low-income persons, it is still not available to millions. And the kind of treatment that millions do receive is often woefully substandard. A study made public in 1973, for example, indicated that if all of the pregnant women in New York had received adequate medical care in 1968, the infant death rate would have been only 14.7 for each 1000 live births instead of 21.9.[8]

In other areas of health, the same kind of thing has been true. An intensive study made by researchers with the Institute of Industrial Relations of the University of California at Los Angeles showed that the Watts section of the city had only 17 percent of the total population, but it had 65 percent of reported tuberculin reactors and more than 40 percent of all cases of whooping cough, amoebic infections, venereal diseases, and rheumatic fever. The death rate was far higher than for any other part of the city. At the time of the riot in the summer of 1965, a commission appointed by the governor showed that only 106 physicians were available for a population of 252,000—a ratio three times lower than that of the rest of Los Angeles County.[9]

Whites in many poor areas have fared no better, since doctors have not been motivated to practice where money is in short supply and health needs are great. In the first part of the 1960s, when poor patients meant only modestly paid doctors, many people resorted to rather desperate measures to lure a doctor to their community. Thus, the inhabitants of Virginia's Tangier Island ended an 11-year search for a doctor in 1965 when a Denver physician heard an S.O.S. on his radio asking for someone to help them.[10] Four years later a Scott Valley (California) Citizens Committee was advertising for a doctor, but without takers. Although the area boasted good school systems, nine churches, "unlimited recreation," and promised a potential net income of up to $50,000 a year, not a single candidate had answered the appeal sent out through all 93 medical schools, the 50 state medical associations, the AMA, the California Academy of General Practice, the Los Angeles County Medical Association, and even the Christian Medical Society located in Southern California.[11]

"No wonder there's a doctor shortage in many low-fee areas," commented a Connecticut practitioner in 1973. In his own state, he pointed out, a hernia repair costs more in New Haven than in Hartford, 40 miles away; and in Connecticut, an office visit costs 50 percent more for patients than it does in Utah.[12]

Even when doctors do accept the opportunities to earn $100,000 and more in low-income areas they often render questionable services, and at high rates. State and local investigations since the advent of Medicare and Medicaid have revealed extraordinary evidence of fraud on the part of doctors, dentists, and others in the health care industry. For example, when a physical check was made by the City of New York on 1300 patients who received dental work under the Medicaid program, it was disclosed that in 9 percent of the cases the work charged for had not been done.[13] In 1969, a Senate investigating committee found that one doctor had defrauded the Medicare program of almost $350,000 by charging for services not given. Another doctor had claimed payments for 21 house calls or office visits to a patient who was in Greece at the time.[14]

In 1975 an investigation by the General Accounting Office led a federal grand jury to look into a multimillion-dollar scandal involving "Medicaid mills" in New York City. Early charges involved such novel medical procedures as "family ganging" and "Ping-Ponging," which were netting the practitioners fortunes. Family ganging, according to investigators, was common: when a mother with a sick child showed up at a clinic, she was told to return with her healthy children as well. All of them would then be "Ping-Ponged," or shuttled past as many as ten practitioners in half an hour—all of whom billed separately for "consultations," "diagnosis," blood tests, and X rays.[15]

It was pointed out that about three quarters of those under investigation were foreigners—"operating on the fringe of the medical establishment, refugees who have been unable to get hospital affiliation." And there is no question that the golden harvest made possible by the medical care system in this country has attracted a number of enterprising doctors from other countries.

In California, a physician who had been writing as many as 169 illegal prescriptions for drugs every day, had received tax money in payment. An emigré from Canada (where he had apparently never had it so prosperous). "Dr. Feelgood" had been billing Medicare and Medicaid for his services to the tune of $250,000 a year.[16]

Even when services are actually rendered, there is no guarantee that the patient will benefit. The extraordinary discrepancies in the quality of care were first called to public attention in 1956 by Dr. Osler L. Peterson. The detailed investigation he and a team of researchers made in North Carolina emphasized how inadequate visits to physicians are when proper time and treatment are not given.

Dr. Peterson said later that he and his group were "totally unprepared" for the extremes in the quality of care that they found. Half of the physicians surveyed were considered substandard in one or more respects, even though the committee had deliberately set *minimum* quality measurements. Of those who were substandard, 62 percent took poor medical histories, 45 percent failed to conduct adequate physical examinations, 67 percent routinely gave antibiotics for viral infections for which they are worthless, 95 percent examined the heart incompletely, 85 percent did not perform necessary rectal examinations. Patients with emotional problems were regarded generally as hypochondriacs to be got rid of as soon as possible (although it is reliably estimated that about 40 percent of all illnesses are psychosomatic in origin).[17] The same findings were made by Dr. Kenneth F. Clute, a Canadian researcher in 1963. There, more than 40 percent of the doctors had failed to carry out such fundamental procedures as taking a proper history or giving a proper examination or performing some basic action such as sterilizing instruments.[18]

Doctors are so concerned with whisking patients in and out of their offices that they don't have time for the essentials. Yet the impact on health is great.

Accurate diagnosis to determine whether treatment is needed, how much and what kind, should not be the questionable activity it now is. We ordinary mortals are convinced of its arcane nature because sickness, like other painful experiences, has an isolating, alienating effect. But, actually, of the well over 2000 diseases known to doctors, only about 200 account for 98 percent of all ailments treated in this country. Since all can be grouped into nine basic categories, the ability of a doctor to arrive at the correct one should be fairly high. Yet today there is no indication that accurate diagnoses are made with any more thoroughness than they were when Dr. Peterson made his study. Several years ago, when a Pennsylvania medical research team made a study, it found that the routine annual checkup obtained by a low-risk group of upper-income business executives revealed fatal diseases such as heart ailments and cancer in only 51 percent of the cases.[19]

If adequate time to perform a detailed medical examination or to prepare a comprehensive history had been allotted, the record would have been otherwise. For, as Dr. Pinckney has pointed out: "What may be the most surprising secret of all the medical arts is that more than half of all diagnoses can be made from the medical history alone."[20] The history gives the doctor information about the particular complaint, events related to and leading up to the illness, relevant past medical experiences, and a careful review of the working of the body systems. In the manner of that master detective Sherlock Holmes, who was actually patterned after a brilliant medical diagnostician, the physician can then sort, categorize, and relate the information. With the help of X-ray, blood, and other objective tests, he can realistically appraise the *causes* of the symptoms, instead of responding merely to the symptoms themselves.

The day is coming, despite the resistance of organized medicine, when the family doctor will put information about a patient's latest complaint into a box on his desk. A few seconds later, the diagnosis will slide out, accurately based on all the facts that have been noted in the past as well as present findings. Since the box will be connected with a computer at a nearby medical center, the diagnosis will represent not merely the individual practitioner's opinion, but that of the best medical experts.

Some efforts to insure proper diagnosis have been made, both in and out of the profession. Some unions and professional groups have been offering, as a membership benefit, special health-testing programs. Mobile units are taken to work centers, and more than 100 medical tests can be administered within 30 minutes.[21] Unfortunately, because of the let's-be-quick-about-this, time-is-money attitude among doctors, there is no guarantee that adequate time will be given for consultation and treatment any more than for examinations. Consider the remarkable visiting record of Dr. 002504, who recently demanded $117,824.50 from Medicare alone in a single year. During that time, he credited himself for 1355 office visits, 154 home visits, 8332 nursing-home visits, 1378 hospital visits.[22] Additionally, he was visiting private patients and patients on the Medicaid program, besides performing surgery, supervising thousands of tests, making X rays, and a whole host of medical chores. His record was not unusual, as Senate investigators pointed out, with "many cases" of what is described as "gang-visiting" of hospital and nursing-home patients.

The dead as well as the living are also victimized by lack of time, as a result of which murders go undetected and natural deaths are sometimes held to be suicides or accidents. According to a study made several years ago, in more than 50 percent of sudden deaths that go to autopsy, the cause of death is determined to be different from the clinical diagnosis made before autopsy.[23] For example, in New York City a middle-aged man who, doctors believed, died of a stroke was found to have been stabbed in the brain with an ice pick that had entered inconspicuously through his eye. An autopsy surgeon in Los Angeles discovered a bullet in the brain of a patient whose death was believed to be caused by pneumonia. More pathologists are generally held to be needed to insure that the cause of death is accurately determined. However, not even that precaution always helps. In Santa Barbara, California, a pathologist was recently forced to resign when the coroner became curious about the quality of his work and the size of his income. He had been paid by the county $28,000 for handling autopsies ordered by the coroner's office between August 1971 and August 1972; $92,000 for his work as pathologist and laboratory chief at Santa Barbara County General Hospital. As an indication of the quality of his work, the coroner cited a number of cases in which no autopsies had been performed, although he had been certified to perform them. In one case, a young man who had died in the county hospital of head injuries from an automobile accident had been called a victim of hepatitis although a subsequent examination indicated that there was no sign of kidney and liver changes.[24]

The quality of care is further decreased because doctors are so highly rewarded for providing unnecessary treatment and for ordering unnecessary operations, which many of them are ill equipped to perform. In his report to Congress in 1972, the Comptroller General cited some startling instances to indicate what a strong inducement money can be in encouraging excessive care. During a 54-month period, one general practitioner submitted claims for 251 office visits and 219 urinalyses for one patient. Only 87 of the office visits and 26 of the urinalyses were held to be medically necessary during a review of the claims.[25]

Prescribing unnecessary medicines has become commonplace, especially when the government is footing the bill. When California's Attorney General made his study of Medicare and Medicaid frauds a few years ago, he found that one pharmacy employing one pharmacist dispensed 290 Medi-Cal prescriptions in a single day (with his share of the take being well over $1100). About 50 percent of the prescriptions were written by two physicians, he said, one of whom saw 75 to 100 patients a day and wrote 100 to 125 prescriptions a day. (For comparison purposes, a major chain drugstore employing seven pharmacists in a 13-hour day dispenses an average of 300 prescriptions a day.)[26]

More than money is involved in providing excessive care and prescribing unnecessary prescriptions. Patients are being asked to submit to X-ray examinations for no reason at all; they are dosed with dangerous and sometimes fatal drugs; they are incarcerated in hospitals and nursing homes, where they are exposed to a whole new set of dangers. Cruelly, they are sometimes forced to continue to exist against their own pleas for a release from torment.

Because of the fee-for-service system of medical care, doctors have been encouraged to regard any removable part of patients, such as the appendix, uterus, gall bladder, tonsils, and other anatomical items, as profitable sources of income. A study made by a Stanford University researcher, Dr. John Bunker, several years ago revealed that in this country 7400 operations (per 100,000 people) were performed annually. As a comparison, in Britain, the rate was only 3770. Dr. Bunker pointed out that when operations were categorized by specific procedures, the comparison showed that the number of hysterectomies was twice as high in the United States; gallbladder removal, hemorrhoid surgery, and tonsillectomy and adenoidectomy were two or more times greater in the United States than in Britain or Wales.[27]

In his study, made in North Carolina in 1958, Dr. Peterson was shocked by the number of tonsillectomies, and said that "Tonsillectomy as it is commonly practiced in the U.S. has the same relevance to medical science as did blood-letting."[28] Yet, over the years, the blood-letting has only increased. Dr. Roger O. Egeberg, Special Assistant to the President for Medical Affairs, said in 1971 he was "shocked to find out in Washington that tonsillectomy is the most frequent operation that Medicare and Medicaid have to pay for."[29] Currently, it is still the most common operation in the United States, with more than 1,500,000 performed each year. Of that number, at least 70 percent are held by surgeons to be of questionable value. Some 300 deaths a year are associated with the operation.[30]

Other studies have made similar findings in regard to other common kinds of operations. As Dr. Ray E. Trussel concluded in his study of hospitals in New York: "Not only are serious humane and ethical issues being raised, but *it is evident that much money is being spent on unnecessary or incompetent care.*"[31]

The Trussell study, made at the request of the Teamsters Union, revealed that one-third of the hysterectomies performed were unnecessary, and questions were raised about the advisability of another 10 percent. Over half of the Caesarean sections were held "questionable." Some of the specific cases were so hair-raising that they caused members of the survey team to depart from the detached language of science in describing them.

"This is the worst case I ever saw," one surveyor reported about a Caesarean section. It had been performed in a "completely out-moded way," he said. "This is a shocking case," another noted bluntly. It involved a middle-aged woman whose physician had refused to tell her what surgery had been performed or to sign her hospital discharge until his bill was paid. According to the findings of the surveyor, "The patient had a small labial cyst, and a mountain, including a laparotomy, was made of it. The proper diagnosis could have been made if the patient had been examined preoperatively under anesthesia. Her pelvis was normal, and at the operation no fibroids or cysts were found, and a normal appendix was removed. The duration of the hospital stay of 12 days was scandalous. She should have been discharged days earlier."

Similar findings were made at the opposite end of the continent in a study conducted to determine medically justified surgical procedures in a community hospital and a teaching hospital. Researchers at the School of Public Health at the University of California at Los Angeles found that only 50 percent of the hysterectomies in the community hospital were justified, as compared with 80 percent in the university teaching hospital; 62 percent of the appendectomies, as compared with 84 percent; only 2 percent of the tonsillectomies in the community hospital were justified, as compared with 80 percent in the university teaching hospital.[32]

That conditions have changed is wishful thinking. In 1974, Dr. Eugene G. McCarthy and Geraldine Widmer, both of Cornell University Medical College's Department of Public Health, reported on an experiment conducted in cooperation with two New York unions. Workers advised to undergo surgery by their physicians were re-examined by board-certified specialists, who found that 24 percent of the recommended procedures were not warranted. Not unexpectedly, unnecessary hysterectomies ranked high on the list; the 32.0 percent found by the Cornell researchers was the same as that found by Trussell and his group. Orthopedic surgery was found unwarranted in 40.3 percent; ophthalmology, 28.2 percent; urology, 35.8 percent.[33]

In recent years, some patients have become suspicious about the need for ordered surgery and have even been seeking verdicts from medical writers in the daily and weekly press. Dr. Walter Alvarez, dean of the medical columnists, offered his readers as "a common type of letter" the following inquiry:

> I went for an annual examination, and the X-ray man, after making me lie down and strain as hard as I could, said I have a tiny hiatus hernia in my midriff. Now my doctor insists I must immediately be operated on for this, but I object because I have no symptoms; so what should I do?

With rather astonishing bluntness, Dr. Alvarez wrote "The answer obviously is, 'Stand your ground, and do not accept a big dangerous operation for which you have no need.' " Pointing out that he had had the same condition since he was a boy, he said sharply that until 10 or 15 years ago surgeons rarely thought about operating for "so slight an annoyance." Today, things are quite different. Some surgeons have told him, he reported, that they have operated on from five to seven hundred people with that condition.[34]

So scandalous is the scope of this (authorities consider that as many as 2,000,000 operations performed annually in the United States are unnecessary) that, in order to provide potential victims with some kind of protection, Herbert S. Denenberg, the Pennsylvania Insurance Commissioner, in 1972 issued a *Shopper's Guide to Surgery: Fourteen Rules on How to Avoid Unnecessary Surgery*—an indispensable booklet for every home library. Filled with practical advice, the booklet also contains some psychological notes explaining the wholesale knifing going on. The surplus of surgeons, as compared with the shortage of family doctors, in relation to the number of patients each will receive, makes surgeons eager to view any patient as a candidate for the operating table. And a good many of their victims are all-too-eager to climb aboard. Neurotic women in America, unlike Europe, have been encouraged to regard surgery as a form of psychotherapy: "Some women have had six, nine, or sixteen major operations in search of relief from their anxiety, malaise, and all-around misery of emotional immaturity."[35] Much of the surgery performed is incredibly incompetent, done by inept surgeons, and even by doctors who have neither the skill nor the training to undertake any kind of surgery at all. Wherever the fee-for-service system prevails, it provides high incentives to doctors to wield the scalpel. Dr. Alex Gerber, a medical educator and practitioner, pointed out to the California Public Health Association in 1975 that the level of surgical quality is far higher in Britain than in the U.S. "One third of the surgery done here couldn't be performed in Britain," he said; "the doctors would be barred from entering the operating room." And the risks are great, Gerber added: "Far more people die in this country as a result of poorly performed operations than in plane crashes."[36]

In Saskatchewan some years ago, where efforts were made to bring the medical profession under control, it was found that family doctors did 73 percent of all appendectomies, 48 percent of all breast tumor removals, 51 percent of all varicose vein operations, and 29 percent of all womb removals. Commenting on that, Dr. Samuel Wolfe, former Saskatchewan health commissioner, told a Canadian Labour Congress:

> The more patients you push through per hour, the more you earn. The more organs you remove, the higher your income. No trade union would tolerate men with equal training, equal skill, and equal hours of work earning greatly unequal incomes. And yet this is exactly what you, as health care consumers are going along with under Medicare payments to the medical profession.[37]

Avarice is not the only reason for the low-level and unnecessary care often rendered. Doctors in the United States, as the world over, suffer more than an average amount of emotional disturbances, which are revealed by the relatively large number of drug addicts and suicides and alcoholics in the profession. In *The Medical Offenders*, Howard and Martha Lewis describe in detail the extent of and consequences of emotionally ill physicians who insist upon and are allowed to practice despite their pathological condition. Drunken doctors hack away at patients, rapists vent their hostilities on sedated women, drug addicts "hype" themselves before entering the operating room.[38]

Doctors without any training at all have been practicing, and some are still practicing who received their licenses 50 and more years ago when real medical education was in its infancy. Newspapers frequently carry "human interest" stories about eighty- and ninety-year-old physicians still plying their trade, without paying too much attention to the niceties involved. Indeed, as long as he possesses a license, and in most states that is for as long as he lives, a doctor in any condition can do anything he pleases professionally, including (blind and halt though he may be) major surgery.

Undoubtedly, however, the most important reason for low-quality care is that doctors have simply been left behind by new developments in medicine. In medicine, as in other sciences, a "generation" passes with such swiftness that the half-life of a medical education is now set at five years. A man who was graduated from medical school ten years ago is "hopelessly" out of date unless he has attended postgraduate courses, seminars, or has made some other consistent effort to keep up. In California, which is one of the better states so far as medical competency is concerned, it is estimated that between 25 and 35 percent of physicians practicing are "hopelessly" behind the times. In terms of care being delivered, that means that the 7000 to 10,000 doctors who have not kept up are inadequately caring for 2,000,000 patients.[39]

A case history used by Dr. Morton K. Rubinstein of the University of California at Los Angeles to illustrate the consequences of outdated care involved a woman who had frequently been brought to a medical school hospital because of increasing leg weakness and back pain over a ten-year period. "She was followed during this entire time by a busy, well-meaning, and popular general practitioner near her home." He considered her problem to be arthritis. Therapy consisted of a variety of medications, but none of them prevented her condition from deteriorating. Although the doctor had never suggested additional consultation, her family finally brought her to the medical school. At that time, he said, she was in a wheelchair, essentially paralyzed from the waist down and had lost complete control over her excretory functions.

If proper diagnosis had been established ten years earlier, it would have been learned that the cause of her weakness and pain was a benign tumor resting on the spinal cord. Unfortunately, by the time the diagnosis was made and surgery performed, it was too late to be of great help, Dr. Rubenstein reported; the tumor had done irreparable damage to the spinal cord.

When a perceptive layman does look into the kind of treatment he is receiving, the findings are likely to be startling. Ray Rayburn, a former YMCA national executive, retired to California in 1946 and became interested in my research about American medicine. He volunteered to provide me with the case history of his family's experience, which he felt could be considered *typical*.

First, he emphasized that his family was not easily displeased, flitting from one doctor to another without provocation. Ray said that in the 30 years the Rayburns had spent in New York City before coming to California, "We had the most expert medical care at reasonable fees and never once did we have to discontinue using a doctor because of poor service or exorbitant charges."

Their introduction to California medicine occurred shortly after their arrival in the Los Angeles area in 1946. The doctor they selected had been recommended by their bank president as "prominent in medical circles and much in demand as a speaker at medical conventions." But the doctor told them he had never heard of the drug used to alleviate Mrs. Rayburn's arthritis by the New York specialist. However, he agreed to give her shots at the rate established by the former doctor. Two years later, when the physician's young partner took over, the bills were higher; at the end of two years, they were nearly double. When the young doctor was questioned about the charge, he said: "It all depends on what I do for the patient. This medicine I'm injecting is very expensive." One of Ray's friends, a drug salesman, told him the doctor paid 30 cents for each shot.

The third experience with a California doctor took place in 1955, when Ray was having digestive difficulty. He was sent to a laboratory for X rays. Soon after, the doctor told him: "You will have to spend the rest of your life on a soft diet. No more roughage for you."

When Ray went to New York a few months later, he took the X rays with him and gave them to one of his sons-in-law, a doctor. He turned them over to a colleague, a specialist in the field, whose opinion was: "If I had a gut like that, I would pay no attention to what the doctor advised; I'd eat whatever I wanted." As a double check, his other son-in-law, also a staff physician at a leading New York hospital, asked one of his colleagues for an opinion. The verdict was the same.

Ray dropped a fourth doctor after he had clocked the entrances and exits being made by the patients. They were being treated and examined at the rate of one every three and a half minutes, at high, high prices. The next doctor, recommended by the local medical society, refused to give itemized bills: "I don't want my patients to know what my charges are."

Another, who seemed concerned and competent, advised Mrs. Rayburn to have her gallbladder removed and recommended a surgeon. Instead of that man, the Rayburns decided to have the operation performed by a Chinese doctor who practiced about 25 miles away. The surgeon had outstanding credentials, but the hospital refused to allow him to operate (until very recently, Orientals have been as unwelcome as blacks and other minorities in Orange County). Only after Ray persuaded the president of the hospital board of trustees to agree, was permission reluctantly given, with the proviso that the Chinese surgeon visit her twice daily, which was an extraordinary demand. The operation was successful, the surgeon's services satisfactory. Not so the behavior of the doctor who had advised Mrs. Rayburn to have the operation: He billed the Rayburns for "assisting" at the operation and for providing hospital care. When Ray protested, the doctor "justified" his charges by saying that if the Rayburns had taken the surgeon he recommended, "there would have been a 50-50 split in the fee."

The same doctor also insisted that Ray get a diabetes test, and he was sent to a medical laboratory owned by 12 practicing physicians. The diagnosis was positive, and Ray was instructed to go to a diabetic clinic in a city 100 miles away to take a three-day course in insulin administration for "somewhere between $160 and $200 for the course." Suspicious by this time, Ray decided to have the diagnosis checked at another medical laboratory. He was assured there that he had no trace of diabetes; the test was completely negative.

After parting company with that doctor, Ray placed his wife under the care of another highly recommended doctor. A few months later, when Mrs. Rayburn complained of violent headaches, they were treated lightly. The doctor continued to dismiss them as trivial although her detailed medical history showed that for years she had had arthritis, high blood pressure, and a bad heart condition. "There is nothing I or anyone else can do for your wife, because there is nothing wrong with her," he told Ray. "It's all in her mind."

Ray then took her to a clinic with a good reputation, where, after a thorough examination, the doctors reported that Mrs. Rayburn's headaches were caused by high blood pressure. Her condition, they said, was "critical."

The next day, Mrs. Rayburn died.

The chronicle continued through experiences with 23 other doctors, most of whom proved unsatisfactory, but all of whom were recommended by medical societies or expert colleagues. Few persons have Ray Rayburn's determination to check on doctors' orders, to question a medical verdict, to investigate the reality of medical care.

The need for quality and cost control had become so obvious by 1972 that legislation to insure that was written into the amendments of the Social Security Act, not by liberals who had been urging it for years but by one of the most conservative Republicans in the U.S. Senate. The law required that Professional Standards Review Organizations, 182 of them across the country, be established to monitor the care doctors provide, either in hospitals or nursing homes, to beneficiaries of Medicare, Medicaid, and maternal and child health programs. The PSROs were to see that care meets professionally acceptable standards, that it is necessary, and that it is provided in the most appropriate place. The law provided that after January 1976, any doctor wishing federal money would first have to sign up with a PSRO.

Viewing it as a cost-control program in disguise and an interference with the doctor's right to do as he pleases, the AMA opposed the bill. However, alarmed by the rising tide of protest about its activities and still smarting from the Medicare defeat, the AMA officials then decided to go along with the PSRO concept—provided the law was amended to make it less onerous by making it easier for local and state societies to become PSROs. Considering the past disciplinary records of the societies, that should not have caused discomfort to any MD, but AMA members had learned their battle hymns too well to accept any threat of supervision and accountability. At the 1974 convention near Disneyland, they rejected appeals by some of their own leaders, by HEW's Assistant Secretary Dr. Charles C. Edwards, and other government officials, and turned thumbs down on the PSRO concept. As a result, the 244-member House of Delegates voted to adopt a schizophrenic position by advocating amendment of the law and at the same time advocating its repeal.[40]

The PSROs are a fact, but since the chances are great that they will be dominated entirely by doctors, there is not much hope that they will be more effective than the audit committees, the tissue and utilization committees and other measures that have been working for the last decade to make health care cheaper, better, and more available. Until the patient realizes how much he can do to write an effective Rx for America's sick system, there will be no permanent improvement in either quality or costs.

4 Unethical and Frankly Illegal

It is often difficult for even the best among us to draw the line between ethical and unethical behavior, as religious and moral philosophers acknowledge in trying to help us. Doctors are more fortunate, at least in regard to their work, since they are required to subscribe formally to a professional code that helps them to determine which is which.

For all of us, the line is less blurred between what is legal and what is not. Yet, when he was confronted by Senator Philip A. Hart not long ago with evidence of widespread unlawful behavior in the medical profession, the best the past president of the American Medical Association could do was to plead: "Physicians are only human beings."[1] All too "human" in many respects, the record suggests. And thanks to the protective shield under which they operate, they are in a position to do more and to get away with more, too.

Doctors complain that their departures from the straight-and-narrow path attract more attention than that given others. They have a point. However, there is more than the usual irony and shock when a physician, whose function is to protect and preserve life, commits a murder or pushes drugs, robs a bank, conducts ruthless experiments on unsuspecting patients, or involves himself in interests that ally him with profiteers and racketeers.

Often, however, their misdeeds go unnoticed because their professional code generally prohibits other doctors from bearing

witness against them and because of the reluctance of legal investigators to name physicians' names. Frequently, if they are indicted, they are given the unusual opportunity to answer criminal
charges publicly. This is a privilege the news media seldom ex-
tends to many ordinary mortals. In 1973, for example, when the
chairman of the board of trustees of the AMA was indicted with
five other businessmen on charges of misapplication of bank funds
in a conspiracy involving nearly $1,800,000, he was given plenty
of time and space in the news media to assert his innocence.[2]

Courts often sentence erring doctors lightly. In one interesting
case in California, a judge offered a doctor the choice of paying a
$10,000 fine or donating 50 days of medical service free to public
institutions over a three-year period.[3] Juries are often reluctant to
inflict disgrace and severe penalties. In *My Life in Court*, Louis
Nizer tells of a case brought by a man whose wife had died after
48 hours in labor and whose unborn child had been asphyxiated
as the result of negligent treatment by a doctor. Aware of the
need for Caesarean surgery since he had been forced to deliver
the couple's previous child by that method, the doctor had left
the woman after 45 hours of agonized labor, promising to return
when he was needed. By the time he returned, she was dead.
After her death, he had violated the rules of the local health
department by attributing her death to heart failure although it
was caused by a ruptured uterus. In the courtroom, he lied under
oath. The jury was unanimous from the first moment of their
deliberations, yet the judge had to declare a mistrial because of a
deadlock. The reason? A number of the jurors feared that evidence of his wrongdoing was "so overwhelming" that if they
formally decided against him, the doctor would be subject to conviction on criminal as well as civil charges and sent to jail.[4]

The most common form of illegal behavior among doctors, as
among citizens generally, is income-tax evasion. Doctors as a
group, however, evade taxes more than other professionals. According to a study reported by *Medical Economics* some years ago,
they evade taxes at least four times more. The article, which contained some interesting case histories about the more imaginative
tax dodgers, was accompanied by a strict note forbidding its re-

production or even paraphrasing "in whole or in part or in any manner whatsoever."[5] (Small wonder that in a subsequent issue a letter from a loyal insider appeared, under the heading "Burn This!" Distressed at finding back issues on sale in second-hand stores, the writer chided: "If the magazine is to stay out of the hands of the public, it's up to the readers to discard copies that are no longer needed with some discretion.")[6]

It is not necessary to buy used issues of *Medical Economics* to acquire some knowledge of the extent to which doctors evade paying taxes. Some years ago, a Cincinnati radiologist made headlines all over the country for failing to report $3,500,000 he had made on the stock market. In *The Great Treasury Raid,* Philip Stern listed physicians among the professionals and small businessmen who had failed to report a total of $7,000,000,000 in a single year. Some of the evasion could be explained by carelessness, Mr. Stern said. A doctor could probably stuff money into his pocket as he went from one house call to another, and forget to enter it in his ledger. (What house calls?) Some was carefully calculated. Mr. Stern told of one doctor who kept a large fishbowl in his office, advising patients that if they dropped cash in the fishbowl, their bill would be only three-fifths the amount of a regular bill. He cited a dentist who was discovered to have $27,000 filed away among his patients' X rays.[7] Indeed, so much cash as well as narcotics and valuable equipment lies around doctors' offices that "plenty" of criminals have made burglarizing them their specialty, according to "No. 76921" of Michigan State Prison, who wrote an article cautioning doctors about their carelessness some years ago.[8]

In Raymond V. Martin's *Revolt in the Mafia: How the Gallo Gang Split the New York Underworld*, there is an extended discussion of the tie-up between gangsters and doctors who funnel cash payments they receive into illicit enterprises in order to avoid paying taxes. Mr. Martin, retired assistant chief inspector in charge of South Brooklyn detectives, told of an instance in which two men, eavesdropping in a Coney Island cabaret, heard a gangster urging a doctor to make a *safe* investment of $20,000: "You might make $100,000 . . . you didn't lose no money with us last time." Martin noted: "From experience, we knew that some doctors and dentists have 'hot money' in the form of cash fees that they do not declare as taxable income. Such money is often available for speculative investment."[9]

Recently the situation has become even worse, thanks to the enormous profits doctors have been realizing from Medicare and Medicaid. In 1970, a Treasury Department representative told a Senate Finance Committee that of 3000 accounts studied of doctors who had received more than $25,000 in payments from the government health programs, half showed "substantial deficiencies." In one case, a doctor had reported an income of $18,000 over three years, neglecting to mention the more than $140,000 he had received from the government. And there were other cases of omissions totaling more than $100,000.[10]

From the standpoint of ultimate social cost, far more serious than tax evasion is the role that doctors have played in the drug traffic. According to former U.S. Commissioner of Narcotics, Harry J. Anslinger, doctors created some of the bureau's biggest headaches. Among the unusual case histories cited in his book, *The Protectors*, is the story of a brilliant deviate physician who was "the real-life version of the underworld doctor" of the George Raft and James Cagney films. As a result of the reluctance of state boards to take harsh action against duly accredited members of the profession, the doctor continued to practice medicine for more than two decades—although convicted of an assortment of crimes ranging from altering the fingerprints of a fugitive to heading an abortion ring and selling narcotics to addicts.

One of the more interesting specialists in Mr. Anslinger's book is "Dr. Oedipus," a physician who also dispensed narcotics to addicts for merchandise. In a single month he issued prescriptions for more than 1000 grains of morphine. His bizarre preoccupation with accumulating merchandise of every variety as payment was related to his abnormal attachment to his mother. (Although she had died years ago, Dr. Oedipus kept her body in the local mortuary so that he could view the corpse; he could not bear to think of her being underground.) The state medical board was finally persuaded to revoke his license. However, Mr. Anslinger noted wryly, so lenient is the treatment of doctors that two years later the board put him back in business again.[11]

It has been very difficult to make cases against doctors. For one reason, addicts don't give away the source of supply. One addict who did reveal the source of supply was Sally Benson, the author of many film and television plays and the novel *Junior Miss.* The talented and gifted woman encountered the doctor who "hooked" her early in 1963, when she was recovering from pneumonia. Unable to reach her own doctor, she called the Los Angeles County Medical Association's referral service and, as a result, asked Dr. Paul Ezra to come to her house. The young doctor did and administered what he called a "magic medicine." (It was, narcotics investigators found, codeine and Demerol.) The "remedy" was so successful that Miss Benson called him again; soon, the doctor was driving his Rolls Royce to her house two, three, and even five times a day at a charge of $40 a visit. The investigators later said that they became suspicious after pharmacists reported that he frequently picked up narcotics prescriptions for various patients: "It is not usual for a doctor to run errands for patients in his Rolls-Royce, was the way they put it. However, it was not until a year later that they were able to get a grand jury indictment, thanks largely to the willingness of Miss Benson to testify that she had become addicted.

The experience had cost her dearly, more than $30,000 during the 18 months of his treatment; it also took a toll in other ways; investigators reported that her daily dosage of codeine rose from 2.5 grains to 20 grains, which was "enough for 20 patients." It ended happily for her; she was able to kick the addiction. And it also ended reasonably happily for Dr. Ezra. He was far ahead monetarily, and he received only a modest sentence for his role as drug pusher: six months in jail.[12]

Doctors have been involved in other famous-name drug-addiction cases. After Judy Garland's death, her husband described her dependence on pills. "She took pills to sleep, pills to wake up, pills to give a good performance, *pills to counteract other pills.*"[13] More than pills, however, she had been hooked on morphine. Harry Anslinger, who had discussed her case anonymously in

The Protectors, described it in more detail after her death and the death of Louis B. Mayer, who was branded "the villain in the piece." Mr. Anslinger said that he had taken a personal interest in her morphine problem as early as 1949 and managed to pry her out of the clutches of a doctor who was himself a drug addict. He said that when he went to the head of the M-G-M studio to ask that the young singer be given a year's release in order to receive treatment in a sanitarium, the movie executive replied: "I've got $14,000,000 invested in her. I couldn't afford your plan. She's at the top of her box office right this minute."[14]

In 1972, the Bureau of Narcotics and Dangerous Drugs placed amphetamines on the list of controlled substances and promised to reduce manufacturing quotas after a number of startling episodes about addiction were revealed. Not the least of them was that Dr. Max Jacobson, who had accompanied President John F. Kennedy to Vienna in 1961 for the summit meeting with Nikita Khruschev, was revealed to have given the "magical medicine" to a list of patients whose names constituted a *Who's Who* of political, entertainment, literary, and social figures. Many of the patients swore by the treatment; some were less enthusiastic. Film producer Otto Preminger, who had been a patient for a short time, said that he stopped taking the treatments because the shots made him feel "terrible." Tennessee Williams' brother told reporters that the playwright spent three months in a mental hospital after Dr. Jacobson's treatments. One patient, a photographer, died as a result of an overdose of amphetamines.[15]

Dr. Jacobson's method of treatment was legal, of course. Efforts have been made, however, to make such treatment illegal in all but some cases of narcolepsy (a condition characterized by attacks of deep sleep) and hyperkinesis (excessive activity among children). Using amphetamines for hyperkinesis is also highly questionable from a medical standpoint. Nevertheless, many schools have been indulging in it so enthusiastically that by 1971 at least 250,000 youngsters were getting daily doses along with whatever training in the three R's they could encompass in the drugged state. Amphetamines were the chief ingredient in the weight-loss drugs prescribed by the "Fat Doctors," who were making millions from unsuspecting patients. Some action has been taken to render that use illegal.

Both amphetamines and cocaine were involved in the case of Dr. David Sachs, noted heart surgeon, who was indicted by a federal grand jury on 80 counts of acquiring and distributing those and other illegal drugs in 1975. Dr. Sachs, who had won the AMA's Outstanding Physician Award, was familiar to viewers of such television shows as "The Bold Ones," "M*A*S*H," and "Mission Impossible." Until shortly before his indictment, he also starred in a weekly medical talk show.[16] (The addiction of doctors to drugs, it should also be noted, is very high—10 to 20 times more frequent than among adults generally.)

The AMA had an opportunity to do something to curb the illicit traffic in psychoactive drugs more than a decade ago, when Senator Thomas J. Dodd introduced a bill to expand federal control over those substances. The bill was a moderate one, requiring only that manufacturers and everyone else except physicians who receive or dispense such drugs, register with the Department of Health, Education, and Welfare. They would be required to keep complete records of the quantities of drugs they handle and make those records available to food and drug inspectors. Opposing the bill were members of the National Association of Retail Druggists, the American Pharmaceutical Association, and the AMA. In a letter to Senator Dodd's subcommittee, the AMA warned that the bill was "restrictive to the degree that it would inhibit and interfere with the manufacture, distribution, and use of these drugs." In typical fashion, it insisted that education and state and local laws—not federal—would provide the answer.[17]

Conditions today indicate how ineffective controls have been. Manufacturers turn out pills by the billion, and popping them has become a way of life, even for children in junior high schools across the country. There is so little concern about their distribution that a couple of years ago it was learned that 1,000,000 uppers and downers a month were being shipped to an address in Mexico that was described as "the nineteenth hole of a golf course."

Restrictive laws of various types have frequently provided doctors with an opportunity to enrich themselves by doing illegally for a high price what might command a more modest fee in the open market. That was certainly the case with abortion laws, which have recently been modified. Many individual doctors lobbied against them. Generally, however, the medical establishment remained silent, allowing members of the profession to take advantage of the laws. They did, on a grand scale. During the 1960s, abortions were being performed at the rate of one to two million a year.

Not all doctors violated the laws in order to make a profit; some believed it humanitarian to do so. Many doctors, however, were more interested in the profits. A hospital intern arrested in New York some years ago was the head of an abortion ring that grossed almost $500,000 a year. A Chicago doctor arrested in the summer of 1965 with two patients had stacks of money totalling $15,711 in his desk drawer and open closet-safe. He could scarcely qualify as an expert, despite the huge fees he was charging. Police had to take one of the young women in his office on whom he had just performed an abortion to a nearby hospital for a repair operation.[18]

Although he is a character in a work of fiction, there is much that is uncomfortably factual about Joseph Heller's Doc Daneeka in *Catch-22*, that neat, cynical Staten Island practitioner who spent his army years mourning over the abortions he could have profited by if it had not been for that draft board:

> I really had it made, I tell you. Fifty grand a year I was knocking down, and almost all of it tax-free since I made my customers pay me in cash. I had the strongest trade association in the world backing me up. And look what happened. Just when I was all set to really start stashing it away, they had to manufacture fascism and start a war horrible enough to affect even me.[19]

Nonfictional is the doctor in *Intern* who indulges in another fairly common racket in which doctors have participated, the black market in babies. The author, "Dr. X," who took refuge in a pseudonym to protect his career, devotes a sizable amount of space to Dr. Jason and his "No informer" cases, who allowed their babies to be adopted. Privately arranged adoptions were not illegal in the state in which Dr. X interned, but he commented: "I'll bet this is one of the places where Jason gets his money."[20] In states where private adoptions are illegal, doctors can make even more. When Senator Dodd appealed for support of a bill he introduced some years ago to halt the "thriving" black market in babies, he cited some dismal evidence that had been presented to his subcommittee:

> We were told . . . of a doctor coercing a teen-age mother to give up her baby to cover hospital expenses, so he could sell it for a huge profit. . . . We were told of a black market sale of a baby who was subsequently found to be a defective. He was thereupon returned to the doctor who, in turn, hired a woman to take the child without notice to its natural mother, and since she was not at home at the time, the baby was simply left in her room.[21]

Far more widespread than such illegal activities have been insurance frauds. These frauds have reached incredible proportions since the enactment of Medicare and Medicaid. The impact on costs of medical and hospital and convalescent care are discussed in detail elsewhere; so is the willingness of the insurance industry to tolerate claims frauds and falsifications. The profession must be kept happy so that insurance will continue to be a private matter, but the premium hikes are always borne by the public.

It is instructive to point out that concern about such illegality has existed for more than a quarter of a century. In New York in the late 1940s, a commission appointed by the state legislature to investigate the handling of workmen's compensation cases made some interesting findings. In four hospitals, it was discovered, 75 doctors listed their services as "specialist" in order to get $100 fees (nonspecialist services commanded only $50). Moreover, the commission found that the doctors being paid the inflated prices were not only not specialists, they were not doing the work at all. In some cases, chief surgeons and medical directors were making as much as $50,000 to $75,000 a year charging for work they farmed out to interns.[22]

Another investigation in New York some time later showed that 1300 physicians were working with ambulance-chasing lawyers to defraud insurance companies in accident cases. One doctor was found to have puffed a bill for a $10 service into $184. Another charged a company for 44 visits to a patient he had seen only once. At that time, an investigator described the extent of medical swindling as "staggering to the imagination."[23]

The situation in New York, of course, was not unique. In 1952, the California Physicians' Service, a doctor-sponsored health-insurance plan, disclosed that 200 doctors in the Los Angeles area were cheating the plan of more than $1,000,000 a year through overuse and flagrant fraud. The Los Angeles County Medical Society promised to deal with offenders promptly. That, of course, was not fulfilled. The only doctor of the 200 accused who was brought into court was, interestingly enough, not a member of the society.[24]

Scandals all over the country involving Medicare and Medicaid programs being looted by doctors, dentists, and other health-care workers have involved hundreds of millions of dollars.

The distinction between what is illegal and what is unethical has been blurred to a great extent for the medical profession by the AMA's flexibility about which is which. Indeed, during an exchange with the director of the AMA's Department of Medical Ethics some years ago about conflict of interest, Senator Hart said sharply: "That doesn't sound like an ethic to me; it sounds like a bookkeeping decision."[25] And many of the ethical standards, he and others have suggested, might far be better cast as statutes. Two decades ago New York Attorney General Nathaniel Goldstein urged, after an investigation of a conspiracy between the doctors and druggists, that the state "make illegal much of what organized medicine now considers unethical."[26] Since then, a good many persons have suggested that it might be equally helpful to have states make illegal much of what organized medicine now considers *ethical*.

What prompted Mr. Goldstein's comment was the fact that

the AMA code at that time specifically held it unethical for a physician to own an interest in a drugstore in the area of his medical practice, unless (as in the case of some rural communities) drugstore facilities were not adequate or available. The Attorney General's investigators found, however, that about a thousand doctors had joined with pharmacists in a scheme to fleece the public. Patients were directed by doctors to drugstores in which they had a financial interest. In some cases, doctors made sure of their victims by refusing to write prescriptions; they insisted that they telephone them. These doctors then could guarantee a steady stream of business at high, high prices. Patients were being overcharged; they were also getting prescriptions for unnecessary medications. Indeed, according to one estimate, 50 percent of the prescriptions written by some physicians were unnecessary.[27]

State and local societies, which had the responsibility for enforcing the Code of Ethics, remained notably mute. But some relief for patients was obtained in 1954 by Mr. Goldstein, who obtained an injunction from the State Supreme Court in New York ordering such activities halted. That was only a temporary palliative, however. Undaunted by the public outrage that greeted news of the conspiracy, the AMA decided that instead of condemning the practice, its House of Delegates would only modify the code to permit physicians to own drugstores "as long as there is no exploitation of the patient."[28]

Why had the AMA modified its stand? Some answers were suggested by a number of witnesses who appeared before the Senate Judiciary Subcommittee on Antitrust and Monopoly in 1964. Paul A. Pumpian, secretary of the Wisconsin State Board of Pharmacy, charged that the AMA policy shift was engineered by physicians who had financial interests in pharmacies. One of them, the owner of a Wisconsin drugstore, was later elected president of the AMA.[29]

The chairman of the AMA's Judicial Council, which has jurisdiction over all questions of medical ethics, said that his group had attempted to reverse the decision in 1962. The matter was dropped after a one-day hearing during which both the recommendation and the chairman were attacked. "They really ground me up pretty fine," Dr. George A. Woodhouse told the Senate subcommittee: "I looked like I had just come out of a meat grinder." Many of those doing the grinding, he added, were doctors with financial interests in drugstores or spokesmen for a group that promotes pharmacies in privately owned clinics.[30]

To illustrate this effect of doctors in the pharmacy business, a case was cited featuring a California doctor who had written prescriptions for indigent welfare patients at the rate of about $10,000 a year. Within a year after he opened a pharmacy next door to his office, the value of the welfare prescriptions he was writing rose to $50,000 without any considerable increase in the number of patients he treated. To halt such practices, California, Maryland, North Dakota, and some other states enacted laws against the ownership of pharmacies by doctors. In others, unfortunately, the "ethical" practice still continues.

A number of physicians as well as most of the Senate investigators were also troubled that little action had been taken against doctors owning drug-marketing firms. Those companies, usually small and geographically limited in their operations, offer prescription drugs and drug compounds under their own trade names, usually products no longer protected by patent. Some merely buy a drug by its generic name and repackage it for sale under a brand name. Although it is considered unethical for physicians to have such interests, many do. At the time of the hearing, at least 140 repackaging firms were known that were owned by doctors. The number is probably much higher. Some interesting revelations came to light about the way in which such ownership influences doctors' prescribing habits. One of the more striking examples involved Carrtone Laboratories in New Orleans, which had 1200 doctors among its 3000 stockholders. Carrtone puts out repackaged drugs under its own trade name, marketing them mainly in the South. In 1961, the doctor-stockholders were chided for their deficiencies: If each Doctor Stockholder had only written three "scripts" instead of one, sales for the month would have increased from $68,417 to $168,000, for profits of more than $65,000.[31]

Some of the doctor-stockholders took a livelier interest than others in their common business enterprise. One of them was a North Carolina practitioner who waxed eloquent in a booster letter to his colleagues. "I look upon Carrtone as a rosebud about to bloom, stockwise," said Dr. Boyce P. Griggs. Call the druggist, he suggested, and urge him to "blanket order all products that you listed and would use in quantity."[32] Another stockholder, this one also company president and dean of the medical school of Louisiana State University, indulged in hard-sell appeal to physicians. "If each individual stockholder would make up his mind to do just a little bit more for his company, the company would start making a sizable profit immediately."[33] (Repackaging is, of course, a small-time operation compared with some of the other conflicting interests of doctors.)

Another business matter the Hart Senate subcommittee took up was the selling of eyeglasses, a big business, with sales of almost $200,000,000 a year. Glasses should be relatively inexpensive items, partly because volume has risen tremendously in the last 30 years. That has been paralleled by simplification in the manufacturing process: lens blanks, which once had to be worked with great skill and infinite hand labor, are now ground by precision machines capable of making minute accommodations. Yet, in relation to manufacturing costs and business volume, eyeglasses continue to be absurdly expensive. (Not everywhere, however, for they are obtainable at very low prices through some cooperatives in the Middle West and at lower-than-average prices through some group-health plans.)

Here, again, physicians have played their part. In 1949, the government filed suit against a number of optical companies and several hundred doctors across the country for violation of the Sherman Antitrust Act. As a result of a consent decree handed down in 1950, the companies were required to withdraw from marketing eyeglasses for at least ten years, to cease price-fixing agreements, and to halt rebates. Physicians, some of whom had been demanding from eyeglass dispensers as much as 50 percent of the price of the glasses they prescribed, were "perpetually enjoined" from accepting rebates in any form, directly or indirectly.

In 1949, the American Medical Association also acted in response to the scandal by making it "unethical" for doctors to dispense glasses. As in the case of the ownership of drugstores by doctors, the AMA soon bowed to pressure. In 1954, it altered the code to permit the selling of glasses if it were a "needed service." (The American College of Surgeons stood its ground, prohibiting members from selling glasses except in hardship cases and insisting they "cannot derive income from merchandising and still be considered on a professional level.") [34]

So many ophthalmologists in the country had come to regard dispensing eyeglasses as a necessary service by the time of the Hart hearings in 1965 that 40 percent of them were indulging in that sideline. Their bypassing opticians and optometrists, neither of whom may diagnose or treat eye diseases, did not bring down the price of glasses for most buyers. The subcommittee was told that a survey in Los Angeles showed that doctors charged about $15 more for a pair of glasses than opticians charged. One witness testified that some ophthalmologists who sold as well as prescribed glasses were realizing daily profits of $600. [35]

Serious concern was later expressed to Senator Hart's subcommittee about the role of doctors in relation to commercial laboratories. Many of them are owned by doctors, who also employ their own technicians and nurses to do routine tests in the office. Many of them are supported by doctors, who pay stated fees of modest amounts for laboratory work; the doctors then bill their patients separately at standard rates, charging up to $15 for a test which cost them $1 or less. For more serious than the financial exploitation is the effect on human life. Senator Hart's subcommittee gathered evidence of needless amputations, deaths, and serious illnesses caused by the negligence and inefficiency of the testing laboratories. Medical authorities like the director of the National Communicable Disease Center in Atlanta, the chief of the division of laboratories of the California State Department of Health, New York City's Commissioner of Hospitals, and others presented evidence showing how fatal errors can be and often are; and it was estimated that *as many as 25 percent of laboratory tests are in error.* [36] To cite one example: a woman had a breast removed because a test incorrectly indicated she had cancer.

Unethical and Frankly Illegal

A good many of the doctors' other business activities are clearly not in the best interests of patients, although doctors are allowed to exercise their own often faulty judgment in regard to them. Few laws now recognize the dangers involved because the vast body of medical legislation that has been enacted was drafted by or with the advice of organized medicine, intent on giving doctors maximum latitude to profit. Since the profession's ethical codes are very permissive and rarely enforced, new laws to protect the public from exploitation are needed.

One of the darker chapters in the history of medicine is that written by Peter Chemberlen and his descendants, whose name continues to be held in deserved contempt after 400 years, despite the remarkable contribution of the family to medicine.[37] A French religious refugee, Chemberlen brought with him to England in 1569 a trade secret he had invented: the forceps. In no time at all, his fame as a superior obstetrician had made him rich. Always he and his son and grandson insisted that the attending physician be dismissed and barred from the rooms where they exercised their miraculous skill. Hugh, the grandson, realized even greater profits from the device than the inventor. He not only accumulated wealth as a practitioner, but as a peddler offering the secret to carefully selected physicians who had money and who wanted to get in on a good thing. His charge to a French obstetrician was the equivalent of more than $10,000.

During a visit to Holland, Hugh sold the secret to the College of Physicians in Amsterdam. The college, in an equally business-like manner, kept the method of delivery of forceps secret, except for graduates of the school, who had to swear to keep it secret. The discovery of the forceps was not made public for 125 years, and then only because two young Hollanders believed it was criminal to deny the world the life-saving knowledge. The two enrolled in the college and took their medical degrees. Then, promptly violating the oath in the interests of humanity, they made it available to all physicians, exhorting them to use it properly.

It was not until 1813, when new owners were going through the palatial home once owned by Peter Chemberlen, that outside eyes saw the source of the family's treasure: four rusty instruments locked in an old chest. With them surely were the ghostly accusations of the hundreds of thousands of women and unborn children, victims of the Chemberlens' modern medical philosophy that ranks profits above people.

5 ...And Inhumane

It was, by strange and bitter irony, an incident at the Jewish Chronic Disease Hospital of Brooklyn that focused public attention on the human experimentation being conducted by medical researchers in this country. There, 22 patients, without their knowledge or consent, had been injected with live cancer cells to determine whether people suffering advanced stages of other diseases could reject invasions of cancer. The furor that followed and that has continued to rage since was started by a lay member of the hospital board, an internationally known lawyer named William A. Hyman. He appeared in the Brooklyn Supreme Court on January 20, 1964 in search of an order to determine what, if any, control there had been over the conduct of physicians in the hospital for which he had assumed a legal responsibility.

The facts in the case were revealed three weeks later by the doctors who had performed the experiment: Dr. Chester M. Southam of the Sloan-Kettering Institute for Cancer Research and Dr. E. E. Mandel, medical director of the hospital. At the Sixth International Transplantation Conference, they reported that 19 of the 22 patients did not have cancer, that nine of the 19 had died since the date of the experiment, July 1963, six months earlier. The report included an oral statement that none of the deaths had been due to the experiment.

However, as was noted by John Lear, science editor of *The Saturday Review: "No pretense was made that the experiment could possibly help these patients, or even that the experiment*

79

would contribute to understanding of the diseases with which the patients were afflicted."[1] (Italics added.)

Meantime, the records Mr. Hyman was demanding continued to be withheld. The executive director of the hospital refused, saying merely that it was not necessary that the patients be told since the cancer cells "are harmless." The court turned him down. A Brooklyn assistant district attorney dismissed his request. But pursuing his fight, without the assistance of medical organizations or institutions, Mr. Hyman finally won a victory from the Court of Appeals of the State of New York 14 months later. At the end of the year, the New York State Board of Regents put the two doctors on probation for a year, with the warning that their medical licenses could be suspended if further transgressions of professional ethics occurred. The charges acted upon were "fraud and deceit" in the cancer experiment.[2]

The story did not end there, however. Within weeks after the Regents' decision, Mr. Hyman was petitioning again—this time to the office of professional conduct of the New York State Department of Education—to protest the dismissal notices issued by the medical director to three staff physicians who, under a summons from the Attorney General's office, had testified against him.

John Lear was not the only one to demand, "Do we need new rules for experiments on people?"

In 1947, the International Tribunal sitting in Nuremberg, Germany, had promulgated the first rule to satisfy moral, ethical, and legal concepts in medical experiments on human beings: *"The voluntary consent of the human subject is absolutely essential."* That means, the tribunal elaborated, not merely that he have knowledge of the hazards and the legal capacity to give consent, but that he be able to exercise the free power of choice "without the intervention of any element of force, fraud, deceit, duress, over-reaching, or other ulterior form of constraint or coercion."[3] The first rule had been written after the whole world had been shocked by the horrors of what had occurred in Nazi Germany in the name of medical science. As a result of the Nuremberg trials, four physicians were hanged for having violated that principle in administering drugs to and performing surgical operations upon Jews, Catholics, and other political prisoners. Nine other participants were sentenced to life terms; three others, who were not doctors, were also hanged.

During the 1950s there seemed little cause for concern about research malpractice, although research, funded largely with federal money, increased greatly. Much of it was carried out in laboratories and required little or no participation by human subjects. But some studies could be carried out only in man, and there were few restrictions. It was possible in America for any physician or even for people without medical training to experiment with drugs on unsuspecting subjects.

Obviously, delicate and complex issues are involved. As Dr. Irwin Feinberg, professor of psychiatry at the University of California at San Francisco, pointed out recently, it is necessary to separate therapeutic experiments conducted in the context of the traditional doctor-patient relationship from experiments which are aimed at acquiring knowledge of potential value to others in general, but which do not benefit the research subjects themselves.[4]

The first category, as he points out, is covered by malpractice and contract law and may, indeed, be part of a doctor's ethical obligation to do what he can to improve treatment. Although risks are involved, the patient's consent must be obtained and there is the traditional legal safeguard: "Experiment at your peril." It is the second category that raises serious ethical, legal, and, many believe, moral problems. Some of the experiments that have been carried on have been of questionable value; some were more concerned with profits of the drug industry, for example, than medical science. Many of them have been conducted with a flagrant disregard for human rights.

As early as 1962, Dr. Henry K. Beecher of Harvard Medical School had presented a bill of indictment in a book called *Experimentation in Man.*[5] However, it was not until after the episode in the Brooklyn Hospital that Dr. Beecher's challenge really began to be heard, that breaches of ethical conduct in carrying out experiments are "by no means rare, but are almost, one fears, universal."[6]

In an article in *The New England Journal of Medicine* in 1966,

Dr. Beecher provided a list of particulars to support his argument that there had been, since World War II, "increasing employment of patients as experimental subjects when it must be apparent that they would not have been available if they had been truly aware of the uses that would be made of them. It seems obvious that hundreds have not known that they were the subjects of an experiment."[7] Among the cases he listed are these.

- In an experiment to study the effects of the thymus gland, which plays an important role in the body's immunological system, on the take of grafts, 11 children aged three and a half months to eighteen years, had their thymuses removed while undergoing heart surgery. For comparison, seven other children in the study were spared. The experiment, he said, yielded only a negative result: there was no difference between groups in the take of skin grafts. (What the ultimate effects on the children may be are unknown.)

- Dr. Beecher pointed out in his preface to another experiment that rheumatic fever can usually be prevented by giving penicillin to treat the recurrent "strep throats" that cause rheumatic fever and heart disease. In one experiment, 109 sick servicemen were denied penicillin; two developed acute rheumatic fever; one, acute nephritis. In a related experiment, 500 servicemen were denied penicillin and given either sulfadiazine or no drug at all in order to compare the effects. The comparison, he indicated, was clear: at last 25 of the 500 developed rheumatic fever; one medical officer put the number as high as 70.

- A piece of a melanoma, a highly malignant cancer, was transplanted from a seriously ill young woman to her mother "in the hope of gaining a little better

> understanding of cancer immunity, and in the hope
> that the mother's production of tumor antibodies
> might be helpful in the treatment of the cancer pa-
> tient." The patient died the day after the transplant;
> the mother died of melanoma 15 months later.

Other doctors, including some of his Harvard medical school colleagues, have taken issue with Dr. Beecher, insisting that the advance of medical science is at stake. That must be considered, and it is not easy to arrive at a judgment in many instances.

At any rate, in 1966 the furor that had been raised and the laxity exposed caused the Public Health Service to establish guidelines for the protection of human research subjects. The revised policy (No. 129) states that the granted institution, usually a hospital or medical school, has responsibility for the protection of research subjects. The guidelines require that an independent review committee determine the appropriateness of the methods used to secure informed consent, and weigh the risks and potential benefits of the proposed investigations. The committee must keep written documentation of its deliberations and of subject consent and maintain surveillance of projects. According to Dr. Irwin Feinberg, however, "few, if any," schools provided the required surveillance once the grants had been approved.[8]

In 1971, because of continuing public demand, new guidelines were approved. They included a discussion of the types of risk which a patient may have to face, including physical, psychological, and social dangers. The guidelines define carefully the difference between therapy and experimentation and provide criteria for informed consent. But more emphasis should be given to the ethical implications of advances in biomedical research and technology.

Take the case of heart transplants. They have been creating a considerable amount of controversy, religious, moral, and legal, as well as scientific, since Dr. Christiaan Barnard transplanted the heart of another man into the breast of a Capetown, South Africa, dentist in 1967 and kept him alive for more than 500 days. Then

Dr. Denton Cooley replaced a critically ill man's heart with an artificial one perfected by Dr. Michael DeBakey, but without having received DeBakey's permission or that of the Baylor Committee on Research Involving Human Beings. The action brought him plenty of glory and a censure; it also intensified a feud which has been the most dramatic in science since the Oppenheimer-Teller battle.[9]

As late as 1973, legal battles were being organized over the definition of death in heart-transplant cases.[10] Scientists and theologians are still struggling with the problem. The public is also still strongly and emotionally divided on the issue.

Some procedures have aroused even greater controversy. Psychosurgery, for example, occupied much of the time during the 1973 Senate hearings. Testimony for a law to bring "nonmedical surgery" under the control of the public rather than boards of specialists or "other vested interests," was presented by a Harvard-trained psychiatrist who teaches at the Washington School of Psychiatry. Dr. Peter Breggin defined psychosurgery, the destruction of normal brain tissue to control the emotions or behavior, as falling into "the class of atrocities, as defined in Nuremberg."[11] (Not included in psychosurgery is brain surgery to treat epilepsy, Parkinson's disease, tumor, stroke, and brain trauma.) He cited a number of recent reports to indicate reasons for his protest. One in 1970 involved a thalamotomy on a woman with "chronic, intractable agitated depression." The authors of the report, Dr. Vernon Mark, Dr. Frank Evin, and colleagues, described the operation as successful, although on the forty-fourth day after surgery the patient went into a phone booth, called her mother to say "good-bye," and downed the contents of a vial of poison she had brought to the hospital with her, killing herself.[12]

Dr. Breggin also took issue with the optimistic reports of Dr. Orlando J. Andy of the University of Mississippi about the variety of operations he has performed on about 40 patients, many of them children. His purpose avowedly is to control the aggressive behavior of children and make them more "manageable." In one case, he operated six times on a nine-year-old boy of normal intelligence, noting that after six operations and signs of gross brain damage, the patient was "adjusted." "Intellectually, however, the patient is deteriorating."[13]

In commenting on other experiments that have been made with psychosurgery, Dr. Breggin discounted some of the reports as grossly inaccurate scientifically and misleading. One involved an epileptic woman "whose violence and her refusal to be reasonable about the dangers inherent in her smoking" led her physician to seek surgical opinion. The report asserted that the results of the temporal lobe surgery were "gratifying."

> She still has seizures but her rages have disappeared. She has set no more fires, and she has become able to function once more as a housewife and mother.

Dr. Breggin held that "nothing could be further from the truth" in his discussion of the only case history used to support the merits of temporal lobe surgery. The violence, he noted, was not associated in any way with her epileptic seizures, and when "cured" of her violence the epilepsy remained unchanged. He added:

> The fact that she is returned to being a satisfactory housewife and mother is again typical of psychosurgery studies. Not only have the vast majority of patients been women, both in the past and in the current literature, but the two most in-depth prolobotomy studies have already told us that psychosurgery is much more effective on women than on men because women can more easily be returned home to function as partially crippled, brain damaged housewives, while there are no social or occupational roles for partially crippled, brain damaged men.[14]

The use of prisoners particularly in relation to psychosurgery and other forms of psychological and biomedical research was sharply criticized by a number of witnesses. Jessica Mitford, in her devastating book, *Kind and Usual Punishment*, said that the waivers that prisoner subjects are usually required to sign, releasing "everyone in sight" from damage claims are "fraudulent, worthless, and illegal." She said that she had found one use of waivers in the Maryland House of Corrections, where the physician in charge told her that they were infecting healthy men there with typhoid and other diseases.[15]

The use of prisoners was also protested by Geoffrey Cowan and Aileen Adams of the Communications Law Program of the University of California at Los Angeles Law School, who visited drug-testing sites in 11 states in 1971. They said:

> We expected at the outset to uncover isolated examples of human abuse; but instead of a few specific scandals, we found a dominant pattern of human exploitation.[16]

In the article they wrote subsequently, they detailed some of the cases. At the Jackson County, Missouri, jail, a cheerful cartoon brochure entitled *Malaria Volunteer* was promising a six-weeks program of "additional food, ice cream, fruit juice, improved quarters," and a $50 cash bonus. Graduates of the program were given a "Certificate of Merit," suitable for framing. The volunteers' job? To submit to infection with a live malaria virus to test new cures being developed by the United States Army. The nurse there told the young researchers: "It also appeals to their sense of patriotism, because they know they're contributing something to the guys in Vietnam."[17]

One of the most shocking instances of prisoner abuse was revealed in the summer of 1969, by Walter Rugaber of *The New York Times*. He charged that federal officials had watched "without interference" while hundreds of inmates in three states were stricken with illness and serious disease, and many of them died.[18] The report, which was introduced in evidence at the hearings held by Senator Gaylord Nelson and members of the subcommittee on monopoly that year, also highlighted some of the most serious problems involved, that affect millions of American consumers as well as the immediate victims. They learned that powerful, potentially fatal compounds have been tested with little or no medical observation of the results. Subjects failed to take some of the compounds, failed to report serious reactions, and failed to receive careful laboratory tests. Yet the "findings" were used as the basis to justify the sale of prescription drugs throughout the country.

. . . And Inhumane

A leading role in the story was played by Dr. Austin R. Stough, an Oklahoma-born general practitioner with large holdings in two corporations estimated to have produced about 25 percent of a plasma byproduct used to protect people against infectious diseases. His experiments with prisoners constituted between 25 and 50 percent of the initial drug tests in the United States.

According to the record, Dr. Stough opened private practice in McAlester, site of the Oklahoma State Penitentiary, in 1957, and soon after began a part-time career as prison physician, with direct access to more than 2000 inmates. He also began to test drugs for pharmaceutical companies, and undertook a major study in 1962 concerning the technique of plasmapheresis. Under that process, the fluid that makes up about 55 percent of the blood is removed and the remaining cells are reinjected. The plasma contains a number of valuable proteins, including gamma globulin, which contains enough antibodies against such diseases as measles and hepatitis to be used against them. It does not, however, contain sufficient antibodies for some diseases such as mumps, whooping cough, tetanus, and smallpox. But antibodies can be built up in potential donors by vaccinating them with those diseases. The gamma globulin thus obtained is known as hyperimmune gamma globulin, which commands premium prices.

One disaster had occurred in Oklahoma after a prisoner suffered great damage when the red cells separated from the blood of another prisoner were reinjected instead of his own. Undaunted, Stough got the right to operate his plasma business in Kilby Prison in Montgomery, Alabama, and two other prisons. A year later, he was also operating a plasma program at the Cummins Farm in Arkansas (which has been held to be one of the worst prisons in the country). Since medical records were sketchy or non-existent and since what goes on behind prison walls is regarded all-too-frequently as confidential, it is not likely that word would have reached the outside world except that an epidemic of viral hepatitis broke out in April 1969 and continued through the next year as a result of Dr. Stough's experiments. Even when the investigation was complete, no absolute number of illnesses and deaths could be fixed. Although only 544 cases were firmly established, the communicable disease center records contain estimates of more than 800. At this point word of Dr. Stough's activities finally reached the outside world. As a result, Oklahoma took over Stough's plasma and drug operation. Alabama authorities halted the plasma program, but allowed him to continue drug testing; Arkansas authorities permitted him to continue the plasma program without interruption.

Prisoners are, of course, not the only victims of large-scale experimentation. And profiteering entrepreneurs are not the only experimenters. The whole country was shocked in 1972 when reports of a federal syphilis study were printed, showing that at least 28 Alabama black men had died of untreated syphilis in the "cause" of medical science. In that 40-year-old "Tuskegee Study" conducted by the U.S. Public Health Service, 431 Macon County syphilis patients had been denied treatment. If the 30.4 percent syphilis-caused death rate established for the first 92 men who died prevails the toll might eventually rise to 107. Moreover, the syphilitic cases suffered more than a high death rate (as compared with the group that had been treated). They experienced "more loss of vision, more manifestations of ill health of all kinds," the report concluded.[19]

Dr. Reginald G. James, medical adviser to the Social Security Administration, recently described his experiences with the Tuskegee Study between 1939 and 1941, when he had been working for the Alabama Public Health Service:

> I was distraught and disturbed whenever one of the patients in the study group appeared. I was advised that the patient was not to be treated. Whenever I insisted on treating such a patient, he never showed up again. They were being advised they shouldn't take treatment or they would be dropped from the study.
>
> At that time, certain benefits were proffered the patients such as treatment for other ailments, payment of burial expenses, and a $50 cash benefit. To receive these benefits, the patient had to remain in the study.[20]

Survivors of the government experiment received some compensation in 1974, when a suit brought on their behalf was settled out of court, with each of them granted $37,500.[21]

Consider a few of the cases cited by the UCLA researchers in their investigative report. The live-virus rubella vaccine for German measles was first tested at the Arkansas Children's Colony, a school for the mentally retarded. The school was chosen because it was in a rural setting. Further, since the 700 students dwell in widely scattered cottages "susceptible" children could be separated from the vaccinated children. Nearly 1500 mentally retarded children at the Willowbrook State School in Staten Island, New York, have been injected with hepatitis virus by physicians over the last 18 years. And retarded children at the Sunland Center at Fort Myers have been selected as candidates for an experiment involving a vaccine for Shigella, a severe form of dysentery that occurs primarily among institutionalized people.[22]

Another scandal came to light in 1974, when the father of two Alabama girls aged twelve and fourteen filed a $1,000,000 damage suit against the federal government and a Montgomery clinic, claiming that the girls had been sterilized without understanding what had been done to them. Office of Economic Opportunity funds had been used to subsidize the operations. The case brought to light that no written guidelines had been promulgated by the Department of Health, Education, and Welfare, which had been financing the program since 1968, with no accounting of the total number of operations (believed to be between 100,000 and 300,-000), with no record of the ages, circumstances, and consent of the patients, and with no policy statement of the clinics and doctors involved. The policies, according to *Newsday* reporter Les Payne, were sometimes both arbitrary and coercive. He cited the case of one South Carolina obstetrician who had sterilized at least 18 women in the Medicaid program. He obtained consent for the "voluntary" sterilization by refusing to deliver a third child for welfare mothers unless they first agreed to submit to the operation.[23]

In addition to the many other ethical problems involved—some of great complexity and not easily answered—the inhumanity of some cases is of a gross order, as Dr. Stough's example demonstrated. While there is a ratio of risks to benefits to consider in many cases, nothing at all can be said for the medical researchers who falsify reports solely to line their pockets. That has been and continues to be the case. After his inquiry into the drug industry, Senator Hubert Humphrey cited the case of a Maryland physician who had received $13,000 in a single year for his assembly-line reports on drugs, which were favorable, of course.[24] And Congressman L. H. Fountain of North Carolina shortly after revealed that at least three doctors had signed their names to articles which had been written by drug company employees or by an agency working for the company. "The articles," he said, "were subsequently used by the company in support of an application for government approval of drugs."[25]

A full professor at the University of Pennsylvania School of Medicine, Dr. Albert M. Kligman, was dropped from the FDA approved list of researchers in the 1960s for his reporting activities. According to an account of the episode in *Time*, Dr. Kligman reported tests on three groups of prison volunteers. But when the FDA checked, prison records turned up only two groups, who were studied for a much shorter time than the researcher had claimed. Moreover, it was charged by the agency, one prisoner had had a severe reaction to the controversial drug solvent that was being tested. That was not acknowledged in the report. The physician was also charged with allowing comparison subjects to take other investigational drugs instead of a placebo, thus rendering the conclusions meaningless. And he is said to have reported blood tests on patients who were not even in the hospital at the time claimed.[26] The FDA official who made those findings was Dr. Frances O. Kelsey, who is best remembered in connection with the thalidomide case, one of the most chilling examples the modern world has known of man's inhumanity to man.

In the summer of 1968, our family sat in an improvised courtroom, an unused workers' social hall, in the small mining town of Alsdorf in Germany, witnessing for a few days what papers all over Europe had been calling the trial for "the crime of the century." The faces, like the issues, were familiar; we had seen and read about them for years. The nine defendants were prosperous businessmen. One was the owner, six were present, and two were past employees of Chemie Grünenthal, a German pharmaceutical firm. These "fathers of families," as they were identified in the biographies handed out by their public relations men, seemed unable to comprehend what their dedication to business had wrought.

Far less uncertain was the prosecutor, whose five-year investigation had culminated in a 972-page indictment against the defendants. Such witnesses as Dr. Widukind Lenz also understood the devastation the defendants had caused. The courageous public health physician whose report to a medical conference in November 1961 occasioned withdrawal of the drug from sale in West Germany had caused worldwide attention to focus on the practices and policies of twentieth-century merchandising. Dr. Lenz had first described the effects of the drug in a letter of protest to the company in 1961 in precise language:

> Since about 1957, a certain type of deformity has occurred in Western Germany with increasing frequency. It is a matter, in the first place, of serious defects in the limbs, especially the arms, which are usually mere stumps with two to four fingers, or none at all. These malformations of the arms are in part combined with serious leg defects; also with absence of the outer ear, closure of the auditory passages, heart trouble, and blocking of the esophagus . . .[27]

Some of the deformed had been there earlier, brought by parents and guardians—"really monstrous," a Swedish journalist assured us. Some of the victims had too far to travel to appear as witnesses. Thousands lived in England, the Scandinavian countries, the United States, and about 20 other countries where thalidomide (Contergan, as it was known in Germany) had been given to their mothers during pregnancy as tranquilizers. Some of the tiny victims could never appear in a courtroom. As an example, some years earlier in Liege, Belgium, a jury had acquitted a young mother, three relatives, and their family doctor in the mercy killing of an armless, eight-day-old thalidomide baby.[28] What was surprising to us was the number of older victims who had been brought to testify or whose testimony was presented by more able persons. They were elderly men and women, chiefly living in nursing homes, who had suffered irreversible nerve damage as a result of being given the drug to keep them calm.

On the basis of his five-year investigation, the company records, and 70,000 pages of testimony from 1200 witnesses, Prosecutor Josef Havertz had charged the nine men with being so eager to turn a profit from the sleep-inducing drug that they had disregarded reports of dangers; that they had lied to doctors who had questioned them; that they did everything they could to suppress unfavorable reports and encourage (with money) reports that were favorable.

As a result of such tactics, Contergan had gone on sale in Germany in October 1957, and was later sold by licensees in 11 countries in Europe, 7 in Africa, 17 in Asia, and 11 in the Western Hemisphere.

It was not sold in the United States, although it was widely used here during a trial run by the William S. Merrell Company, which was seeking to obtain government approval of its license to merchandise it. At least 19,822 persons, including 3760 women of child-bearing age, were given thalidomide by their physicians, who were participating in the experiment. (Actually, it is not really known how many persons took the drug since FDA agents turned up 36 additional doctors who were not participating in the experiment but who had thalidomide in their possession and prescribed it for patients.) [29]

That it was not sold here was due entirely to the efforts of a stubborn woman doctor in the FDA, Dr. Kelsey, who refused to accept the Merrell evidence as conclusive. What troubled her chiefly, despite the glowing reports made by doctors, some of whom the company had labeled as "very materialistic in outlook," was that experimental animals had not been made sleepy by the drug, as humans were. There was, really, no need for haste, she reasoned. The drug was not intended to provide relief for serious disorders, merely sleeplessness.

She continued to hold off, skeptically, despite what Senator Kefauver described as almost incredible pressure. On fifty separate occasions, Merrell approached her and her superiors, cajoling, harassing, even threatening. She was still resistant in 1962 when Merrell withdrew its application for the drug, after Dr. Lenz had destroyed Grünenthal's elaborately constructed facade behind which it was extracting money for misery. At the urging of Senator Estes Kefauver, President Kennedy awarded her the Distinguished Federal Civilian Service Medal.[30]

The story is still being played out in various countries. Two years after it began, the trial ended inconclusively in Alsdorf. Criminal charges were dropped; the company agreed to set up a fund of $27,300,000 for the 5000 and more affected children in West Germany, and another $1,100,000 for about 300 cases of nerve damage to adults.[31] Grünenthal got off lightly compared with some of its licensees in other countries. In 1973, for example, a British High Court judge approved a $50,000,000 penalty against the Distillers Company to compensate the 443 victims and their families in that country.[32]

In 1973, as Dr. John Lister noted in the *New England Journal of Medicine*, thalidomide had become "a party issue," with Labourites calling for immediate legislation to deal with the problem, including the establishment of a trust fund and asking for additional millions to be made available by the government for children with severe congenital deformity, whether or not due to thalidomide.[33]

In his article, Dr. Lister noted the family problems that had resulted. Mothers had taken the drug in confidence of its safety; nevertheless, they often had "a real sense of guilt" that they had created family stress. Another "distressing problem," he said, was the normal or above normal intelligence of the children . . .

> that made them acutely aware of their disabilities and presented peculiar educational problems. The long-term frustrations of difficulties in finding employment and in many cases of being debarred from opportunities of marriage had yet to be met.

And all that for bonuses to officials and added dividends for stockholders.

6 The Sleeping Sentries

Freedom, according to the AMA, means absolute liberty for doctors to go on doing as they have been doing, without interference of any kind from any one. When uncomfortable questions are raised about incompetence and unethical behavior, they are shrugged off with the familiar: "Well, only a tiny minority. . . ."

That is far from the case. As many as one-third of the country's practicing physicians are held to be hopelessly outdated in their knowledge of modern medical practice.[1] Another 5 percent are held to be unethical in their activities. Recently, even the AMA acknowledged that a sizable number of doctors are "deviant." Each year the profession loses about 600 of them, (which is equivalent to the annual output of six medical schools) from excessive use of alcohol, from narcotics addiction, and from suicide. And the number of deviants continuing to practice is much higher.[2]

Nonetheless, the AMA continues to insist that "we can police ourselves." And state and local affiliates echo that sentiment, asserting that all public complaints against doctors are carefully investigated—despite open acknowledgement of the existence of a conspiracy of silence—and "erring members are appropriately admonished and disciplined."[3]

Professional self-policing might be a rational way of managing medical affairs since patients are not likely to know what does constitute competence and what is ethical, medically speaking. Patients in the North Carolina study, referred to in detail (see pp. 49–50), were pleased with even the most substandard care they

94

had received. Even though 40 percent of the persons surveyed in the Teamster study were found to have received only fair or poor treatment, the patients "overwhelmingly" believed that they had been provided with "the best of modern medicine."[4]

During the last ten years, however, the attitude has changed markedly. When the Secretary's Commission on Medical Malpractice made its comprehensive study in 1971 and 1972, it questioned families about negative medical experiences. A surprising 42.5 percent of the heads of households questioned reported that they, their spouses, or dependents had had a negative experience.[5] Errors in judgment on the part of the doctor and errors in skill were most frequently cited as chief faults. Not surprisingly, the higher the social status of the family, as measured by education, income, and occupation, the more dissatisfaction was expressed with the kind of care received. Persons lower on the socioeconomic ladder were less likely to blame the doctor for experiences that resulted badly.

Ideally, doctors are in a better position to protect patients from the incompetent and deviant physicians who presently constitute a hazard to public health. They have an obligation to do that. Even the American Medical Association's Principles of Ethics imposes that duty on them. As strong on forms of behavior and as weak on truly moral concerns as Polonius's farewell exhortation to Laertes, the Principles of Ethics stress that doctors are not to solicit patients, pay or receive commissions for referrals, charge more than patients are able to pay, reveal professional confidences, accept jobs that may impair the free and complete exercise of medical judgment and skill, associate with persons who do not practice a method of healing based on science, and neglect patients they have accepted. In addition to the "Do Nots," they are also advised to improve knowledge and skill, seek consultation when necessary, and uphold the dignity and honor of the profession. Until 1957, they were also told that doctors should expose, "without fear or favor, incompetent or corrupt, dishonest or unethical conduct on the part of members of the profession."

Apparently the AMA regarded the Principles as too much of an interference with physician freedom, for in 1957 the strong admonition was amended on recommendation of the House of Delegates to read: "They should expose, without hesitation, illegal or unethical conduct of fellow members of the profession."[6] There was really no need to weaken the urging. The AMA has always seen to that by insisting that exposure of and action against members must be taken at the lowest possible level, where it is sure not to be taken. It has also fostered the widespread belief among doctors that the most unprofessional action they can perform is to indulge in disparaging remarks about fellow practitioners.

Doctors learn early how to solve the dilemma and live with their professional conscience. *Intern*'s "Doctor X" received a memorable lesson early in the game. A cocktail waitress had been forced to undergo a painful and costly ordeal because during an operation "some jackass couldn't tell the saphenous vein from the femoral artery." Her complaints of suffering were ignored for several days; finally, as a result of the original blunder and continuing negligence, her leg had to be amputated below the knee. Then gangrene set in; an above-the-knee amputation had to be performed.

The young woman was, as Dr. X noted on that occasion, "just about at the end of her tether emotionally." She had already been charged $3000 for hospitalization and surgeons' fees for what had been represented to her as "uncontrollable complications." She could probably have won a $100,000 malpractice judgment, Dr. X felt, if someone had told her the truth. No one did. No one offered to pay the doctor and hospital bills, as far as he knew. His colleague, Hank, explained the system:

> You just can't nail the man for making the mistake, and as for negligence, there isn't another doctor alive that isn't negligent one way or another every week of the year. So how can you crucify this guy just because he happened to get caught? You go pointing fingers and you may find yourself in a very slippery spot sometime with a whole lot of fingers pointing at you.[7]

Like a well-instructed young intern, Dr. X did not point any finger. He did worry later "exactly where medical ethics come into a picture like this. Or whether they come into it only when it's convenient for the doctors."[8]

With such an attitude, it would be madness to imagine that individual doctors will point out incompetent colleagues or that patients will soon come to recognize them. Because they know they are in short supply, few doctors have any concern about unsatisfied customers. The waiting rooms of quacks, charlatans, and imposters are jammed, and there are queues of eager standees willing to take the nearest vacant seat in the office of even the sloppiest and shoddiest practitioner. The rigid scrutiny of ability and ethics that goes on in the great teaching hospitals, the outstanding group-practice plans, and in organizations like the Mayo Clinic is nonexistent in fee-for-service practice.

Efforts to educate the public to demand quality and honesty have not met with any but cool receptions in the profession. As one doctor pointed out recently in relation to the realistic medical "guide" books that have been appearing, the education of the public is a desirable trend. Few doctors would entrust their lives or those of members of their family to a doctor without careful investigation of his training and competence; laymen have been asked to do just that. Yet, as one pointed out recently, calling a doctor about whom you know nothing at all "is like spinning the revolver cylinder before pulling the trigger in Russian roulette." Yet doctors consider it "unethical" to halt the dangerous game by publicizing dangerous colleagues.[9]

An interesting case occurred in 1973 in Los Angeles after the *Times* carried an admirable article about the need for doctors to update their education in order to keep abreast of developments in medicine. Dr. Morton K. Rubenstein, a professor at the University of California at Los Angeles and a distinguished neurosurgeon, cited as important forward steps the proviso by the Oregon Medical Association that membership is contingent on continuing post-graduate education and laws now in effect in a few states requiring doctors to up-date their education in order to have their licenses renewed.[10] The article was restrained and gave a factual, reasonable discussion of conditions in California and other states. Dr. Rubenstein is in an excellent position to appraise matters and a man who had spent years organizing courses and seminars for doctors. The response in the Los Angeles County Medical Society *Bulletin* was remarkable. It ran full-scale diatribe by Dr. Leonard Kurland, a copy of a letter he had written to the *Times*. That was prefaced by an editorial note emphasizing that the *Bulletin* does not "normally" reprint letters sent to other publications concerning articles published in them, "but an exception is being made in this instance to present Dr. Kurland's answer in behalf of the profession."

The letter, itself, offered not a single fact to refute Dr. Rubenstein's claim that many practicing doctors were "hopelessly outdated." Instead, it called the article a "scare" piece that was "dishonest in the bargain." The psychiatrist attacked Dr. Rubenstein and his criticism in a scarcely scientific vein:

> There is plenty that is wrong with the practice of medicine and a good part of what is wrong is the same as what is wrong with our society. We've bad-mouthed traditional values and the largest victim has been personal responsibility. . . . The problem of keeping up is mainly the problem of throwing out the deluge of junk articles that are written by the highly subsidized government grant doctors at the universities. . . .[11]

Dr. Kurland's heat was not a limited matter. Dr. Rubenstein got "a lot of hate mail" from other doctors, he told me some weeks later. But the excessive warmth of the psychiatrist does allow for some interesting speculation since the psychiatric profession has come in for some of the sharpest criticism in recent years, occasioned by such public events as the trials of Sirhan Sirhan and Jack Ruby and by such private tragedies as that experienced by the James Wechsler family. After their young son killed himself, the Wechslers wrote a book about it chiefly to warn others about "being intimidated by professional counsel."[12]

That the county medical society should have participated in the attack is not surprising, considering past actions of the more than 1900 county medical societies in the country. The precedent for their response to criticism from within the profession was established, as has been noted in an earlier chapter, in 1900 when the Chicago Medical Society censured the two doctors who had publicly exposed the widespread fee-splitting racket in that area.

Actually, the Los Angeles County Medical Association has been better than many others in receiving criticisms arising from within. It has had for several years an actively functioning peer review committee that investigates questionable insurance claims to determine whether the physician was involved in questionable medical practice, whether he was at fault, or whether he was "out of the scope of his practice."[13] The committee, which was set up because of the difficulties doctors were having in obtaining malpractice insurance, has done something to upgrade quality.

A memorable illustration of professional policing involved an aged surgeon who was causing no little concern in an Alabama hospital. Physically and mentally he was in bad shape. He was almost completely unable to hear, his vision was poor, his memory was so erratic that he often could not even find his car in the hospital parking lot. Although his condition was commonly known, no action was taken until one doctor, apparently unable to stifle professional conscience pangs, decided to act. At a staff meeting at the hospital one day, he moved that the surgeon's privileges be withdrawn. Only one person voted in favor of it—the elderly surgeon himself, whose hearing was so bad and whose mind was so clouded he hadn't the foggiest notion of what he was voting for. All the rest of the staff elected to allow him to go on unchecked.[14]

In response to popular demand and increasing threats of legal action, many local medical societies decided to establish grievance committees in the 1950s. Patients who believe themselves victims of incompetent and unethical doctors were encouraged to bring their gripes to the local medical societies for redress. The grievance committee, made up of members working on a volunteer basis, would hear them out and take appropriate action against offenders. Theoretically, it was a good idea; and some of the societies found themselves doing a brisk business, handling more than 1000 cases a year for everything from requests for fee adjustments to charges of negligence and gross incompetence. Practically, however, the public relations watchdogs had little power other than to exert "moral suasion" on offending doctors. The severest action any of them could take was censure, suspension, or expulsion from the society. Even then, societies kept most of those actions secret.

Despite those precautions to protect the profession's good name, the societies continued to display almost incredible timidity in dealing with colleagues who have indulged in illegal as well as unethical activities. One of the more extreme cases reported involved a doctor who was found guilty of selling narcotics to high school students. The grievance committee voted to expell him; then it suspended the sentence.[15] That pattern prevails throughout the country. Although convictions of high crimes and misdemeanors have been relatively frequent, grievance societies have almost never acted extensively to protect the public. Between 1957 and 1967, the Philadelphia Society suspended two physicians and expelled one.[16] A California state senate committee investigated medical inadequacy in the 1960s. They found that in 1961 only one doctor in the country had been expelled from a local medical society, although a number of society members had been convicted in the same year of offenses ranging from murder to income-tax evasion.[17] However, even if a doctor is acted against, there is no guarantee of the effectiveness of the action. The doctor expelled in 1961 was able to continue his medical way of life without interruption since he owned his own hospital. (Being barred from hospitals is the most serious consequence of expulsion from a local medical society).

Another deterrent to action is the fear of suit. Some years ago, the Academy of Medicine of Cleveland and the members of its grievance committee were sued for $700,000 by an ophthalmologist. The grievance committee had merely suggested to the doctor that he lower his fee in one case. The doctor went to court to recover the fee and was awarded it in full. After being called before the ethics committee of the society, which told him the fee was still too high, he filed suit against the grievance committee and Academy directors on the grounds that his character and reputation had been damaged. He also insisted that his practice had suffered a $200,000 loss of referrals from other physicians.[18]

Medical societies often are reluctant to censure their members because they fear they may be taking on somebody who may cause trouble. In one case reported by Howard and Martha Lewis, the members of an ethics committee decided that they could not take action against a doctor "because of the prominence of the accused in the society and in the community." They referred proposed action to the full membership. The other members were no less intimidated; they sent the case to the state society, which, also concerned about offending a prominent doctor, asked the AMA's Judicial Council to make a decision. Charges were returned with the brief note that it was up to the local society: "If local societies fail to curtail unethical practices, ethics lose their effectiveness."[19]

Bowing to pressure from the insurance industry, a number of medical societies have established screening panels. They are composed of equal numbers of doctors and lawyers who hear medical, dental, and legal malpractice claims, plus a chairman who may be either a doctor or a lawyer. The screening panels might have had a happy effect on the quality as well as the cost of medical care, but the Secretary's Commission on Medical Malpractice made a comprehensive study in 1971 and found that *only* one of the committees made positive use of information it received to improve medical care. This was the Honolulu County Medical Society, which is, importantly, one of the few committees with a "public" member: Monsignor Kekumano.[20]

Yet such screening panels do have a powerful weapon in the recommendations they can offer to doctors to determine the kind of malpractice insurance coverage doctors can obtain through the local medical society, which is sometimes the only available source. If erring and aberrant doctors are causing rates to soar, other members may feel differently about their conduct. And if the offenders find themselves without insurance, they would be encouraged to shape up.

The record of the state societies is very little better than that of local groups. On the national level, the AMA has maintained a position of state's rights and local control.

The agencies that are legally empowered to act against incompetent and unethical doctors are the state boards that administer the state medical practices act. They do not have to worry about suits since they are public agencies, nor about costs since they are financed by public money. They have meaningful sanctions; they can revoke licenses. Yet there is about as much likelihood that the boards will deal with doctors as there is that the county and state medical societies will act, or the AMA. That is because medicine, like law and some other untouchable professions, has managed to achieve the dream of all monopolists: it writes its own statutes and administers them, too. Instead of being a protective barrier against the special interests of organized medicine, the boards are almost invariably extensions of it.

In most states, boards of medical examiners have been established to grant licenses to practice and to administer the state law in accordance with the public interest. The members are supposed to be men of wisdom, learning, skill, and with enough integrity to detach themselves from narrow professional interests in order to serve the people. Frequently, however, they are simply official lobbyists, proposed by state medical associations. Armed with authority to make rules for their own guidance and efficiency, they have commonly used that power to encourage such monopolistic practices as eliminating competition, fixing prices, and failing to insist upon reasonable standards of conduct by doctors.

In fairness to the boards, it should be pointed out that the medical practice laws enacted in most states with the counsel and consent of the medical establishment are not conducive to protecting the public from incompetent and unethical doctors. Some state laws even prevent licensing boards from investigating cases of mental incompetence. Some years ago, an Ohio official protested that the board could not take official action even in known cases of insanity until court action was completed or the licensee voluntarily entered an institution.[21] In mid-1973, only three states had laws insisting that licensees update their knowledge; only a few have laws to insure that doctors mentally and physically incapacitated by age retire from active practice.

Although more action is needed to implement existing laws, state medical boards have been notably passive. In a typical year, about 75 licenses are revoked by medical boards in the United States. Yet, as *The Medical Offenders* points out, as many as 20,000 licensed doctors are thought to be severe disciplinary problems.[22] About a third of the disciplinary actions are taken in California and New York; 11 states have taken no action at all. Actions that are taken are sometimes unpredictable. In the 1960s, the Missouri Board of Registration for the Healing Arts refused to license a well-qualified practitioner because he believed in pacificism and was a conscientious objector. But Dr. Harold Will Lischner's credentials were impeccable. A graduate of the University of Chicago Medical School, he had taught at the University of California, the University of Missouri, and the University of Pennsylvania. He was a diplomat of the American Board of Pediatrics, which would normally qualify him for a Missouri license. He had license to practice medicine in California and Pennsylvania at the time he applied in Missouri. The *Newsletter* of the Society for Social Responsibility in Science did point out later there were a number of what the board considered "debits." Among them was Dr. Lischner's attitude about the AMA. He considered it an undemocratic organization that "has been very, very arbitrary in its total opposition to any consideration of programs of social support of health care." He also criticized the AMA for racial segregation.[23]

The St. Louis Civil Liberties Committee rushed to the defense of Dr. Lischner, pointing out that "by this bizarre standard Albert Schweitzer would be refused permission to practice medicine in the State of Missouri." So did the Attorney General, Thomas F. Eagleton, who refused to handle the case for the Board. Although he said that he disagreed with the views of Dr. Lischner: "His espousal of those beliefs presents, in my opinion, no legal grounds for denying him a license to practice the healing arts in Missouri. Under our system, one need not sacrifice his right to adopt unpopular or even intellectually erroneous views in exchange for a license to practice a profession."[24]

An extensive investigation into the activities of a state board was made in California in the 1960s by Senator Walter W. Stiern, dismayed by evidence of negligence and fraud. The findings of his committee were such that he promptly introduced legislation to protect people from doctors whose practice constitutes a menace to public health. He had learned that the California law, which seemed such a comprehensive one, hedged in the 12-man board so that it was almost powerless to act. Seemingly, the law provided everything that could be asked. Practically, the law was another matter, for the practice of a mentally ill doctor could not be restricted, however obvious his deranged behavior might be. He could continue to practice unless he had been committed to a state hospital or adjudicated insane, measures not likely to be taken against a doctor. Even if a doctor were convicted of a crime, he could continue to practice until the matter was finally disposed of. In all, as Senator Stiern pointed out:

> Neither the Board of Medical Examiners nor any other agency of government has authority to restrict the right to practice medicine of physicians who engage in unethical medical practices or whose mental conduct amounts to gross negligence or gross incompetence, no matter how harmful to patients the physician's conduct may be.[25]

At the time of the hearing, at least 1500 doctors in the state were estimated to be operating in a grossly substandard manner; yet during the preceding year, complaints had been filed with the board against only 80 doctors. Those doctors and 60 others whose cases were still pending from 1963 had been charged with and most had been convicted of serious offenses, including murder. Most of them had been apprehended by state and federal law enforcement agencies for such felonious activities as violations of the narcotics laws. Of the total number, 27 had been completely forbidden to practice, which was a very high number, incidentally, in relation to the rest of the nation. Another 50 were placed on probation; 15 had their licenses suspended for mental illness.[26]

A number of legislative reforms introduced by Senator Stiern were approved in 1965. The board was empowered to act against a mentally ill doctor who represented such a danger to himself and others that he is "in need of supervision or restraint." The board was also given authority to require diagnostic examinations and additional medical training for physicians. Importantly, it received authority to restrict, revoke, or suspend the license of physicians whose conduct constitutes gross incompetence, gross immorality, or gross negligence. Examples of negligence that were specified were fee-splitting, overcharging, ordering unnecessary hospitalization, performing unnecessary surgery, failing to call a consultant when needed, failing to carry out adequate diagnostic procedures before treatment, prescribing improper medication, and failing to keep up with advances in medicine. It also strengthened the provisions of the act in relation to making false reports. False reports were extended to cover not merely documents "required by law," but to insurance claims and any other document directly or indirectly related to the practice of medicine.

Another measure authorized the state board to establish five review committees in each of the state's appellate court districts to conduct hearings and to recommend disciplinary actions. Final decisions would continue to be made by the board. The legislator believed that the review committees would provide relief; professional "insiders" would encourage voluntary compliance, and their public standing would remove them from the "economic and social ties" that have rendered purely private monitors ineffectual.[27]

The measure had the endorsement of public health leaders and medical educators, in addition to many hospital leaders and lay persons. District committees were promptly appointed; the stage was set for action. What happened? Very little. A majority of committee members were appointed by local affiliates of the AMA, which had been decidedly cool to the idea. If the medical society grievance committees and hospital staffs did not turn over complaints, the review committees had no basis for action.

Not surprisingly, a report by a Nader study group called for a national regulatory board on the grounds that "in 1970, no such review mechanism worthy of the name yet exists."[28]

The modest improvement begun by the legislation that was enacted in California in 1965 was enhanced several years ago when the Board of Medical Examiners, along with other state boards, was placed under the California Department of Consumer Affairs. In 1972, for example, California revoked the licenses of

33 doctors, suspended 12, and placed 58 on probation—more than the total of all the other states. In 1973, the licenses of 52 doctors were revoked, after they were found guilty of incompetence, moral turpitude, fraud, misuse of drugs, negligence, and other forms of malpractice.[29]

Sample cases included: a surgeon based at a major hospital who was found "grossly negligent" in treating patients and who had been using dangerous drugs for seven years; a physician who was ingesting 50 milligrams daily of a "relaxant" drug even when performing surgery. Another surgeon had his license suspended after court conviction on charges of defrauding an insurance company of $14,733. One was given five years probation and prohibited from performing operations; during his probation, he is required to see a psychiatrist and file regular reports with the board. Licenses of three doctors were revoked after their conviction of having raped women patients who were under anesthesia or hypnosis.

The number penalized represented only a small number of those against whom complaints were filed. During 1973, 2081 complaints were charged against professionals in the healing arts —only slightly below the number filed against TV-electronics repairmen and well above collection agencies and private "detectives."

As long as policing is a job for insiders, there is little likelihood that the peer review committees will be effective in weeding out the doctors whose performance constitutes a danger to public health and to financial security. And many outside watchdogs have done little better. The insurance carriers have been in an excellent position to identify dishonest and incompetent doctors, but they have done little—even Blue Cross and Blue Shield. Indeed, they have done so little that in 1972 the Pennsylvania Insurance Commissioner said he told Blue Shield:

> We would not give it a nickel's worth of premium increases, today, tomorrow, or *ever* until it put into effect some of the reforms and economies we were talking about, including the forty-four guidelines, with priority given to greater consumer control of its board of twenty-seven,

then dominated by eighteen doctors and other health providers.[30]

Even the private insurance carriers, whose boards are not dominated by doctors, have been operating on the basis that "we'll-take-care-of-you-if-you-take-care-of-us."

The General Accounting Office investigation of Medicare and Medicaid payments to doctors revealed shocking laxities on the part of carriers. Although they are required to make postpayment investigations to determine that the claims paid have been for necessary services, only some of the carriers did and *only a few* did any follow up. For example, the report noted that during 1970, 539 physicians whose services exceeded quarterly postpayment norms were identified by one insurance carrier; of that number, only 12 were investigated. Another company had produced, under its postpayment review system, a listing of 645 physicians in a single month warranting further investigation. *None* of the 645 had been investigated.[31]

Insurance officials agreed with GAO investigators that "further action was needed"; however, they excused their inactivity on the grounds of lack of staff and higher priorities. Since billions in tax dollars are involved and since millions of Americans may be receiving unnecessary treatment of hazardous nature, it is not easy to understand the insurance industry's priority rating system.

The federal government is hampered from acting because of the "confidentiality" barrier that organized medicine has imposed all along the line. Until 1970, the names of "problem" physicians working with the Medicare program could not be made known to the state agencies responsible for Medicaid. Thus, a doctor found dishonest and incompetent by one program could continue to serve patients under another. A few of the cases will illustrate the Alice-in-Wonderland approach:

· In December 1966, an investigation by a state Medicaid agency showed that a doctor had submitted claims for home and office visits that were not made.

Rather than face legal proceedings (none were instituted!), the physician voluntarily withdrew from the Medicaid program on January 30, 1967. However, he continued to submit claims under the Medicare program, receiving payments of about $112,000 from 1967 through 1970 .

- Another physician was barred from the Medicaid program on March 31, 1966, because of the discrepancies between his claimed number of visits and the number verified by patients. On June 1, 1968, the physician was reinstated under the Medicaid program with a warning that any additional abuses would result in his being permanently barred from the program. The doctor was also participating in the Medicare program, under which he was paid about $99,000 from 1967 through 1969. As a result of a patient's complaint, an investigation was made in 1969 and the case was referred to officials of the Social Security Administration, which is in charge of Medicare. While the case was pending, Medicaid payments continued to the doctor—who had already been suspended once for his fraudulent activities.

- In another state, 14 physicians were suspended from the Medicaid program between 1966 and 1969 for fraudulent billings. When the Medicare carrier became aware in 1971 that those physicians "warranted special scrutiny," they had collected large sums—all during the 53 months in which they had been suspended from Medicaid.[32]

Surely what is crooked under one program is crooked under the other.

Much could and should be done to prevent the conspiracy of silence in the medical profession from exacting the terrible toll it now does in terms of money and health.

At the national level, dishonesty could be minimized by private and public insurers' insisting that doctors whose claims show unusual patterns of service are investigated and identified. Those who indulge in fraud and provide unnecessary services should be barred from every program involving public money.

Also at the national level the quality of health care could be enhanced if all candidates for a license were required to pass a national examination and to show cause why their licenses should be renewed. The wide variations that exist from one political unit to another cannot be justified in the twentieth century. And wide variations do exist, not merely in relation to moral character, but in such critical matters as graduation from an approved medical school and internship in a board-certified institution.

Some of the inequities have been overcome because many states issue licenses only to those applicants who have passed the examinations given by the National Board of Medical Examiners. Drafted by highly qualified medical educators, the examinations meet or surpass the standards of any state. As a result, state boards would be able to devote more time to disciplinary actions. And reform of the disciplinary procedure should include open meetings at which the public would be represented. Local grievance committees and insurance carriers should be required to pass on to the board legitimate complaints. Hospitals and other health-care institutions should also establish grievance procedures to help patients with their problems. The names of doctors violating standards should be sent to the state board for further investigation and action.

One of the significant recommendations made by the Secretary's Commission on Medical Malpractice was that an Office of Consumer Affairs be set up in each state with financial assistance from the federal government. The office would provide patients with a forum for their complaints. In making the recommendation, the Commission pointed out such an office would have the happy effect of minimizing malpractice suits:

> If the patient has no one to go to except a lawyer, the problem will either develop into an adversary claim or

result in another instance of rejection. It is still characteristic of medical care that the patient *trusts* the doctor
probably to a greater degree than he trusts a member of
any other profession or business. To bring suit requires
him to make a complete turnaround, to switch from a
position of trustful expectations and confidence to one of
distrust and accusation. Most patients are apt to do that
only with reluctance, yet no other avenue of redress may
be open. Even this one may be closed if his claim is too
small to be of interest to an attorney.[33]

Such an office, headed by a Commissioner of Consumer Health
Affairs, would be in an excellent position to upgrade the quality
of care since it would establish and maintain records of health-
care complaints and related health-care factors and would act as
a source for a central data bank. As the Commission views the
possible job, the office would periodically issue public reports
concerning information gathered by its officers in order to suggest
ways of improving the health-care system.

The AMA must come to acknowledge that what is good for
the patient is also good for the doctor. If real protection were
assured, the boast that American medical care is the best in the
world might become meaningful. Meantime, since it is not and
since the doctor—unlike some of the remedies he prescribes—
is not required to wear a warning label, the courtroom continues
to be one of the few means an individual has for insisting that
health care be fairly priced and of reasonable quality.

7 Malpractice and Medical Justice

In the lexicon of organized medicine, few words carry more loathsome connotations than *malpractice*. And few persons are regarded with greater loathing than Melvin Belli, Louis Nizer, Jack L. Sachs, Patrick F. Kelly, Albert Averbach, and other legal "kings of torts." So intense is the hostility that when the National Commission on Medical Malpractice held hearings in New York in 1972 a doctor became so badly upset when he saw an attorney involved in a suit against him that he erupted in the hearing room. He swore that he "would not look at television that night for fear of seeing the lawyer." Another doctor told the committee that the malpractice problems he had experienced had persuaded him to "retire earlier and seek medical employment which involves less patient contact."[1]

Even doctors who have never known what it is to appear in a courtroom suffer intensely, living under a sword of Damocles. As one of them told the Commission:

> As a physician, I live in an aura of fear—fear of suit. Fear contributes to hostility. . . . It may be hard to believe, but we are a frightened profession. The doctor feels put upon. He feels nude on the corner of the Main Street of life. He tries to cover himself with pride, and even occasionally arrogance, only to find himself being castrated.[2]

Doctors' fears are understandable, considering the sensational headlines given to extravagant demands of six- and seven-figure awards:

PATIENTS WIN $3 MILLION
IN MALPRACTICE SUITS

QUADRIPLEGIC, 6,
WINS $1.2 MILLION
OVER TREATMENT

$500,000 SUIT FILED IN
ETHER DEATH OF GIRL

Medical journals have been no less sensational in playing up threats of malpractice. As yet, the medical establishment has not attempted to curb their reporting, though it has attempted to make it illegal for newspapers to report the amount being claimed in damage suits. Reasonably indicative of the emotional content of some articles in professional journals are titles like "Today's Malpractice Threat Isn't Just Talk," "Hospital's Insurer Sues ex-Intern," "Seven Mistakes Led to a $160,000 Verdict." An article warned doctors that not even their widows and children will be spared. Another article made an emotional appeal, pointing out that a Pennsylvania lower court had ruled that a physician's estate could be sued for malpractice after he had died.[3]

Rising insurance rates—even though premium payments are passed on to the patients—are considered further proof that patients are naturally litigious, just waiting for a chance to get in there and sock it to the man in white who was misguided enough to have provided medical treatment. But doctors have been carefully coached in how to avoid suits. Some years ago, for example, the California Medical Association hired a research psychologist, Dr. Richard Blum, to investigate and report on malpractice suits and why and how they happen. Following that, he was asked to devise a test to determine the "unreasonability" quotient of prospective patients. And within a short time, hundreds of doctors were administering a ten-minute examination, which they could grade in about two minutes. In this way they would weed out the amiable patients from the "failures" likely to bring suit.[4] Naturally, they were free to reject the latter.

The "Patient Aptitude Test" was not popular among patients, who were not given an equal opportunity to test either the reasonableness or competence of their examiners. Nor was Blum's report very popular in medical circles since the establishment has preferred to ignore the psychologist's findings that "suit prone" doctors are as responsible for the growth of malpractice actions as "suit prone" patients.

One of the more important aspects of the malpractice syndrome is who benefits. Lawyers obviously do. The "contingent fee" arrangement under which most malpractice attorneys operate has been partly responsible for the haphazard and sometimes excessive judgments. The fees of attorneys handling cases under the Federal Tort Claims Act against the government have been limited by statute to 25 percent; in nonfederal cases, attorneys collect as much as 50 percent; sometimes more.

For some aggressive and skillful lawyers, malpractice litigation has become a bonanza. For most, however, it has been somewhat less. After making a detailed study of malpractice claims in 1970, the Commission found that less than 1 percent of the cases closed amounted to more than $100,000. Most were for less than $3000. On the basis of the Commission's findings, plaintiff lawyers averaged $63 an hour, which is far less than most medical doctors consider their services worth. Moreover, that sum represented only earnings for time expended in actual prosecution. No consideration was made of the time and research involved by lawyers listening to would-be plaintiffs state their case and investigating the possibility of making a legal case.[5] Many lawyers have found malpractice suits to be so unprofitable that they will no longer touch a case that involves less than $25,000. Some set $50.000 as a minimum. It should be pointed out in fairness, however, that there are lawyers not motivated solely by monetary motives to take malpractice cases. Some lawyers have taken on the medical profession in outrage against the profession's refusal to deal with the enemy within.

113

George Bernard Shaw pointed out in *A Doctor's Dilemma*: "Every doctor will allow a colleague to decimate a whole countryside sooner than violate the professional etiquette by giving him away." Sophisticated jurists have agreed. Some years ago, Judge Alfred C. Clapp of the Appellate Division of New Jersey's Superior Court said, after a woman who had suffered permanent paralysis as a result of inept diagnosis and treatment was unable to get a single doctor in the state to testify for her, "malpractice is not answered by an attempt to throttle justice."[6]

Melvin Belli said that his first malpractice case opened his eyes to "this incredible conspiracy." He had been retained to sue a physician who had prescribed enemas and cathartics for a young man suffering from classic appendicitis symptoms. The appendix burst. The young man died. In addition to the patently wrong treatment the doctor prescribed, he was, according to the attorney, intoxicated when he made the house call. Although seemingly a *prima facie* case, Mr. Belli said that he lost it. "Not one of this drunken doctor's colleagues would testify in court to what he had obviously done. Worse, five doctors testified in his behalf, including the head of one of our largest university hospitals."[7]

Just as some lawyers benefit from malpractice, so do the insurance companies to an even greater extent. Although not legally necessary, insurance against malpractice claims is in fact imperative for doctors, dentists, hospitals, and other individuals and agencies involved in health care. That has created a tremendous demand for this insurance, but only a relatively few giant companies dominate the field. One study indicated that only *four* firms control up to 50.8 percent of the market as measured in premium volume; *ten* firms control up to 86.2 percent.[8] Figures of that type indicate a dangerously monopolistic situation, which is perhaps true in view of the fact that premium payments have been skyrocketing. Physicians' premiums rose from $7,600,000 in 1960 to $48,700,000 in 1970. Premiums for surgeons went from $19,700,000 to $206,700,000. Total figures for 1960, including premiums paid by dentists and hospitals, amounted to $61,100,-000; by 1970, the total amount of premiums being paid had soared to $370,600,000.[9] Since then, they have taken off into orbit. A report early in 1975 indicated that the average doctor in New

York State had been paying $7000 a year for malpractice insurance in 1973; that doubled in 1974; and premiums for 1975—just in case the insurance companies decided that they would insure doctors—would be $41,000.[10]

Only a small amount of the money collected by insurance companies as premiums makes its way to injured patients. According to Professor Robert Keeton of the Harvard Law School, much less money is paid to claimants in health insurance cases from premiums than to those involved in cases arising from automobile accidents—only forty-four cents on the dollar. It is estimated that *only between 16 and 17 cents of the premium dollar ends up as benefits to victims of medical injuries.*[11]

The insurance companies protect themselves further by charging very high rates to those specialists who are very likely to have claims made against them. For example, physicians who do not perform surgery or who ordinarily only assist in surgery pay only one-fifth the amount charged anesthesiologists, neurosurgeons, obstetrician-gynecologists, orthopedists, otolaryngologists, and plastic surgeons.[12] And the insurance companies further protect their own profits by picking and choosing the doctors they will insure. As recently as 1970, the Commission pointed out, doctors in Hawaii, Utah, Oregon, and Nevada found themselves in a crisis when malpractice insurance carriers decided to restrict coverage in those trouble areas. Fortunately, the insurance industry was persuaded to restore the malpractice insurance policies. The insurance industry can and does take advantage of its position to whip up a new crisis whenever it feels a rate hike is in order; one of them got underway shortly after the beginning of 1975, when a number of companies in New York, Maryland, California, and other states with frequent suits announced that it was costing them too much to continue present arrangements.[13] The doctors retaliated by following out on strike the anesthesiologists, who had been hardest hit. A crisis of major proportions occurred and continued until the state threatened drastic intervention.

The medical establishment also preys on the fears of doctors that they will be sued for malpractice as an effective way of bringing into line doctors who might oppose the programs and policies of the county, state, and national associations. To do this, the associations have offered bargain-rate insurance with built-in protection against policy cancellation as long as the doctor follows the policies the societies endorse. The medical societies also try to induce doctors to conform with their programs and policies by encouraging the notion that the increase in malpractice actions is all the fault of plaintiffs' attorneys who have made "ambulance chasing" a respectable legal activity and of emotionally disturbed patients who find malpractice suits a way of venting their hostilities on hard-working doctors doing the best they can as they travel the lonesome and righteous road. The societies thus are partly responsible for the broad gulf between *us* and *them*, a gulf so broad that at least half of the doctors in the country have declared that they would not render emergency aid despite the protection offered them by Good Samaritan laws enacted across the country.[14] There is non-involvement with a vengeance.

Malpractice cases have provided some benefits, aside from large settlements. One of Melvin Belli's favorite stories involves an instructor in a California medical school who used to ask his students to name the man who did most for medicine within the past century. As they went through the list of medical greats, he put down their guesses sharply: "No, Melvin Belli, because the son of a bitch has made medical men conscientious about their courtroom testimony and has made lawyers learn medicine."[15] A number of medical men would go far beyond that. Dr. Milton Roemer of the University of California at Los Angeles School of Public Health and Dr. David Rubsamen, editor of the *Professional Liability Newsletter*, are among the many who believe that the threat of malpractice suits has made doctors learn medicine and practice it with reasonable caution and skill.

It is instructive to examine the myths that have arisen about malpractice and that circulate wildly among doctors.

Myth Number One has it that court calendars are crowded with suits and that half the doctors in the country are spending much of their time defending themselves instead of practicing medicine. It is true that there has been an increase in the number of suits.

The first court action in the United States taken against a physician for medical malpractice dates all the way back to 1794; but until 1930 they were practically unheard of since surviving an illness was held to be a near miracle. In the 1930s, however, expectations about doctors' services heightened, and, as a result, there was a notable increase in the number of malpractice suits, first in California, and then in Ohio, Texas, Minnesota, and the District of Columbia. The number of suits has grown since. That is not surprising since more people are seeing more doctors and many of the widely heralded new therapeutic measures involve great risks. The warning signals went up, hoisted by persons like C. Joseph Stetler, then director of the AMA Law Department, who declared in 1958 that: "In some localities the likelihood of being sued is becoming so great that the practicing physician must recognize that it constitutes a definite occupational hazard."[16] Figures like the ones he quoted have been used since. Nationally, one out of every seven AMA members had been sued; in some localities, one out of every four. Many doctors have become firmly convinced that those are the probabilities.

However, when HEW Secretary Richardson's Commission studied the risk that doctors ran of being sued for malpractice, the facts proved otherwise. Basing its figures on the 14,500 claims-producing incidents reported in 1970, the base year for the study, there is *less than one chance in 100,000* each time a physician or dentist treats a patient that an incident will occur that will give rise to a medical malpractice suit, actually only *one out of every 158,000 patient visits to doctors.*[17] Even those figures do not represent the complete story. If the number of reported incidents, which prompted the opening of 18,000 claim files in 1970, were divided among the 382,000 doctors, dentists, and hospitals at risk, it would appear that one of every 21 health-care providers was the object of a malpractice claim in 1970.

Although doctors in some areas are more likely to be sued than those in others, most doctors have never had a medical malpractice suit filed against them, and those who have have rarely been sued more than once, the Commission reported. In Maryland, which was outranked only by Tennessee and California in the percentage of claims increases in 1970, a ten-year study showed that 84 percent of the physicians in the state had never been sued; 14 percent had been sued once; 2 percent, more than once. Likewise, hospitals in some areas are more likely to be sued than those in other areas. If the number of claims were divided equally among the nation's 7000 hospitals, each would be sued twice a year. But this is not so; most hospitals, no matter what their size, have no claims filed against them at all. Fifteen percent of the hospitals accounted for more than half the claims filed.

If organized medicine, the insurance industry, and hospital associations saw to it that suit-prone individuals and institutions shaped up, they could do much to lower the cost and improve the quality of medical care. Instead, they perpetuate the myth that suit-happy patients are to blame. And that leads to *Myth Number Two, which holds that most suits are groundless.* That is not so, as the Commission's report and other investigations have shown. "With the exception of a few psychotics and outright frauds," the report noted sharply, "most people do not file claims for compensation unless they have been hurt."[18] Every study to date, it said, indicates that there are many times more medical injuries than there are claims. The Executive Director of the Secretary's Commission, Eli Bernzweig, recently pointed out that according to the AMA study, for every patient who files a suit *"there are probably ten times as many who never become aware of the fact that they have legitimate fault claims under our system."*[19]

Even if they were aware, many—perhaps most of the patients—are in no position to do anything about it. Supporting Mr. Bernzweig, Dr. David Rubsamen pointed out that many who have legitimate claims of negligence and who do seek legal aid are not accepted. "A patient may have lost a month's work and be out of pocket a thousand dollars for medical expenses because of the doctor's negligence. Assume he is now completely recovered and feels fine. That month of work lost and the thousand dollars for medical expenses is a heavy burden for a man making five hundred dollars a month. But no first-class attorney in California will take that case because the malpractice insurance carriers will not settle, and it just costs too much money for the plaintiff's attorney to try them."[20]

During one of the Commission's public hearings, a New Orleans woman testified that she had consulted a local lawyer for advice after having suffered a "foot drop," a foot condition due to lesion of the peroneal nerve, following a hysterectomy. He told her that she would have to advance $300 just to get the case started; another $3000 advance would be needed to obtain the necessary out-of-state medical expert witnesses. The possible judgment? $10,000. When the witness heard that, she dropped the whole thing: "We would have been gambling, and I'm not a gambler."[21]

Myth Number Three has doctors and the public convinced that the fastest route to becoming a millionaire is to institute a malpractice suit. Here, again, the facts are otherwise. Newspapers have given prominent space to the half-a-million-plus demands that are sometimes made. Medical journals also have played up extravagant claims. But in its study of the 16,000 malpractice claims files closed in 1970, the Commission found that only 3 percent of them resulted in awards of $100,000 or more. Even more revealing were other findings: 21.1 percent received a total settlement of less than $500; 65.2 percent received less than $5000; 78.6 percent less than $10,000. Those cumulative figures do not include the 45 percent of claimants who received nothing.[22]

And in the few cases in which huge sums are paid, the legal action often goes on for years, as in the case of Mrs. Ellen Holl, who finally won a $1,500,000 judgment in Florida in 1972 from a hospital and two doctors. In 1959, Mrs. Holl had been paralyzed by an improper dosage of drugs. For the next seven years, according to testimony, she lived—but like a vegetable. Her husband left her and her three children. Her mother took care of her and the children, with the help of welfare payments. She began to show some improvement, and by 1967 was able to talk. In that year, an attorney working with the family got the award from a Dade County jury. Victoria Hospital began to pay its share of damages: $500,000. The two doctors appealed, tying up the money until 1972. Mrs. Holl did not live to know that she was a millionaire. She died just after the Florida Supreme Court ruled that there was no cause to review the case.[23]

Myth Number Four encourages the delusion that it is easy to win a suit once a good lawyer has been found. As Mr. Stetler himself pointed out in his book, *Doctor and Patient and the Law,* it is still very difficult to prove negligence. Ordinarily, no inference of negligence is permitted from a "mere" diagnostic error, nor from the wrong method of treatment. Generally, no inference of negligence is permitted "merely" because the treatment is unsuccessful or produces such untoward results as infection and death. Among specific instances he cites in which no negligence was inferred: the puncture of a patient's bladder during a hysterectomy, the puncture of a bile duct during a gall-bladder operation, the displacement of a vertebra during a tonsillectomy, and plastic surgery which left the patient's face more disfigured.[24]

Doctors are protected by a special rule of law, which protects professionals from becoming fair game for every dissatisfied client. They are not required to effect a cure or even an improvement; they are simply required by law to employ reasonable skill and to exercise their best judgment, however inferior that may be. The law holds that the patient takes his chances when he submits himself to the care of a doctor. There is an implied contract between them which, as Louis Nizer points out in discussing his malpractice cases, enables the doctor to tell the patient: "Medicine is not an exact science. I will use my experience and best judgment. You take the risk that I may be wrong. I guarantee nothing." Nizer, one of the most distinguished trial lawyers in the country, considers this rule of law to be such a defensive cloak for doctors that "it is almost impossible to win a malpractice case against them."[25]

The need to obtain an expert witness is a formidable obstacle. As Nizer has noted: "I do not know whether it is a compliment to the medical profession to say that it is almost impossible in most states to induce a doctor to testify against another doctor."[26] For years, it was. If a doctor did testify against another, he ran the risk of being read out of the medical society, dropped from hospital lists, having his malpractice insurance canceled, and being ostracized by colleagues. A few doctors risked and experienced those very real threats as a matter of principle, but not a few have come to do it for money. It is, after all, far more profitable to provide expert testimony for a plaintiff for $400, $500, and more than to serve under subpoena for a few dollars. Recently, a number of doctors have taken up the practice of law, as malpractice attorneys.

Tort actions against a physician also require proof that in his treatment he violated the standards of his locality in providing care. His treatment cannot be measured against learned or gifted levels, merely the *average* treatment provided by the *average* doctor in his community or in a similar community. Not only lawyers, but doctors themselves object to this since it does not do enough to upgrade standards. Dr. James W. Bush of the University of California said of that: "What I am concerned about is how to stimulate legitimate medical innovation and how to distinguish what is clearly nonstandard and then label it as such so that it doesn't persist in health care just because fifty per cent of the doctors are still doing it."[27] And Dr. Roger Egeberg, Special Assistant to the President for Medical Affairs, added: "So we say, 'What is standard in the community is the norm.' But . . . there are some communities where tonsillectomies are standard. I think the weakest argument for what constitutes malpractice is that it 'deviates from the standard.' "[28]

Lawyers have found themselves depending in malpractice suits on the doctrine of *res ipsa loquitur*, "the thing speaks for itself." That doctrine derives from a nineteenth-century English case in which a customs officer tried to obtain compensation for being hit on the head by some sacks of sugar which had fallen from the window of a warehouse. Reasoning that sacks of sugar are not a normal pedestrian hazard unless there has been negligence in their handling, the judge responded favorably to the plaintiff with the comment of *res ipsa loquitur.* What is held to be a classic example of the application of that doctrine in this country involved an eastern surgeon, charged with having left a hemostat in a patient on whom he had performed an appendectomy. The trial judge was of the opinion that no expert witness was needed to testify that normal surgical procedures do not include leaving instruments in patients. He sent the case to the jury on a charge of *res ipsa*, and the jury responded by awarding the victim $9500.[29]

Doctors' protests that the doctrine of *res ipsa loquitur* guarantees a victory for the patient is not verified by court cases. Some physicians have been defended successfully by the excuse that there was the need for haste. More than one surgeon has been able to convince a judge that he left some gauze in a patient's abdomen because speed was imperative in order to protect the patient's life. (And an amazing variety of items have been left in patients after operations: sponges and gauze are the most common, but the list also includes pieces of bone, drains, needles, instruments and parts of instruments, broken glass, and towels.[30]) Nevertheless, there are very real grounds for protest about the doctrine. Contrary to most Anglo-Saxon justice it puts the burden on the defendant to prove himself innocent. And it has been extended to medical accidents that do not really involve negligence, but result from a rare chance.

There are other very real objections to malpractice actions. They are costly. Patients are now paying between 20 and 50 cents of every $10 they give the doctor for his malpractice insurance premiums; they are paying 50 cents a day for malpractice insurance when they are hospitalized. They are also paying for unnecessary hospital stays and office visits, and exposing themselves unnecessarily to X rays because doctors say that they have to indulge in *negative defensive medicine* through fear of suits. Doctors also cite the danger of being sued for malpractice as a reason for their reluctance to accept paramedics and assistants to relieve the doctor shortage.[31]

The AMA's opposition on that ground is not to be taken too seriously, however, since it has opposed most efforts to compensate for the shortage of medical men. According to the Commission report, "there does not appear to be any indication that the use of allied health-care personnel . . . has led to any significant problems of medical malpractice liability or malpractice insurance coverage."[32]

Another principal problem for patients is that it is really too chancy and too costly to sue a doctor in order to obtain medical justice, as indicated above. Recently, some interesting alternatives have been developed. A number of county, state, and federal district courts began to adopt impartial medical witness plans. The witnesses examine the records and reports and attempt to help the litigants work out a fair pretrial settlement. Bar associations in a number of places have objected to this since the witness is selected usually by the local medical society. Also, screening panels have been set up by medical societies either independently or with bar associations in order to determine whether a claim has merit. If the panel agrees, it will provide the claimant with an expert witness; if it does not, he must agree to drop the claim. There are undoubtedly some advantages; psychotics and frauds can be dismissed at this point; the proceedings are short and inexpensive. On the other hand, there are disadvantages. As the Commission pointed out, many medical malpractice cases involved more than one defendant. If a hospital, drug company, or manufacturer of medical devices were to be named as a codefendant and refuse to submit to the judgment of the screening panel, the panel could do nothing for the claimant.[33] Moreover, the patient would have no guarantee that even if lawyers were to join screening panels that his best interests will always be protected. The code adopted by the Bar Association of San Francisco, the San Francisco County Medical Society, and the San Francisco Lawyers' Club some years ago seems to have been principally designed to improve the practical working relationships between the two professions. Nowhere in the code is the patient mentioned, except as the payer of fees, and it holds among other things that:

> The public airing of any complaint or criticism by a member of one profession against the other profession or any of its members is to be deplored. Such complaints or criticism, including complaints of the violation of the principles of this Code, should be referred by the complaining doctor or lawyer through his own association to the appropriate association of the other profession; and all such complaints or criticism should be promptly and adequately processed by the association receiving them.[34]

An alternative to litigation that does hold considerable promise for claimants against doctors is arbitration. This device would be particularly effective if consumers were represented on the arbitration panel and if the findings were made public, as they are now in 40 states. Arbitration is being tried out in several Pennsylvania counties, where the courts have initiated a requirement that all claims against physicians be presented for arbitration that involve less than $10,000. The panel's decision is not necessarily final; either the physician or the patient may demand a court trial. But it is inexpensive; and it is speedy.

In addition to imposed arbitration, patients can ask for contract arbitration to settle claims against their doctor. This is usually required by union contracts to settle grievances, and it has the advantage of saving time and money and allowing for the use of experts in the field of controversy. Both hospitals and insurance companies are experimenting with contract arbitration. In California, patients are required to accept the procedure of contract arbitration as a condition of admission. The patient, of course, ultimately has a right to reject the condition. If he changes his mind, he has until 30 days after discharge to cancel the agreement. Some insurance carriers are now offering reductions in premiums to doctors holding their malpractice policies who are willing to obtain advance written agreement of a minimum percent of their patients to arbitration.

Those experiments are too new to provide significant findings. However, one contract arbitration arrangement that seems to have worked out well is that developed by the Ross-Loos Medical Group in Los Angeles. It is obviously regarded as effective both by members and the doctors' organization, judging merely by the increase in membership since Ross-Loos was founded more than 40 years ago. As a condition of membership, a binding arbitration agreement is required. Recently, a study was made showing that only three of the 35 claims Ross-Loos has dealt with since 1964 alleging malpractice actually went to formal arbitration. In one case, the claimant won $70,000; in two others, the medical group won and paid nothing. All of the remaining were settled in advance of arbitration. Importantly, in a significant number of the cases closed compensation was awarded—although the records indicate that they would have been extremely unlikely candidates for court action.[35]

If all medical practice were on the level of Ross-Loos practice, contract arbitration might well be the answer. Meantime, malpractice suits are a necessary evil, although limitations should be set for attorney fees and making monthly payments to the victims—instead of lump sums—would do much to curb excesses.

8 War for the Hospitals

The power struggle between organized medicine and hospital interests over control of the nation's health-care facilities has been waging for decades. Occasionally, a slash in the gauze curtain has allowed the public to witness the causes for and the nature of the conflict.

One such episode occurred some years ago in California, when fragments of a confidential report about doctors' treatment of hospitalized patients appeared in the press. The California Medical Association, which had commissioned the report, was understandably upset by some of the revelations. One of the more dramatic portions of the report described two surgeons conducting a fist fight over a patient on an operating table. The battle ended when one was knocked down and his colleague was left in possession of the helpless "trophy."[1]

Hospital authorities maintained an air of calm about the affair. The president of the Hospital Council of Southern California shrugged in answer to inquiries about that episode and others: "I can see no reason why the survey should be an indictment of the hospitals, as we have no control over the doctors."[2]

In the summer of 1965, the cold war erupted with fury during hearings on the Medicare bill conducted by the Senate Finance Committee. The AMA angrily accused the American Hospital Association of seeking "aggrandizement for its members, ever-widening control over the provision of medical care in this country." The AHA president promptly denied that hospitals were attempting to exercise "unrighteous dominion over doctors." He

126

urged the establishment of a truce, deploring the notion that "one mature organization should be using the public press to condemn another."[3]

The seemingly minor issue that had precipitated the conflict was whether or not specialists on the staff of hospitals should be permitted to bill Medicare patients separately for such things as X-ray treatments and pathology tests or whether the hospitals should charge for them as "institutional services." Behind that was the major issue of fee-for-service medical care, the right of doctors to decide how much, what kind, for whom, the basis of organized medicine's power.

Refusing to concede the people's right to participate in regulating the facilities in which they have invested billions, brushing aside the new sciences of hospital planning and management, ignoring the potential of modern hospitals to serve as centers of community health, organized medicine has adamantly decreed that hospitals continue to be "repair shops" for the sick and injured. The doctors hold that the publicly supported facilities should be treated as workshops where doctors can ply their trade for private gain.

That was the position organized medicine had taken 10, 20, 50 years before. But the stakes had increased enormously, and have continued to increase. The assets of the nation's hospitals were $7,791,000,000 in 1950; by 1970, assets were valued at $36,159,-000,000.[4] Annual revenues have skyrocketed: in 1950, Americans were spending $3,851,000,000 on hospital care; by 1970, annual expenditures were up to $27,961,000,000. And in those years, daily service charges rose by almost 600 percent.[5] Since then, the wildly upward spiral has continued. In 1972, for example, when a 6.5 percent increase was established as a ceiling for wages and profits, daily hospital rates rose by 11.6 percent. In a petition to the Cost of Living Council for relief, the Health Research Group associated with Ralph Nader, pointed out that consumers were obliged to pay more than $745,200,000 because reporting requirements failed to contain hospital price increases. They protested:

> In the face of mounting evidence of hospitals depositing

millions of dollars in non-interest bearing bank accounts, hospital pathologists "earning" $200,000 per year or more, and massive conflicts of interest in hospital purchasing—this blatant attempt to defraud consumers and further cripple their ability to afford health care must not go unchallenged.[6]

Any effort to impose ceilings on hospital costs involves the imposition of a ceiling on physicians' fees, and the challenge was not successful. Nor is there much immediate likelihood that a challenge will be, as long as doctors are in a position to dictate to hospitals. Their threats in 1965 against hospitals hiring salaried practitioners were repeated in 1974 about hospital utilization review committees. They were successful then as they had been many times before—in New York, Seattle, Washington, D.C., Los Angeles, Detroit, St. Louis, and other places, when the boycott weapon was used in the attempt to destroy prepaid group practice plans.

In 1961, the public and even more sophisticated legislators had little notion of what was involved. They did not understand that Medicare, Medicaid, and other public programs were intensifying the AMA's stranglehold over American medical care. They guaranteed to pay, without any control over cost or quality, whatever the doctor ordered.

The hospitals did have a better idea. Although doctors receive only about 20 percent of the health-care dollar, they control about 60 percent more since they are essentially in charge of hospitalization and other supporting services. As Dr. I. S. Falk pointed out recently, in making that estimate:

> The hospital responds to the physician's needs and orders, though typically he is not an officer or employee of the institution and is not responsible for the financing of its costs or for its legal obligations to society. And all this operates in a framework that gives medical care as a whole an open-end lien on the fiscal resources of society.[7]

Instead of resisting, the hospitals decided to hop aboard the gravy train. Together doctors and hospitals could make the most of what amounted to an unrestricted license to loot.

Hospitals receive most of the personal health-care expenditures, accounting for more than a third of the money spent. During the 1970-1971 fiscal year, private expenditures for hospital care were $14,871,000,000; public expenditures were $14,757,000,000, a total of $29,628,000,000.[8] Official estimates that the amount may be trebled by 1980, to reach a high of $92,600,000,000 now seem mild.[9] Cost increases in 1974 soared to 20 percent, suggesting a 1980 bill of almost twice that amount.

What this means in the lives of individuals, aside from the continuing tax burdens they are forced to bear, is r-u-i-n. Consider just a few of the stories told by witnesses to the Senate Subcommittee on Health during nationwide hearings in 1971 and reported in *In Critical Condition*. The witnesses represented all social, educational, and economic backgrounds; all of them illustrated how catastrophic illness can be.

In Denver, the wife of a bank president testified that her family had been forced to seek support from relatives because of bills incurred as a result of her husband's injury in an automobile accident. Their Blue Cross insurance did cover all but $875 of the $12,000 bill for his three-months' stay at Lutheran Hospital. But it covered only a small portion of the costs at Craig Rehabilitation Hospital, an institution built almost entirely by voluntary contributions of Denver citizens. The man was forced to make a $5000 deposit before he was admitted, and was told the day before he entered that costs would be $3000 a month. At the time of the hearing, the family's savings had been exhausted, no insurance benefits were available, and "There's no end in sight."[10] If it had not been for their parents, they and their three children would have been added to the welfare rolls.

In Ohio, a factory worker told of his plight. With insurance benefits exhausted after his wife had several operations because of kidney failure, he was at the end of his rope. She died shortly before the hearings in Ohio were held, but her husband still had a hospital bill of $5200. His take-home pay was $140 a week; he had two children to support.[11]

In Nashville, Tennessee, the Subcommittee was told of a university professor who died at the age of forty-six of cancer of the brain. His widow was left with bills amounting to $20,000. There was "additional irony" in that story since about six months before the man died he had been offered a position in Israel, their original home:

> Had they lived in the country of their origin, which has a completely different system of medical care, this entire tragic event would have had no financial consequence for her whatsoever, because under the system of medical care in Israel all medical bills would have been paid.[12]

Official estimates of daily hospital rates, ranging up to $150 by 1973, are meaningless. The stories told the Subcommittee indicate that $150 covers only the basic care of a bed and board and whatever nursing attention the patient can get. An official of the New York sanitation workers' union spelled out some of the "extras" at a hearing by a state legislative committee recently. A ten-year-old boy was taken to one of the hospitals in the city at 3:20 one morning. The child died 19 hours later. The bill presented to the grieving parents for services rendered was $1717.80: $105.80 for drugs, $184.80 for X rays, $220 for inhalation therapy, $655 for laboratory work![13]

In the winter of 1973, a man with whom I have worked for some years told me of his hospitalization experience. As he was walking up the stairs to his house early one evening, a neighbor called a greeting. Turning to answer him, his foot slipped and he fell against the iron railing flanking the stairway. His arm hurt badly that night; by the next day, the pain was so severe that he went to a doctor. The doctor clapped him into a hospital, where he remained for eight days. An extraordinary battery of tests was given to him for what was later diagnosed as a pinched nerve. The bill for his stay was more than $4000. Sometimes protest is made. Recently, a California county administrator turned down claims by a hospital and two physicians, who turned in bills for more than $10,000 following the death of a patient who had been in their hands for 70 hours. An insurance company paid $6,672.40 for the two operations and the three-day stay; it rejected the claim for the rest; that was then passed on to the county administrator to be levied against the man's estate—which was worth less than $4000. "I don't think you should charge $11,000 or $12,000 for dying," the administrator said. "I want the claims proved. That's quite a hospital bill for only a couple of days."[14]

Costs are assigned all out of proportion to services rendered. And costs for services rendered are arbitrary, varying wildly from one hospital to another. Some years ago, the Commission on Financing Hospital Costs found that in North Carolina hospitals the price of a grain of streptomycin ranged from 50 cents to $6. In Oklahoma, it found that one hospital charged ten cents for a pill; another charged $5 for the same pill.[15]

A Los Angeles manufacturer told me of his experience with a large community hospital. After his mother's death, he was given a statement that he owed nearly $5000. He returned the statement with a note that he would not pay the charges until he was given an itemized accounting. After some discussion, the hospital administrator grudgingly agreed to that, and several weeks later he was presented with a sheaf of papers. When his accountant went over the charges, he found that the price for a single aspirin tablet had varied from 80 cents to $1.50; the same test cost $7.50 on one day, $13 on another, and $15 on still another. "This is ridiculous," he fumed. "If we ran our business this way, we'd be ruined in a week."

Recent investigations of Medicare and Medicaid gouging make it clear that overcharging is going on quite a massive scale. The General Accounting Office made a survey in 1972 of payments to hospitals of which about 70 percent of the $7,500,000,000 paid in 1971 under the program were made. It found that 12 of the 14 institutions studied in depth had overcharged the government.[16]

Hospitals not only insist that they be regarded as businesses, but as ones with special privileges. Unlike airlines, restaurants, and other enterprises that serve the public, they insist on the right to pick and choose their customers. As a result, as Senator Alan Cranston has pointed out, *175,000 people die needlessly each year because they are unable to get adequate medical care in an emergency.*[17] A West Virginia woman told of her experience in a hospital emergency room after a second heart attack:

They wouldn't even let me in the emergency room, because I was on welfare. It took me an hour and a half before I could get hold of a nurse. Then she treated me like I was a dog or something—take you out in the hallway and strip you down and give you a shot in the hallway, and turn you loose, like you was a wild animal or something.[18]

Paul Johnson of Chicago told of his ordeal shortly before Christmas in 1969 after his ten-year-old son had a heart seizure. He drove him to the nearest police station to ask for an escort to County Hospital. The policeman assigned said that he could not go out of the district and suggested that they go to St. George's Hospital. He led the way. When the Johnsons arrived the father was subjected to intensive questioning about his ability to pay, his employer, and similar matters. The doctor in charge of the emergency service, Mr. Johnson reported, said of the child, who was being held by his older brother: "He couldn't be sick with a heart condition if he is able to scream and holler like that." And when the distraught father pleaded for help, the doctor retorted: "If you don't like the service here, take him somewhere else." In desperation, Mr. Johnson did. He drove past a number of hospitals along the expressway: "I was afraid to stop. I think the same thing would have happened if I had stopped at one of the other hospitals. I might as well try to make it to the County."

They did. At Cook County Hospital, he did receive attention. After examination, the doctors decided to put a pacemaker in; but the child went into a coma and died before they had a chance to insert it. Questioned by Senator Kennedy, Mr. Johnson acknowledged that he had heard from St. George's Hospital later; he had received a bill for use of the emergency room and for the services of a doctor.[19]

Because many hospitals turn away patients who may pose "financial problems," the emergency rooms of county and city hospitals are jammed. Medicare opened hospitals to about 20,000,-000 people, as did Medicaid, covering an almost equal number. Yet these programs did nothing for other millions. Papers all over the country carried word of the way of things at Jackson Memorial

Hospital in Miami, Florida, after two men in wheelchairs died in the emergency room. Four hours passed before any of the nurses or physicians noticed the corpses.[20]

Pressure by medical and hospital groups on legislators to skimp on appropriations for public hospitals has resulted in scandal after scandal in cities across the nation: New York's Bellevue, Chicago's Cook County, and Houston's Jefferson Davis Hospital, after the publication of Jan de Hartog's *The Hospital.* The Dutch writer and his wife had anchored their houseboat with delight in a bayou near the richest city in the world, as Houston likes to boast. They were eager to savor again the "instant welcome" they had found on another trip; and by way of making a reciprocating gesture, they volunteered to work at "J.D." The needs of the city-county charity hospital staffed with public nurses and residents and interns from Baylor University had been called to the de Hartogs' attention by newspaper reports, including one about 16 babies dying of a staph infection in the maternity ward. The hospital turned down their request to work as volunteers, making it clear that outsiders were not welcome. But the couple persisted; so did other members of their Quaker meeting. Once inside, they found it a nightmare out of Hieronymus Bosch. He later described the Emergency Room as it had appeared to him at 2 AM on the Saturday of his first weekend on duty as a volunteer aide:

> By then, the place was a chaos. The floors were slippery with blood and vomit, littered with soiled linen, dropped instruments, discarded bottles of Novocaine, torn gloves, paper wrappers of sterile gauze flats and the blood-soaked flats themselves, dropped regardless after the litter baskets had started to overflow. There had been no time to clean the stretchers between patients; blood-soiled mattresses had been flipped over and hastily covered with another sheet, as long as there were sheets. After that they were not even turned over any more; each man lay in the blood of his predecessor.[21]

Jan de Hartog's quiet note that "J.D." was "probably no more backward, politics-ridden, or neglected than similar institutions of charity all over the country" has been borne out in many other places. And the response of hospital staffs and politicians has been invariably hostile. For example, in the 1960s when some VISTA workers in Newark became familiar with the county hospital's conditions, they issued a detailed report of their findings. "Their report was so shocking that there were red faces all over town, mostly in City Hall," noted an article in the *Christian Science Monitor*. Not unexpectedly, the removal of the VISTA workers from the hospital "followed quickly."[22]

Occasionally, however, legislators rebel as in Los Angeles after the Watts riots in 1965. That ghetto, which has a death rate 22.3 percent higher than the rest of the city, was woefully short of physicians and hospital facilities. Of eight privately owned hospitals there, only two met minimum standards of quality.[23] When it was proposed that a branch of the county hospital (which has become an excellent health-care center because of its association with the University of California Medical School) be established in Watts, Watts' doctors and businessmen insisted that government funds be used to construct a $10,000,000 private hospital there. The president of the Golden State Medical Society, which represents 300 black physicians, argued "We want to encourage self-esteem and self-sufficiency in the community, and we feel that giving the community the responsibility of supporting its own hospital will instill those qualities."[24]

At that time, only 14 percent of the men and 18 percent of the women in Watts had any kind of health-insurance coverage; 24 percent of the people in the area were receiving public assistance. Just how persons in such circumstances would derive self-esteem and self-sufficiency from the kind of hospital that had the right to reject all but paying customers so perplexed even tax-conscious officials that they vetoed the private hospital plan. The Martin Luther King Hospital, which was erected instead, is a model hospital. It provides a wide range of social services in addition to excellent medical and surgical care; it is truly a community health center.

Black Americans have been notoriously victimized by the exclusionist policies of hospitals. So have other ethnic minorities. In 1973, two physicians with the Office of Civil Rights told a House subcommittee that the HEW agency had been "unsuccessful" in insuring that hospitals did not discriminate against minority patients who receive Medicare and Medicaid funds.[25] But plenty of white, middle- and even upper-income persons have suffered and even died because they were not able to obtain treatment before producing a down payment and guarantee of the rest of the bill.

The reason for the chaos that has resulted from the hospital-as-business attitude is partly that the concept of a hospital as a comprehensive community-health institution is such a new one. "Within living memory, an age-old institution has been transformed from a hostel for sick poor into a medical center for everyone," Dr. Michael M. Davis pointed out correctly some years ago.[26] Fifty years ago it was as unusual for a moderately privileged person to be born in a hospital as it was for him to be buried from an undertaking parlor. *Nice* people would not be caught in either—dead or alive.

The first hospitals in the country were simply poorhouses, where some care was given to sick inhabitants. Bellevue Hospital, for example, had its origin as a six-bed infirmary in the "Publick Workhouse and House of Correction of the City of New York" in 1736.

During what Dr. Henry E. Sigerist, the medical historian, has called the second period of hospital development, "real" hospitals were founded as places in which medical treatment was given to the indigent sick whether or not they were normally public charges. They were, he said, "infinitely better" than many of their European counterparts; they also instituted a new businesslike note. Benjamin Franklin conducted the initial fund-raising campaign for the Pennsylvania Hospital, which was considered the first true hospital in the United States. He had decided that patients were to be charged for care they received in order to foster "self-respect."[27]

As cities burgeoned, the quality of the hospitals deteriorated. In *House of Healing*, Mary Risley notes that even after reforms were made in Bellevue Hospital in 1870, "New Yorkers fought like tigers, if they had the strength, to avoid being sent there when they were ill."[28] Toward the end of the century, however, advances were made in medical science that included asepsis, new surgical techniques, and innovations in medical treatment. These advances created an awareness that hospitals could be more than death traps for the indigent and hopelessly ill. Hospital building suddenly became as fashionable for America's rich as constructing summer palaces at Newport or embarking on the Grand Tour of Europe. The Rockefellers, the Astors, the Vanderbilts, the Morgans were persuaded by physicians like Dr. J. Marian Sims and Dr. Simon Flexner to donate huge sums. Edward Harkness alone donated more than $34,000,000 to Columbia-Presbyterian Hospital in New York. Actually, the motives of all were mixed. Some of the donors were inspired by personal tragedies; some by humane concerns. All of them appreciated the tax write-offs; all of them benefited from the good public relations they generated. To become known as a hospital benefactor was to silence criticism about all kinds of unsavory activities and to acquire social prestige. Religious and secular organizations grew interested in setting up hospitals; even the moderately well-to-do and the frankly poor were persuaded to donate, through Red Feather and United Way campaigns.

After World War II, the public was encouraged to make even greater contributions through the Hill-Burton program for building and equipping private as well as public hospitals. Between 1947, when the program was started, and 1971, $3,700,000,000 in federal tax money had been spent to construct and equip health-care facilities. Almost no strings were attached in the way of reasonable regional planning and quality of care being provided. But that amount, as has been noted, is but a small part of the donations hospitals received. Most of the $36,159,000,000 in hospital assets as of 1970 were contributed by the public; much of the $27,961,000,000 annual revenues were given by the public to support both public, nonprofit, and frankly profit-making hospitals.

The term *nonprofit*, it should be emphasized, is used very loosely by hospitals, as it is by cemeteries and other profiteering enterprises. The nonprofit organization that operate the hospitals provide a respectable facade behind which speculators can siphon off enormous profits by controlling such money-making aspects as pharmacies and gift shops. A man I know, who had been devoting a good bit of time as a volunteer on health-care projects, was horrified a couple of years ago to find out just how businesslike a nonprofit hospital can be. His wife was in the intensive-care unit of one of the largest and finest institutions in Los Angeles, for which he had for years been helping to raise funds. When the air-conditioning broke down one stifling summer day, he decided to go to the gift shop to buy some packets of the dampened paper towels that travelers find so convenient. Downstairs in the gift shop, he noticed that it was remarkably cool. "Oh, yes," the woman in charge enlightened him. "we have a backup system here. After all, with the flowers and the chocolates. . . ."

As profit-oriented as many nonprofit hospitals are, however, far worse have been the proprietary hospitals. A World War II phenomenon, the private institutions are mostly owned by doctors, and they have become "hot" investments—attracting major corporations and such unlikely outsiders as Debbie Reynolds, the movie actress.[29] The administrators of these hospitals can make a fortune by providing only minimal services and the doctor-investors can guarantee full occupancy.

Years ago, Sinclair Lewis described in *Arrowsmith* how profitable those medical factories can be, with their "lyric faith" in the value of separating people from any anatomical item that could be removed at a profit.[30] More recently, Seymour Kern's *The Golden Scalpel* describes in even greater detail how patients are victimized by money-hungry doctors who pool modest cash sums and modest talents to construct private hospitals in order to parlay small investments into fortunes. In an article on the same subject, Mr. Kern cited the case of one proprietary hospital in California that had been built at a total cost of $517,000. Only $117,000 represented a cash investment, yet the annual net profit on the 50-bed institution was $129.542, or a 124 percent annual return on cash invested.[31] Sales brochures prepared by the American Hospital Management Corporation estimate that operating profit would pay for a hospital in less than five years. One promised that the initial investment would be returned within less than three years.[32]

Since the advent of Medicare and Medicaid, the business of private hospitals has boomed. In the winter of 1973, Victor Cohn of the *Washington Post* described how one enterprising obstetrician-gynecologist near the national capital had organized a hospital-building scheme that could net him half a million from construction and half a million a year thereafter from operating the hospital. A prospectus submitted for approval by the Maryland Securities Division by Dr. J. Allen Offen spelled out the ways in which money could be made for the benefit of the 100 prospective "limited partners" he hoped to attract, at an initial investment of $26,250 each.[33]

To carry out his goal, Dr. Offen formed Parkway Hospital Partnership. He and his own Parkway Development Corporation were to be the general partners, placing him in sole control. The Partnership would build, own, and lease the hospital to Intercity Hospital Corporation, which would operate it. Dr. Offen is president of Intercity and, for a $16,121 contribution, its controlling stockholder. The hospital was to be built on land bought by a company in which Offen owns a 40 percent interest, then sold to another firm owned by Offen and his son for a huge profit. As a result of additional buying and selling and reselling, which developers call "pineappling," Offen and other land investors would have $1,000,000 in cash from less than 20 acres of land that originally cost less than $6000 an acre.

Additionally, Dr. Offen was to get, according to Mr. Cohn's analysis of the prospectus, (1) a $200,000 fee for services in development and construction; (2) any saving if building costs were less than $11.500,000; (3) a 20 percent share of hospital profits; (4) a general management fee of "up to $120,000 a year" when profits justify it; (5) about $360,000 profit from the land sale; (6) an unstated share of what could be a very large income from the lease of the hospital's X-ray, laboratory, pharmacy, and other possible services, and 39,000 square feet of "patient referral areas," apparently doctors' examining rooms.

There are many ways in which hospitals owned by doctors can be made to turn a profit; that is why many of the largest chains have deliberately followed a policy of selling stock to local physicians. Perhaps most important, as will be considered later in more detail, the physicians can insure a full house. Additionally, as the Senate Finance Committee learned during its investigation of Medicare and Medicaid costs, doctors who are owners can derive large bonuses by charging large fees for visiting practices, by ordering sometimes almost incredible amounts of laboratory tests, X-ray treatments, and medications provided by hospital pharmacies. One, for instance, received $14,220 from the government for hospital visits to 74 patients during a single year. As hospital owner, he was paid $37,597 for laboratory tests for the patients, $11,016 for diagnostic X-ray treatment, and $16,135 for drug injections. All that was in addition to other services he rendered as a physician.[34]

Recently, doctors who are owners of private hospitals have developed a new gimmick by converting their hospital to a nonprofit status to increase profits. The Senate Committee described how profitable such a nonprofit arrangement can be. A group of doctors owning a hospital with a depreciated replacement cost of $2,000,000 claim that its fair market value is actually $4,000,000, which would include the good will that had been accrued. They could sell it for that sum to a nonprofit corporation which they had organized and which they control. The purchase price is paid from the excess of cash flow over expenses. The entire income, let us say of $200,000, becomes tax free and is applied toward payment of the inflated $4,000,000 purchase price. The enormous returns are thus not subject to ordinary income-tax rates.[35]

Costly as that kind of financial manipulation and tax-dodging is, at least it is legal. That cannot be said of many of the ways in which the private hospitals particularly exploit government programs, insurance funds, and individual patients by means of double-billing, overservicing, and exacting kickbacks from druggists, technicians, laboratories, nursing homes, and even undertakers.

Fraud has been rampant since the inception of Medicare and Medicaid. But it was not until 1973 that federal officials prosecuted the first large hospital fraud case. In that case, the administrator admitted and was convicted of conspiring with other corporation officers of defrauding the Social Security Administration by making false entries in hospital ledgers and charging as "reimbursable" costs $45,000 for such items as season tickets to Los Angeles Angels baseball games, country club memberships, art objects, and direct payments to the board of directors between 1966 and 1969.

Because we have tolerated the idea that hospitals can be just like any other business rather than all being public service institutions, rational planning has been minimal. Thanks to the casual way in which federal and state money has been tossed around, "overbedding" has reached dangerous proportions in many parts of the country. The Department of Health, Education, and Welfare has estimated the national surplus amounts to about 6,000 beds. More recently, Ralph Nader's Health Research Group petitioned that agency to impose strong regulations on hospital construction. According to the Nader Group's findings, federal programs of hospital construction cost consumers $2,000,000,000 in 1975 for an estimated 100,000 unused beds. Consumers additionally paid $6,000,000,000 for a quarter of a million beds "filled by patients who should not have been hospitalized in the first place or who stay in the hospital too long."[36]

The large public facilities continue to be overcrowded; in some metropolitan institutions with an open-door policy even hallways are jammed with sickbeds. Proprietary hospitals are also well filled. And why not, since doctors can and do see to it that their patients are hospitalized whether they need it or not. Doctors on the staffs of nonprofit hospitals can also help to keep the doors open in that manner, although their record is considerably better and for that reason a number have been forced to close their doors. The extent to which the practice of unnecessary hospitalization prevails was revealed not long ago by an expert witness testifying before a Senate subcommittee. He said that *at least 30 percent of the people admitted to hospitals should not be in them at all.*[37]

Some of the methods used by hospitals, including convalescent hospitals, have been ingenious in the extreme. In 1975, for example, a class-action suit was filed against eleven hospitals and their operators, doctors, and other staff members, along with the County of Los Angeles and an enterprising promoter. The latter worked out of what is called the "drunk court," persuading judges to give him custody of elderly men charged with drunkenness who would agree to obtaining rehabilitative care. According to the suit, the men were then plopped into the various hospitals where they were told they would have to stay and where they were subjected to "injections, medications, physical abuse . . . [that] resulted in severe injuries, in some cases causing loss of consciousness, allergic reactions, shock, and in one or more instances resulting in death."[38] Cost of the "treatment" was subsidized by the taxpayers.

Most seek more "respectable" ways of filling beds, ordering extended examinations, rest cures, and unwarranted operations, and no one is the wiser. Although hospitals qualifying for funeral funds must have utilization committees to determine that none except medically necessary cases are admitted, the law is so loose that it requires only *one* member of the committee to have no financial interest in the hospital.[39] Not even that standard is met, however; when the Social Security Administration recently checked out the Medicare program, it found that 47 percent of the hospitals were not reviewing any admissions.[40]

As a consequence, unnecessary operations have become so common that a few years ago the Pennsylvania Insurance Commissioner issued a *Shopper's Guide to Surgery* to protect consumers against knife-happy doctors bent on anatomical raiding expeditions. He pointed out that they were performing as many as two million unwarranted operations a year.[41] No one really knows the exact total, although in the famous study made by the leaders of the Columbia University School of Public Health, it was found that as many as a third of the operations in various categories were completely unnecessary.[42] Hysterectomies, appendectomies, tonsillectomies have been performed arbitrarily by the millions. One of the more recent popular operations has been the unnecessary removal of female breasts.

What makes the situation even more depressing is that consumers have been kept almost entirely in the dark about the hospitals where the abuses are most likely to occur. The quality of hospitals fluctuates wildly, yet, thanks to AMA policies, laymen are not made privy to how one doctor's workshop differs from another. (Commissioner Denenberg pioneered an effort to inform the public with his *Shopper's Guide to Hospitals in the Philadelphia Area*, the kind of booklet which should be duplicated by every insurance commissioner in the country.)

Instead of clapping people into hospitals for minor and imaginary reasons, doctors should make every effort to keep them out. *Hospitals are dangerous places.* That they are stems largely from the AMA's determination to keep them private workshops where doctors can ply their trade in their own way without any concern for cost or quality control. The AMA has fought hard to keep doctors from practicing "corporate medicine," from working on a salary, as ordinary mortals usually do. The quality of care is at its best where doctors do practice "corporate medicine" in the great university teaching hospitals, in the group-practice hospitals like those owned by the Kaiser Foundation and the Group Health Cooperative of Puget Sound. Quality is lowest in the proprietary hospitals, where no realistic controls are imposed on the doctors. In the Columbia University study made for the Teamsters, it was found that two-thirds of the patients in hospitals that had not been accredited by the Joint Commission (most of them proprietary) received no better than "fair care"; 43 percent of the patients received "poor care."[43]

Doctors send patients to hospitals that are not equipped to treat them, at a great cost in life and health. In a study made public recently it was revealed that although most of the 170 hospitals in the Los Angeles area accept cancer patients, only 19 of them had been approved for cancer treatment by the U.S. College of Surgeons. Generally, it was estimated, if patients were directed immediately to the proper facility, between 10 and 20 percent of cancer victims could be saved. That is the average. In the case of some specialized types of cancer, the difference between life and death is much greater. For example, only 5 percent of the children suffering with acute leukemia in this country now make it beyond the five-year survival period. Yet 50 percent of the children survive who are treated at some highly specialized centers.[44]

Millions of middle- and upper-income Americans have learned, along with the poor, how serious the consequences of the AMA ban on salaried physicians in hospitals can be. Emergency rooms have, until recently, been staffed entirely by interns and residents. The AMA made exceptions of them and also of foreign-trained doctors. As a result, thousands of the latter poured into hospitals in major cities across the country. By 1965, conditions were so bad that a physician said that if a person was injured in a car crash along the Merritt Parkway between New York and New Haven, his chances of being cared for first by a foreign medical school graduate were practically certain. Subsequent hospital care might also be provided, with sometimes disastrous consequences. In one New York hospital, for example, a foreign medical gradu- ate removed a young man's lung even though he was utterly with- out qualifications to perform the operation. The young man was an autopsy case within 48 hours.[45] In one of the most publicized disasters, Martyn Green, the actor-singer star, lost his leg after he caught it in an elevator in a parking lot. Emergency aid was sum- moned, but the Indian doctor who arrived with the ambulance had not even remembered to take his medical equipment. Never- theless, he decided to act—hacking off the actor's leg with a pocket knife borrowed from a policeman standing nearby. The public outcry over that bit of butchery became louder after other investigations. One study disclosed that 11 major hospitals in New York were without a single American or Canadian medical school graduate. At Harlem Hospital, interns and residents in- cluded a number of practitioners who had failed the examinations given to foreign medical students. Dr. Ray E. Trussell, who had directed the Teamster study, was appointed Commissioner of Hos- pitals in New York. Braving the AMA ban, he hired fulltime physicians trained in the United States to supervise work in all the city's hospitals. Operating costs rose by only 10 percent; the quality of care improved immeasurably.[46]

The AMA finally bowed slightly to pressure and agreed that

doctors could be hired to staff emergency rooms in a few selected hospitals in each area.

Other dangers make it imperative that patients be kept out of hospitals unless it is absolutely necessary for them to be there. The chances of becoming infected with a disease in a hospital are great, affecting as many as 5 percent of hospital patients and annually increasing their stay by 1,800,000 to 3,600,000 days.[47] The chances of acquiring a drug-induced disease are between 10 and 30 percent.[48] And if that figure seems minimal, remember that one of every seven persons in the country is scheduled for hospitalization this year. Hospitals are dangerous on other counts. The Secretary's Commission on Medical Malpractice revealed that about 88 percent of the incidents that give rise to suits occur in hospitals. The operating room, not unexpectedly, headed the list; but the patient's own room ranked second as the location of claims-producing incidents—ahead of the emergency room, the intensive-care unit, and other places where injuries might be expected to occur.[49]

A priority objective is to get hospitals out of the stock market and into the business of helping patients to get well, and to do that at a reasonable cost.

No tax money should be given to any hospital builders until the absolute need for another hospital has been established. Indeed, many experts believe that a moratorium should be declared to prevent any further hospital construction whether publicly or privately supported until a coherent plan for every area in the country has been worked out.

Planning should be based on the model of those European countries that have worked out a fully integrated system of delivering health care. Under these systems responsibility is delegated to regional health councils that coordinate all health-care resources within a particular area, insuring available and comprehensive services for everyone in it and guaranteeing quality care. In Sweden, for example, the "sun" in this "planetary" system is called a regional medical center. It is the central facility for a population of a million people. Around each of the regional medical centers gravitate: (1) four central hospitals serving about a fourth of the population; (2) district hospitals, which serve 60,000 to 90,000 people; (3) health centers, each serving a population of 15,000. Some efforts to effect such a system have been made in a number of places in this country, with good results. For example, the Bingham Associates Fund, centered in the New England Medical Center of Tufts Medical School in Boston, established a working relationship with 56 small hospitals in Maine and Massachusetts.

It is irrational for two or more hospitals in a single location to have and maintain some of the very costly and very expensive services separately that are now customary. Mergers could and should be effected of the hospitals and of the specialized services they provide. A notable effort has been made in Seattle, where a single obstetric center was authorized to handle the maternity cases that six downtown hospitals had been providing previously.[50] Similar steps should be taken in regard to some kinds of cardiac, kidney, and cancer units so that in one area vital facilities would not be unused, while in others they are nonexistent.

Hospitals built to provide short-term care should not be used as nursing homes or convalescent centers. Yet it is estimated that about 25 percent of the patients in the country are being treated in facilities excessive to their needs. An HEW study showed that if patient needs had been matched with facilties' services, about $3,000,000,000 would have been saved in 1970 alone.[51] Some patients now in acute hospitals should be in longterm facilities, in nursing homes, or even at home. Ambulatory surgical centers can save millions of patient days; so have neighborhood health centers and fuller utilization of outpatient departments.

Proper accounting measures would also help to reduce costs. So would public disclosure of expenditures, including those of administrators and the trustees. Presently, there is almost no accountability, as a Pennsylvania newspaper publisher recently noted. In questioning the management of Altoona Hospital, a 430-bed institution in the economically depressed area, he acquainted readers with copies of 50 hospital expense accounts, liquor bills, dinner checks, travel vouchers, and other documents that caused no little stir.[52]

Consumer representatives must be given a place in hospital management and planning to insure that cost and quality are realistically controlled since doctors, hospital administrators, and boards of trustees have for the most part failed to do that.

The government must police doctors and hospitals to insure that unnecessary hospitalization and unwarranted treatment are not given at taxpayers' expense. An effort to establish a utilization review program by requiring preadmission certification failed recently, when the AMA and the AHA threatened to sue the government. A compromise, requiring review within two days after a patient is admitted, went into effect (partially) in 1975. It was estimated that if fully operative, the review and cost controls would save millions.[53] Government agencies at all levels must also act to insure that the results of tissue studies, now considered an in-house secret, are used to rate hospitals. And those ratings should be made public since people's lives are dependent on the knowledge.

In 1972, the American Hospital Association issued to its 7000 member hospitals a 12-point "Bill of Rights" for distribution to patients. It covered such fundamentals as the right to "respectful" care; the right to complete information about their condition and the treatment from the physician; the right to privacy; the right to know about human experimentation affecting their care or treatment; the right to examine the bill; and to expect "reasonable" continuity of care. The action to inform patients that they have rights was a commendable one, although it was a long time in coming. But hospitals have a long way to go toward breaking the control of profiteers in and out of the medical profession before patients will be able to rest easy in their beds.

People to Burn

We came upon an old lady locked to her bed by means of a leather belt and whose neck was fixed in a metal contraption which resembled the stocks of early Puritan settlements. Her scalp was matted and filthy and her hospital gown was covered with food stains. . . . She told us she was 98 years old. . . .

A few minutes after we rang, the door was opened by a disheveled nurse, whose breath was noticeably alcoholic. The hallway was dark and dirty, the one water fountain not working, the urine stench overpowering. On several bedside tables stood open wine bottles for "medicinal" purposes. In this 27-bed facility, 23 beds were occupied. . . .

One two-bed room was dark and the inspector asked why. Both ladies were blind. One of them complained that she had glaucoma, was in pain, and that her doctor had not been to see her "since July" [five months before]. The nurse was visibly infuriated and told us that the patient was a "troublemaker" whose mind wandered and who had no sense of time. We checked the medical chart; the patient had glaucoma and had not been seen by a physician since the previous July. . . .

We passed a door which the consultant did not notice in the dark, but which the inspector did. It was locked (a violation) and a patient was in it. The inspector asked the nurse to open the door and she replied that the patient was a mental case who would attack us. We insisted that the door be unlocked. The stench was so overpowering that the consultant became nauseated. An old lady in a

*thin cotton nightgown was lying on a bare urine-soaked
mattress in a deeply drugged stupor. The floor was caked
with dried vomit which appeared to be old. The walls
were flecked with dried excrement. The woman appeared
malnourished and her hair was matted. The chart did not
contain a record of a doctor's visit for the past several
months, nor an order for medication. . . .*[1] (Italics added.)

The findings of a Board of Charities Commission in nineteenth-
century England? The sensational revelations of a turn-of-the-
century American muckraker? No, merely a staff report on *Health
Care Services for the Aged* prepared for the California state legislature by Lillian B. McCall in 1965. The grotesque images that
emerge from Mrs. McCall's carefully detailed account of conditions in some of the more than 1000 nursing homes in California
become even more horrifying when we realize that California has
been a "paradise" for the aged, with almost unequalled pension,
social welfare, and health benefits. California, at the time the
report was presented, was paying nursing homes up to $280 a
month to care for elderly ailing persons needing public assistance.
By contrast, Delaware was paying $75 a month; Florida, $100 a
month; Kentucky, $115. Many states paid nothing.

Earlier warnings about the conditions in nursing homes throughout the country were provided by public and private investigators.
Ruth and Edward Brecher, in a comprehensive series of articles
in *Consumer Reports* in 1964, also described the way in which
patients were being "subjected needlessly to physical restraints"
and dosed excessively with sedatives and tranquilizers, which
served as a "psychic straitjacket." Fed woefully inferior food,
patients were often locked up at night like criminals with no one
left in attendance.[2]

Eleven years later a fuller account of American nursing homes
was given at a series of hearings across the country held by the
Subcommittee on Long-Term Care of the Special Committee on
Aging of the U.S. Senate. The evidence pointing to a need for regulation and control was staggering. Indeed, to read the subcommittee's 908-page compilation of findings, *Conditions and*

Problems in the Nation's Nursing Homes, is to journey into the the heart of darkness.

Across the country, there was widespread agreement that something had to be done about the anachronistic and brutal method of caring for the senile and the sick, turning them over by the millions to the counterparts of Mr. Bumble, the villainous entrepreneur in *Oliver Twist* who operated on the simple theory that the weaker the gruel, the scarcer the meat, the fewer the employees, the greater the return. Indignation was rife about the twentieth-century Bumbles, who had been created by public apathy and medical avarice, along with legislative short-sightedness and stupidity.

They were a new breed of entrepreneur. Traditionally, caring for the aged and for the sick in this country, as elsewhere, had been "a good work," that is, a charitable activity. Families assumed the burden of providing for their own; those without families became charges of hospitals, almshouses, and "old folks homes" sponsored by religious and fraternal groups and by local governments. That pattern was first broken as the result of an action taken by the New York state legislature in 1930. It enacted an old-age security measure providing a 50 percent state subsidy for pensions granted to aged persons by local governments. The legislature, wishing to discourage the use of public almshouses, stipulated that pensions would not be granted to inmates of such institutions. The intention was admirable; unfortunately, the legislature failed to act upon a complementary recommendation that the state itself build modern institutions to provide the kind of care that was needed, that almshouses were not providing.

Five years later, when the federal social security laws were drafted, New York was adopted as the model.[3] As a result, there was a general exodus from state hospitals and almshouses by persons eager to get pension benefits and "go it alone." The law encouraged all kinds of small businessmen to seek a share of the millions in pension money being distributed. Private establishments for Old Age Assistance beneficiaries mushroomed across the country, advertising themselves as convalescent homes and nursing homes. Many, most, were simply converted dwellings, with beds set up in parlors and dining rooms after available bed-rooms became too crowded to shelter additional patients. The OAA payments were not adequate to provide the care that many of them required; but the new industry was not daunted; a profit could be made by providing less care or none at all.

In the 1940s the need for facilities to provide for the aged increased. Business boomed in what has been called "the blackest era in American care for the aged."[4]

In 1950, the federal government took steps. OAA payments were extended to residents of public medical institutions, except mental and tuberculosis hospitals. That prompted some states to enlarge existing facilities and to build new ones, some of superior quality. Importantly, it required each state to establish a licensing agency to elevate standards. However, licensing laws were generally ineffectual since they were not enforced by a single agency. In California, for example, authority has been divided among the departments of Social Welfare, Public Health, and Mental Hygiene. Consequently, the excellent state health and safety code has been almost useless to protect nursing home patients. The bureaucratic attitude toward the resulting abuses was summed up some years ago by the chief of the Department of Public Health's Bureau of Hospitals, who said in response to questioning at a hearing: "In general a third of the nursing homes are in full compliance with the minimum standards or exceed those standards." California legislators understandably expressed astonishment at the inversion of figures. Obviously, if only one-third of the nursing homes were in compliance with minimum standards, two-thirds were not.[5]

Even in states where a single agency had the authority to enforce standards, violations were frequent. After a fire in an Indiana nursing home took the lives of 20 elderly persons just before Christmas in 1964, a reporter for the *Indianapolis Star* said:

> In the case of the Fountaintown disaster, we found that the health facilities council inspector, a registered nurse, had made official notification of the fact that the administrator of the nursing home was very hostile, very unfriendly about the inspection, and had informed her that

he always threw communications from the department of health in the wastebasket. He did not pay any attention to them.[6]

Neither federal nor state governments made any meaningful effort to discourage such Bumble-ing. It did nothing to reward the nonprofit voluntary nursing homes of excellent quality. They were further penalized by Federal Housing Administration policies. Only the profit-makers could obtain FHA-guaranteed loans; only the profit-makers could obtain reimbursement for costs of building and maintaining infirmary facilities.

The American Hospital Association decided to act in 1957, recommending that a listing and accreditation program be set up for nursing homes, as has been done with hospitals. Homes were to be surveyed periodically, and lists of those which met standards would be published. Persons seeking a nursing home would thus gain some assurance about such important matters as adequate qualified nursing service, physical plant safety and sanitation, proper licensing. Standards also specified that the food served patients meet their nutritional and dietary requirements, that narcotics and other medications be issued only with physicians' orders, that health records be maintained, that laboratory and hospital in-patient services be available. The standards also required full disclosure of nursing home ownership, a delicate point.[7]

The program worked out by the Joint Commission on Accreditation of Hospitals was widely hailed as a significant measure. Aged, chronically ill persons and their families who had found "blind" shopping for a nursing home a dreary, guesswork affair were delighted. So were health and welfare leaders, who saw it as the beginning of quality control. Representation in administering the program was to be broad. In addition to representatives from the AHA, the AMA, the American College of Surgeons, and the American College of Physicians, which make up the Joint Commission, others represented the American Academy of General Practice, the American Dental Association, the American Nurses' Association, the American Psychiatric Association, the

Association of Rehabilitation Centers, the Federation of Licensed Practical Nurses, and the National League for Nursing. Also included were members of the two national organizations of nursing home owners and administrators: the American Association of Homes for the Aging, made up of administrators of nonprofit nursing homes; and the American Nursing Home Association, representing owners of the commercial establishments.[8]

All of them were willing to join forces to clear up the national scandal, with two notable exceptions. The American Nursing Home Association, not unexpectedly, objected to the "too demanding" national standards and the regulation by "outside" agencies. Like most trade associations, it prefers to regulate itself and that the basis of regulation be suitably vague and general. More unexpectedly, the AMA's Board of Trustees voted to oppose accreditation by the Joint Commission. Since the commission needs a three-fourths majority to pass on such matters and since the AMA has seven of the 20 voting memberships in the commission, it could and did veto the program. Greater shock was felt a few months later, when the AMA and ANHA announced that they were jointly sponsoring a National Council for the Accreditation of Nursing Homes, with the AMA supplying 90 percent of the "seed money" needed to get that started.[9] After conducting the Senate hearings across the country, which revealed the full horrors of the treatment of elderly persons cooped up in what social workers have called the "pre-mortuaries," Senator Frank E. Moss accused the AMA of having abolished the greatest hope for remedying the shortage of nursing homes and improving their quality. One consequence, he noted, was the increase in thousands of elderly persons being "railroaded" to mental institutions because there was not other place for them.[10] In some states, as many as a third of the patients in mental hospitals were aged patients whose only "problem" was that they had no other place to go.

In addition to the denunciations of the measure, there was general speculation about the reasons for the AMA's action. When Consumers Union asked the AMA for a list of the "important factors" in the decision a year later, the reply "failed to mention even one."[11] Indeed, one of the principal reasons for the Moss subcommittee's country-wide hearings a year later was to learn those reasons. As Senator Wayne Morse said bluntly during one exchange:

> I think this committee has to dig in and find out why the American Medical Association and the Nursing Home Association feel that it is in the public interest to give, if they have it, the policies that you outline here which, for want of a better descriptive term, I would call sort of monopolistic control of accreditation in the country.[12]

One reason, of course, is the AMA's absolute opposition to any attempt to regulate the quality of care given by physicians.[13] Another reason cited was that the American Nursing Home Association also represented physicians' interests. It is no secret that the huge return of 30 percent and more that can be realized annually on a nursing home investment has attracted doctors as well as former garage mechanics, motel owners, housewives, and board chairmen of conglomerates to enter the business. In the 1960s, the number of doctors in that line of business was estimated to be as high as 10 percent of all practitioners.[14] Many have joined the ranks since. It is difficult to tell how many are, since doctors are not at all eager to have their interests publicized, a reason why "full disclosure of ownership" was proposed in the standards. Patients and relatives might get the "wrong impression" if they knew the doctor had a financial stake in the home he recommended. If the doctor owns the home with others, his fellow investors also prefer to have his interests kept low key, since even the rather flimsy Code of Ethics promulgated by the ANHA requires that: "No financial inducements of any kind shall be offered to any personnel or organization for the purpose of attracting patients to a nursing home."[15]

Nonetheless, so many doctors have been secretly involved that after their investigation the Brechers called it "a festering scandal that warrants prompt attention from the American Medical Association, county medical societies, and state licensing officials."[16] Actually, it warranted intervention by the government since none of those agencies would be likely to act.

Not the least reason for the AMA's rejection of the accreditation program was suggested by representatives of the American Hospital Association. An article in *Modern Hospital* suggested that the AMA had joined the nursing home association to "deal AHA out" because of the latter's support of Medicare. Both the AMA and ANHA had favored retention of the Kerr-Mills plan, instead, which turned over money for nursing home care, but did nothing to improve the quality.[17] In this instance, however, the AMA had gone too far for even the most malleable legislators. Congressmen allowed that portion of the Medicare law to stand that required nursing homes to meet certain standards before they could accept patients under the government's program. The Joint Commission was named as an example of the kind of national body needed to do the accrediting; the AMA-ANHA National Council was ignored. Shortly after Medicare was signed into law, the AMA bowed to the inevitable and reversed its policy. It authorized its representatives on the Joint Commission to vote for a single accreditation program to be administered by that body.

But the damage done by the AMA's three years of obstruction and the continuing pressures applied to government agencies by that organization and the nursing home trade group are still felt. The only real change that has occurred is that Mr. Bumble has become Bumble, Inc.

By July 1, 1967, six months after the extended-care benefits of Medicare and Medicaid went into effect, only 740 of the 4,160 facilities which had been certified fully met the conditions of operation. Some of the others certified did not even meet the requirement of having a qualified charge nurse for each tour of duty.[18] Another 9000 were operating without any concern for federal standards; about 7000 were passing themselves off as nursing homes although they were only "intermediate care facilities" and provided almost no services at all, though often at high prices.

A principal reason for the inclusion of nursing homes in the health laws was to cut hospitals' costs and reduce demand for their services by patients who needed only a modest amount of supervision and treatment. But because the law was written to make it mandatory for persons to be hospitalized at least three days before they could be admitted to a nursing home, hospital admissions increased. Demand for nursing home care skyrocketed. Why not? The first 20 days were "free," and most of the cost of the remaining 80 days were allowed. And demand was accompanied by a stiff rise in prices. The insurance industry's estimate of a $12.60 daily rate fell woefully short; the average daily costs in 1967 were $18.16; by 1970, they were $24.35 a day.[19] People found themselves paying much more than that for "extras" tacked on to the basic board and room bill such as aspirin at 50 cents a tablet, or special mattresses at $45 a month. Congressman David H. Pryor, who spent some of his weekends after arriving in Washington as a volunteer at a nursing home, reported that once he was clipping the toenails of an 80-year-old veteran and the man begged him not to let the attendant see him do it; when it was done by the home, the charge was $7. He was afraid they would not like him to have it done by a volunteer.[20] Understandably revolted and outraged by what he saw, the young representative from Arkansas demanded remedial action. Congress, he pointed out, had appropriated money to assist state and regional planning agencies to "rationalize" the numbers, types, distribution, and quality of new health facilities so that modern medical care could be delivered in an effective and economical way. But Congress, he charged, had simultaneously "frustrated those aims by enticing investment capital into the industry on a huge scale, with a virtual guarantee of business and profits."[21]

The nursing home business, which had such humble beginnings, became a booming industry. Between 1970 and 1971, the income of the industry was more than $3,400,000,000, and that was expected to increase to $4,600,000,000 by 1975.[22] Federal, state, and local governments in 1970 paid $2,027,000,000; private expenditures were $1,338,000,000.

Word quickly got around Wall Street that in the nursing home business there was no way to lose. Nursing homes began to go "public." By 1970, 70 nursing home chains were selling stock, and mutual fund companies were snatching up shares by the millions. The number of beds began to increase wildly: 750,000 in

1969, as compared with about half that number eight years earlier; and another 90,000 were being added annually. Reports of nursing home chain revenues were dazzling. Beverly Enterprises, which had opened 27 homes in six years, reported a revenue increase from $3,200,000 in 1967 to $17,451,000 in 1968. "Outsiders" began to move in. International Chemical and Nuclear bought a 31-home Ohio chain with revenues of $3,000,000 for an estimated $45,000,000, which was 209 times the company's fiscal 1968 earnings. CNA Financial Corporation, ITT's Sheraton unit, and Cenco Instruments also got into health care. And bemused investors were buying stock at prices of 50 and even 100 times earnings, three to six times more than a blue chip commands in the market.[23]

There was almost no way to lose, particularly when investment companies sold a major interest in each home to groups of local physicians who could, and sometimes did, see to it that all the beds were filled.

Not all the hopes were realized. In 1973, the Justice Department charged Jack L. Clark, an Oklahoma City builder, and two other officers of the Four Seasons Nursing Centers of America, Inc., with having criminally defrauded investors of $200,000,000, one of the largest stock frauds in recent history. Also indicted were two partners of Chicago's Arthur Andersen & Company, one of the eight largest accounting firms in the country, and Glenn R. Miller, third ranking official of Walston & Co., a large Wall Street broker and underwriter.[24] The debacle also involved prominent Republican officials in Ohio, some of whom had been given hefty compaign contributions for helping to arrange a $4,000,000 state loan less than four months before the nursing home company filed bankruptcy proceedings.[25]

Despite that scandal, investment in nursing homes continues to be a very good thing, thanks to government laxity at all levels. It is a particularly good thing for the corner-cutters. The situation was stated bluntly by the president of a Baltimore-based chain in an interview with a *Time* reporter a couple of years ago. Richard Rynd, a former scrapmetal dealer, expressed little respect for a competing home that employed registered nurses rather than aides, who were receiving $1.30 an hour. "No wonder it loses money," he said. Like most other operators, his homes had no full-time staff physicians or dieticians, and each home had only one registered nurse on duty at a time. However, as was pointed out, his homes exceed Medicare's staffing standards, which require only one registered nurse in a home and permit licensed practical nurses to take charge when the nurse is off duty.[26]

In addition to cutting corners, a good many owners often pad their revenues by such measures as cheating on billings and such special rackets as forcing pharmacists and X-ray technicians to kick back sizable sums. A good many of them have even worked out arrangements with undertakers.

The extent to which unscrupulous doctors, dentists, and other health-care providers are joining forces with nursing home owners to loot the public treasury is indicated in two separate reports of the Medicaid nursing home program in California in 1968. Investigations were made by the state Attorney General and by the U.S. Comptroller General's General Accounting Office. They found unnecessary services were common. In four counties studied intensively by the GAO, between 20 and 35 percent of all patients receiving nursing home care were not in need of it.[27] They could have been treated in an intermediate-care facility or they could have been at home. Since MD certification is needed, obviously doctors were involved in the abuse. Moreover, since Medicare patients bring nursing homes greater revenues than Medicaid patients, nursing homes were having Medicaid patients "qualified" for Medicare benefits by shipping them to a hospital for three days and then returning them to the home. Doctors must also authorize that.

Not only was a high percentage of the care unnecessary, but in many cases care was not given at all. Medi-Cal consultants were approving requests from nursing homes for payment even though the patients had been discharged from the establishment or had died. And the number was not small. The GAO study showed that nearly 10 percent of the recipients included in their study had not received the services claimed. The number of days for which nursing homes were paid after patients had died or been discharged ranged up to 21.[28] When questioned about it, nursing-home owners said that clerical errors were responsible for the overpayments; insurance agencies insisted that the claims had been paid because they had no way of knowing that a patient had died or been discharged.

The owners of nursing homes were also making illegal fees because of the lack of supervision over the two programs. Between one-fourth and one-eighth of a group of patients studied in the four counties had proven twice as valuable to the owners as ordinary patients; they were being paid for by Medicare *and* by California's Medicaid. One nursing home received a duplicate payment of approximately $50,000 by its double-billing practices.

Even more shocking abuses were noted during the California Attorney General's investigation. Although kickbacks are prohibited by Medicaid regulations, state investigators found it "a common practice" for pharmacists, therapists, X-ray technicians, and laboratory clinics to give kickbacks ranging as high as 35 percent of the fee.[29]

Doctors with an interest in nursing homes or who are on retainer as "house physicians" have a captive audience to exploit to their bankers' delight. In many cases, they *oblige* nursing homes by signing blank prescriptions to be filled in by the home. In one instance, a "drug" prescription blank was used by a nursing home to order a wheelchair for an ambulatory patient. In another instance, investigators found 75 blank prescriptions signed by a doctor. Expensive drugs are often ordered with the blanks, particularly when the nursing home has an "arrangement" for profit-sharing with a pharmacy, and the drugs can also be sold to private patients. Nursing homes reciprocate by relieving the doctor of "unnecessary" chores. The Attorney General noted that although physicians are required to complete forms describing the conditions of persons who seek admission to a nursing home, they sometimes simply sign the forms and allow the nursing home to conduct the necessary physical examination and fill out the forms.[30]

Pharmacists and nursing homes have worked together to loot the public program. In return for substantial kickbacks, pharmacists have been filling prescriptions with expensive brand-name drugs instead of generic equivalents, charging higher rates for drugs than are charged to ordinary customers, misusing "pre-printed" prescriptions, and, in some cases, submitting totally false claims.[31] Even worse, between 20 and 50 percent of medications are said to be given erroneously.

Dentists have also joined the crowd of profiteers. In one county, more than 50 percent of the requests to perform treatment for patients in one nursing home were rejected on the ground that the treatment would not benefit the patient.[32] Even though the request to perform elaborate procedures on dying patients might be turned down, the dentist, like the doctor and other profession-als, is entitled to and does charge for mass examinations, "gang visits," as they are frequently described. Optometrists, therapists, X-ray technicians also can use nursing homes to exploit patients, with the understanding that their fees will be shared with the owners. Not long ago when I was visiting an elderly person in a "Grade-A" nursing home, the niece of her roommate expressed surprise and indignation about a bill for physical therapy for a month. The woman had been charged $150 for six treatments she was supposed to have been given, although at the time she had not been in the nursing home at all.

Public money is further used to enrich nursing home proprie-tors by their misappropriation of patients' incidental expense al-lowances of $15 a month. In one case reported by the California Attorney General, a nursing home was in possession of $2000 which belonged to persons who either died or were discharged from the home.[33] And aside from all those opportunities to profit, many nursing homes have been requiring beneficiaries of Medic-aid or their relatives to make under-the-table payments as a con-dition of admission and stay.

California has been by no means alone in this. When the mem-bers of the U. S. Senate Committee on Finance made a survey a couple of years ago on the finances of nursing homes, they found similar abuses and frauds all over the country. In New York, for instance, a nursing home charged the government $3240 for "physical-therapy" treatments for 58 Medicare patients in a single day. The treatment received by 20 of the 58 patients involved being lined up in wheelchairs while they moved their arms and legs. That nursing home during the year received a total of $372,000 from the government for physical-therapy treatments for Medicare patients.[34]

The Senators learned that the Associated Physicians of Cook County Hospital, which is a nonprofit group of teaching and supervisory doctors in Chicago, took in $1,600,000 in 1968. Some of those Medicare fees went to pay for an annual banquet and for doctors' parking. Of the 747 cases for which the group was paid, the doctors gave no treatment in 129; in others, interns or resident physicians performed the services.

A study made by the Senate Finance Committee on physicians who owned nursing homes in Texas revealed "unusual" patterns of service for Medicare patients. The committee was particularly concerned about the frequency of visits to the institutionalized patients and the amounts billed for them and for injections and laboratory services. One doctor, who received a total of $117,824 from Medicare, had submitted bills for $83,020 for nursing home visits to 104 patients and $10,461 for laboratory tests for them.[35]

In the summer of 1974, auditors in New York checking some nursing home accounts ran into unwarranted claims against Medicaid for more than $4,623,000. The government had been billed for a yacht, personal servants, family cars, vacation trips, jewelry, tuition for owners' children at college and even in nursery school! The state audits covered the billings of only about one out of every ten nursing homes in the state for the 1969-1970 period; and after disclosure was made, a Manhattan assemblyman estimated that more than $24,000,000 in Medicaid funds could be recovered if additional homes were checked.[36]

Not many more controls exist over quality than price. In an appeal to colleagues to do something to improve matters in the country's 23,000 nursing homes, Congressman Pryor recently spelled out some of the particulars:[37]

• The National Fire Prevention Association ranks nursing homes at the top of unsafe places to live.

• Actual health care is almost nonexistent. In Minnesota, the average physician care per patient in 100 nursing homes amounted to two and a half minutes a week. In Topeka, Kansas, three-fourths of the nursing home patients checked had not seen a doctor in six months.

• Drugs are commonly used to make patients "easier to handle." More Medicare money is spent on tranquilizers than any other type of drug.

• Help is in short supply, mostly untrained, often harried, and sometimes brutal. He quoted from a friend's letter describing the cruelties he witnessed while trying to find an extended care facility for his father: "All in all, it made me think that when the time comes, there's really no substitute for a nice clean head-on collision." (In another investigation it was revealed that one Chicago nursing home had been recruiting employees from a skidrow flophouse.)

• Food and sanitary conditions are often abominable: "rooms filthy, roaches in glasses, dirt in water pitchers, and indescribable conditions in bathrooms."

Some of the individual testimony Congressman Pryor heard almost defies belief. One patient, confined to a wheelchair, had been forced to sit in her excrement for hours on end; a "spunky" woman was mercilessly beaten into submission every night at bedtime and her bruises were attributed to falling; patients died prematurely of neglect. One of Congressman Pryor's informants, Joe Hamm, told him about a blacklist for "insiders" who protest. As a result of his having written to the governor of Michigan describing conditions he saw on his nursing home job, Mr. Hamm said, he can't get a job with a nursing home in Detroit.[38] Not surprisingly, Congressman Pryor called for a full-scale investigation of the nursing home industry.

Not surprisingly, colleagues applauded his efforts—and did nothing.

Subsequent efforts to investigate nursing homes in other areas have done little to correct matters. In 1973, California Assemblyman Leo T. McCarthy, chairman of the Joint Legislative Committee on Aging, introduced a series of eight bills designed, among other things, to keep as many elderly people as possible in their own homes and to break up the "partnership" that he said existed between the nursing-home industry and the state. Assemblyman McCarthy had the support of just about everyone: senior citizens groups, other legislators, radio, newspapers, television, interested people who came forward to bear witness about the "intolerable conditions" he protested.

Naturally, the trade association rushed forward to defend itself, insisting that whatever partnership might exist was only in the interests of seeing that "every regulation and standard should be enforced." Moreover, said the president-elect: "In addition to stringent state and federal controls already strictly enforced, our association maintains its own standards, ethics and peer review committee in which inspection reports of members and those applying for membership are reviewed, and, when indicated, membership is withdrawn or application denied."[39]

That defense might have been more convincing if one had forgotten that less than two years earlier the treasurer of the American Nursing Home Association, immediate past president of the state association, along with his wife and accountant, had been indicted on charges of having bilked the Medi-Cal program out of $97,613 over a three-year period.[40] And the appeal about the state's concern might also have been more convincing if, toward the end of 1973, it had not been revealed that the first disciplinary investigation ever had been undertaken by the state's nine-man Board of Examiners of Nursing Home Administrators. As a result of that investigation, the owner of six facilities was placed on two year's probation for charges of gross negligence. Although those facilities had been disqualified for Medicare patients years earlier, patients on the state welfare program were being sent to them.[41]

The struggle to obtain long-overdue reform was intensified in 1974 by public and private champions of the aged victims by bumbling cruelty and avarice. Following up on the 1970 report by Ralph Nader's Group, a Cleveland community-planning consultant—Mary Mendelson—revealed in a book called *Tender Loving Greed* the hell in which many of the nation's senior citizens were living out their last days. And Senator Moss's special subcommittee issued another devastating document—*Nursing Home Care in the U.S.: Failure of Public Policy*. The 5000-page document expanded on earlier subcommittee reports and severely scored industry as well as the government for appalling conditions . . . abuse and physical danger as well as unsanitary conditions and miserable food. Good homes, he charged, are in the minority, thanks not only to profiteering owners and unfit staff members, but to the DHEW's attitude of "neglect, indifference, and ineptitude."[42]

The industry rationalized deplorable conditions and pleaded—successfully—for more time, at least until 1976; hopefully, never.

In 1975, however, a number of public scandals erupted that made apparent that the time for reform was at hand. The Moss committee held public hearings in New York, where the investigation centered around a group of nursing homes owned by Bernard Bergman, a 63-year-old Hungarian-born rabbi without congregation. Witnesses included a New York hospital physician who said that patients from the nursing home were frequently brought into the hospital emergency room dehydrated from lack of water and dangerously infected from bedsores. New York health department inspectors testified about filthy conditions, and the secretary of state and an assemblyman alleged that the nursing home owner had not only mistreated patients but had defrauded the stage of Medicaid funds by submitting false and inflated bills.[43]

In Los Angeles, County Supervisor Baxter Ward offered a full-scale public hearing into nursing home abuses after reports that no investigation had been made when six nursing home patients were held by the coroner to have died "at the hands of another other than by accident"—the coroner's euphemism for suspected murder. Patients were moved from six nursing homes and felony complaints were issued against 12 persons after witnesses sickeningly described the treatment accorded patients. Routine punishment at one involved chaining incontinent persons to their beds for days at a time, "teaching them" by allowing them to lie in their urine and excrement; a woman patient who attempted to escape from the facility had her foot broken—as punishment—by a male attendant, who stomped on it. A young mentally retarded male patient was strapped to his bed for months; during the evening hours he was sometimes freed by staff members who amused themselves by having her perform "tricks" like those performed by a dog.[44]

Senator Moss took advantage of the momentum created by the New York and California scandals to introduce reform legislation. A bill introduced into the Senate by him and a similar House measure proposed by Edward I. Koch of New York was designed to correct nuring home problems by strengthening enforcement of federal standards and realistic penalties; it also sought to upgrade training of unskilled workers—now providing between 80 and 90 percent of patient care. Importantly, the legislative proposal expanded federal funding of alternative types of care that could keep many older persons out of nursing homes.

Pioneer projects, public and private, have shown what can be done. In communities across the country many senior citizens are living at home because of the "Meals on Wheels" programs. Volunteers carry to them low-cost nourishing and appetizing meals prepared by commercial restaurants or church groups. The delivery also checks daily to see that recipients are well; it provides them with meaningful contact with other people. Another effective means of keeping seniors out of nursing homes is the "Homemaker" programs in California and some other states; domestic aides are made available to elderly persons to help them for a few hours a week with household chores and marketing. Another promising program is the neighborhood "day care centers," along the lines of those provided children of working mothers. Many of the participants live with relatives who cannot provide constant care and companionship; some, however, live alone. Almost all of them would otherwise be in nursing homes since they suffer health problems that include heart disease, multiple sclerosis, stroke, blindness, and even mild senility. Psychologically, the centers have been a boon; physically, too.

There is no question but that the government will have to get tough—with lives at stake and with federal funds now paying more than half of the annual $7,500,000,000 nursing home care bill. If proprietary homes can't comply with standards, public ones must be built to take care of the need. Citizens committees will have to insist that government agencies regulate—as some are now doing—by publishing ratings of nursing homes so that the selection of a facility will not be mere luck.

Doctors must acknowledge their obligation, as Senator Moss and his subcommittee have pointed out: "Until physicians accept greater responsibility for the care of nursing home patients, the endless stories of negligence, poor care and abuse will continue."[45] But in this, as in many other areas of social concern, they will need outside help. Following the Senate subcommittee report in 1975 that doctors were ignoring their responsibilities in regard to nursing homes and, therefore, partly to blame that at least half of the nation's facilities were substandard with one or more life-threatening conditions, AMA reaction was swift. Dr. Frederick C. Swartz, chairman of the AMA Committee on Aging and a member of the Nursing Home Accreditation Council, said: "I think, by and large, that the medical care the average nursing-home patient receives is adequate for his needs."[46]

Insuring decent care for the aged is, as the Senate subcommittee pointed out, everyone's problem. The question is whether older people in the country are given the opportunity to live out their lives with dignity or are allowed to be victimized by the Bumbles in and out of white coats.

10 Prescriptions and Profits

"It is fortunate that physicians find themselves allied with nature. Otherwise, it might be unbearable to see so many examples of how little effect the drugs prescribed have on the course of an illness."[1] Less fortunate than that alliance pointed out some years ago by a couple of pediatricians is the alliance between organized medicine and the drug industry. As Senator Gaylord Nelson said recently: "There is no end to the ingenuity of the drug industry in exploiting the American people."[2] That exploitation could not occur without the willing complicity of American doctors.

One of the stock comic situations in all literatures involves the wily underling who, piously styling himself "your humble servant," gulls his master and benefactor into surrendering his power and prerogatives. If they are ample enough, the comedy may evolve into a tragedy of magnitude. Such is the case with the drug industry. The medical profession's willingness to allow the industry to assume its role as chief prescriber for the nation's sick has looted American purses; it has also placed in jeopardy American lives.[3] Worthless, dangerous, even deadly drugs are being sold to unwary consumers frequently for astronomical prices.

Investigations by legislators concerned with antitrust matters for more than a decade have left no doubt about the awesome nature of the profits being realized by the ethical drug industry, which turns out those pharmaceuticals obtainable only on prescription. A relative newcomer to Wall Street, the ethical drug industry was lifted into orbit during and after World War II by one dazzling breakthrough in medical science after another. In 1939, not a single drug manufacturer in America boasted a sales volume as large as a department store like Macy's in New York or Hudson's in Detroit.[4] By 1959, three of the six largest corporations in the country were drug companies; 13 of the 50 largest.[5] And the most rewarding. A Federal Trade Commission study released in 1970 showed the drug manufacturing industry to be the most profitable in the country, outranking such runners-up as computers, automobiles and trucks, radio and television equipment. The 12 largest drug companies reported an average profit of 18.8 percent.[6] By the beginning of 1973, profits had soared. One company, Upjohn, reported an increase in profits of more than 53.3 percent; American Cyanamid and Eli Lilly were well over 20 percent.[7]

According to the *Fortune Directory*, the drug industry has ranked first or second among all industries in the country in the return on equity and sales since 1961. Individual success stories have the belief of even the most dedicated gamblers on the stock market. For instance, the Schering corporation earned net profits of $32,000,000 five years after the firm had been bought for only $29,100,000. Smith, Kline & French earned net profits of $132,-200,000 in 11 years, which were *12 times the entire worth of the company in 1949*.[8]

During the rise to riches, the industry's reputation altered in an equally dramatic fashion. Drug making and peddling has always been regarded suspiciously by medical scientists, particularly in America, where the "golden age" of quackery was so gross and so extended that the medicine show became a national symbol for fakery. The contempt felt by the medical profession for the industry was summed up by Sinclair Lewis in *Arrowsmith* in 1925: a bacteriologist who joined a drug house was considered to have "gone wrong"; professionally, he was "dead."[9] Many medical schools prohibited faculty members from working with drug firms; the American Society for Pharmacology and Experimental Therapeutics ruled in 1927 that "entrance into the permanent

employ of a drug firm shall constitute forfeiture of membership."[10]
Yet in less than 25 years an extraordinary "cure" had been effected. So friendly had the relations of organized medicine become
with the drug industry that doctors were applauded and handsomely rewarded for working with it, even though they were
guilty of practicing "corporate medicine." Graduates of Yale,
Harvard, Johns Hopkins, and other top-ranking medical schools
were vying for jobs. Dr. Austin Smith, the editor of the *Journal
of the American Medical Association*, said in 1957 that the drug
houses had some of the "best" medical men. Several years later,
he joined the group and subsequently became president of the
Pharmaceutical Manufacturers Association.

To appreciate the radical nature of that change in attitude by
the medical profession, which has become the principal defender
of its traditional enemy, it is instructive to consider briefly the
ancient and frequently dishonorable history of pharmacy. Its real
beginnings—the powdered root, the crushed leaf used by some
ancient priest to drive the devils out—are among the mysteries of
prehistory. In recorded time, it began some 4000 years ago, when
a Babylonian healer-priest carefully pressed into a clay tablet the
cuneiform instructions for making a dozen medicinal preparations
that included such esoteric ingredients as the amamashdubkaskal
plant and the kushippu bird. Egyptian, Greek, Roman, Near and
Far Eastern doctors and divines added some remarkable recipes
to the international pharmacopaeia during succeeding centuries,
compounding magic and myth with science and skill.[11] Occasionally, astonishing successes were reported: the physician to Harun
al-Rashid of *Arabian Nights* fame so impressed the ruler with his
medications that he was rewarded with a fortune estimated at
$7,000,000. Others who were less successful in those days of eye-
for-eye medical practice paid for their fanciful concoctions with
life and limbs.

Since the days of Hippocrates, doctors who belonged to the
rational school of medicine had protested the activities of drug
dealers and dispensers. During the Middle Ages, doctors trained
at the universities that were being opened in England and on the
Continent became so enraged about the purveyors of "wondrous

cures" that they had laws enacted to prohibit apothecaries from dabbling in medicine. In Nuremberg, citizens who consulted quacksalvers were banned along with the quacks themselves. But it was impossible to stop the traffic, and many of the shrewder physicians joined the apothecaries to add to their incomes.

An occasional genius attempted to set things straight. Paracelsus in the fifteenth century denounced doctors as liars, murderers, and cheats; their cure-all remedies, he said, were the worthless concoctions of fools. Thomas Sydenham in the seventeenth century urged colleagues to exercise restraint in writing prescriptions; this is not to be wondered at since the pharmacopoeia reads like a collection of sewage, featuring such items as live worms, urine, moss from the skull of an executed criminal, sexual organs, and animal excrement.[12] So few improvements were made in pharmacy over the next two centuries that, in 1860, Dr. Oliver Wendell Holmes warned Harvard students that if the whole of *materia medica* was jettisoned and sunk to the bottom of the sea, "it would have been all the better for mankind and all the worse for fishes." Some of the botanicals and biologicals used had value, but generally prescription was a risky matter. One of the more honest manufacturers indicated that in offering a guarantee: "$500 in case of death if you use this medicine."[13]

Within two decades some important steps were taken to provide a basis for scientific medications. In 1880, Louis Pasteur's successful vaccines established the germ concept of infectious disease and launched the age of microbe hunters. At the turn of the century, Paul Ehrlich opened the way to chemotherapy by discovering that certain dyes had an affinity for certain tissues and thus could be used as "messengers" to deliver packages of germ-killing chemicals into afflicted tissues. Paracelsus had found arsenic a remedy for syphilis, but that was also a deadly poison. Ehrlich set about finding a way to deliver the poison only to the murderous cells; on his 606th try he met with success; salvarsan became known as the "magic bullet."[14]

The next major breakthrough in chemotherapy came a quarter of a century later. Following up on the work of Ehrlich, Dr. Gerhard Domagk, a bacteriologist with the I. G. Farben combine, also developed a dye that delivered germ-killing chemicals to afflicted cells, leaving healthy ones untouched, a red dye that contained sulfonamide: *prontosil.* Having experimented with thousands of mice, he performed his first experiment with a human being in 1934. His daughter, desperately ill with blood poisoning, had been given up by doctors. Fearfully, he administered a dose of *prontosil* and waited. She recovered completely.[15] Another experiment was made in 1936 with 38 mothers afflicted with childbirth fever in Queen Charlotte's Hospital in England. They, too, responded. It was first tried on this side of the Atlantic with some seriously ill persons at Johns Hopkins Hospital. When Franklin D. Roosevelt, Jr., who was in grave condition in a Boston hospital, also improved at once after being given the drug, sulfanilamide (as it became known) made headline news all over the world.

World War II gave tremendous impetus to the development of the chemotherapeuticals and to the new antibiotics, those extraordinary extracts of organisms that "peel" the skin from germ cells and destroy infections caused by other organisms. Sir Alexander Fleming had discovered penicillin in 1928, when he returned from vacation to his laboratory at St. Mary's Hospital in London. During his absence, one of the dishes in which a variety of germs had been left to breed had been "spoiled" by a mold. About to throw it away, he noticed that the mold was separated by a ring from the wildly proliferating germs in the dish. He cultivated the mold and isolated penicillin. That remained a laboratory curiosity because of its instability until 1938, when a group of Oxford University researchers attempted to obtain enough to experiment with its effect on a human. Frustrated by war priorities, they nonetheless managed to round up enough bedpans and clinical crocks to produce a few hundred gallons of broth; from that they extracted a few grams of powder. The first therapeutic injection was given to a London policeman, near death from an infection. He rallied dramatically. But the supply of penicillin was exhausted before the infection was routed, and the bobby died. Sir Howard Walter Florey, one of the Oxford scientists, came to the United States in 1941 to seek help in getting penicillin into production. The government sponsored a crash program, and within three years anti-biotics were in wide use.[16]

Unconcerned by the scientific processes involved and deeply moved by the dramatic triumphs over death and disease, people spoke in awed terms about the *wonders*, the *miracles* that had occurred. And marvelous they were: the chemotherapeutics like the sulfa compounds, the antibiotics like penicillin. Hormones also were evolved which enabled medicine to control the func-tions of body and mind and emotions. Antihistamines were isolated that provided protection when the body's normal defense mech-anisms failed. Psychoactive drugs were discovered that gentled or stimulated on demand. Scientific reports became paeans of praise as the laboratories produced means of sanity, health, and life. They were justified by statistical estimates indicating that in 1965 3,500,000 persons living in the United States owed their lives to new drugs.

That is the moving side of the drug story. But there is also a squalid aspect: the profiteering in drug making.

Great scientists have frequently made their gifts with rare gen-erosity. When Marie and Pierre Curie were asked to patent their techniques in order to profit by them, they were shocked: "It is impossible. . . . If radium is to be used for the treatment of di-sease, it is impossible for us to take advantage of that."[17] A noble procession has marched under their banner, but for the indus-trialists, the discoveries were another matter entirely—a matter of "your money or your life." Paul Ehrlich's "bullet" possessed more than one kind of magic. He turned over his patent rights to the Leopold Cassella company of Frankfurt. The firm, which eventually became part of I. G. Farben, struck it rich.

The intolerable consequences of the German monopoly on many necessary drugs became apparent during World War I, when they were either eliminated entirely from the American market or be-came prohibitively expensive. The price of salvarsan, for exam-ple, rose to $100 a dose.[18] Scientists here set about duplicating the drugs. In Philadelphia, a chemist reproduced the 606 compound in six months; a University of Illinois chemist developed a process for making procaine and barbital (German novocaine and veronal). Prices plummeted.

But while scientists were breaking down German monopolies, chemical and pharmaceutical company officials were striving to create new ones on this side of the Atlantic. Like many other segments of the economy which pay lip-service to the American free enterprise system, the drug industry has not allowed its appreciation of a good idea to stand in the business way of a "good thing." The drug industry has, by taking advantage of every legal loophole and by perpetrating criminal actions, successfully established all the essential elements of monopolistic control. It has concentrated power in a few hands, enabling the giants to dominate the marketplace and bring possible competitors into line. It has controlled prices through secret "fixing" agreements and by lobbying through laws that make it illegal for consumers to know how much they are being overcharged. It has corrupted and captured government agencies financed by the public to protect them against exploitation and hazard. It has stimulated a tremendous demand, all out of proportion to need. And it has cloaked all those activities with a thick whitewash of advertising and publicity, persuading victims that the doses administered are for their own good.

None of those successes could have been fully realized without the aid of the medical profession. Consumers may exercise free choice about many products. They may shop around for a cheaper equivalent or find a substitute or do without. So far as ethical drugs are concerned, however, they are captives. They must buy what the doctor orders. They may not shop around for a cheaper equivalent; they cannot substitute another *type* of drug.

The industry defends the exorbitant annual bill of more than $11,000,000,000 for prescription drugs by insisting that high prices are necessary because of the great risks involved and because research is so costly. Neither of those arguments holds up, as even insiders themselves acknowledge. George Squibb, grandson of the founder of E. R. Squibb & Sons, told a Senate investigating committee in 1967 that, "The risk is very little in the pharmaceutical field."[19]

Other experts have agreed with him. Dr. Willard Mueller, chief economist for the Federal Trade Commission, reported to Senator Nelson's subcommittee that, "Losses, or even low profits, are practically unheard of among large drug companies. In this respect the drug industry is practically unique among important American industries."[20] Rand Corporation economists supported that, asserting that the risk premiums for drugs are "very low" and that the explanation for profits "must be sought in factors other than risk."[21]

Similarly, arguments about the huge amounts of time and money the pharmaceutical industry claims it needs for research must also be discounted, as much as $10,000,000 and ten years to bring a new drug to market, it says.[22] But that is an illogical argument since profits are calculated only after all costs have been deducted, including those of research. Moreover, the difference between the drug industry estimates of research costs and the estimates of more objective sources, such as *Standard & Poor's Industry Surveys*, are very great. The research expenditures of some of the large firms in the industry in 1970 and 1971, in terms of the percentage of sales, are shown in the table.[23]

Much of the research carried on by the industry has nothing to do with finding new cures and treatments. Instead, as Congress-

COMPANY	1970	1971
Abbott	5.9	6
Baxter	5.3	5
Bristol-Myers	3.8	4
Johnson & Johnson	4.0	4
Lilly	10.3	9
Merck	9.2	8
Morton-Norwich	2.6	3
Pfizer	3.5	4
Richardson-Merrell	4.4	4
Schering-Plough	5.3	6
Smith Kline & French	9.0	10
Syntex	12.0	11
Upjohn	10.6	10

man Benjamin J. Rosenthal pointed out recently, it is aimed at "adapting existing drugs for competitive purposes."[24]

Moreover, American taxpayers are actually paying for most of the research costs. By 1965, the government was spending more than $1,000,000,000 of the $1,700,000,000 total.[25] Far from realizing any benefits from this in terms of lower prices, consumers have been charged high prices for drugs by the profiteering drug companies. For example, all of the money needed for the development of the Salk vaccine was provided by the people of the country. But as one drug manufacturer reminded the Kefauver subcommittee: "The profits from the $53,000,000 sales, at wholesale level, were shared by only five large concerns."[26]

An even grosser example was called to public attention by Senator Russell Long, who took up Senator Kefauver's battle against granting private patent monopolies on the results of research paid for by taxes. In a speech on the Senate floor, he said: "When the desire to make monopoly profits at the public's expense can adversely affect the health of our children, it is time to call a halt to this immoral practice." He cited as illustration a kit that had been developed to prevent mental retardation in babies. American taxpayers spent about $750,000 to finance research for methods to detect an imbalance of phenylketonuria (PKU) in new-born infants. If PKU is diagnosed in a baby during the first month, the afflicted child can be spared permanent brain damage by a special diet. Working on a government grant, Dr. Robert Guthrie of the University of Buffalo developed a simple test and made a kit for testing. "Guthrie tests" were considered so important that they were made mandatory in Louisiana, Massachusetts, New York, Rhode Island, and a number of other states. Hospitals were producing the kits needed for the tests for $6. What aroused Senator Long's ire was that Dr. Guthrie filed for a patent before he submitted the required report to the U. S. Public Health Service. Shortly after, he entered into an exclusive licensing agreement with Miles Laboratories. The company, which then had the exclusive rights to manufacture the kits, proceeded to charge what Senator Long called the "exorbitant" price of $262 for the same kit that hospitals had been turning out for $6. "If this is not blood money at the expense of the taxpayer," Senator Long said to his colleagues, "I should like to know what is."[27]

Patent monopolies are, of course, a principal reason for unreasonable drug prices. The United States is one of the few major nations which gives patent protection to drugs. Fifty-four other countries deny them on the grounds that they are not in the public interest.[28]

Not only are drug patents awarded more freely in this country than any other in the Western world, the lucky owners are given 17 years in which to exploit consumers, to charge whatever the traffic will bear without fear of price competition. There is little question about the impact of patents on costs. Penicillin is a case in point. After World War II, when there was genuine competition to produce unpatented penicillin, the price plummeted. The drug which was sold at $20 for 100,000 units for injection in 1943 was selling in 1956 in equivalent tablet form for only 20 cents. After that "unhappy experience," many manufacturers decided to concentrate on patented specialties. Seymour Harris has pointed out in *The Economics of American Medicine* that as a result of the monopoly positions they gained and agreements among a few producers and sellers, "prices declined relatively little."[29]

Relatively few of the epoch-making drug discoveries of the past few decades have been made by American drug companies. As one University of California Medical School expert pointed out: "far from leading in drug progress, it appears that our [U.S.] industry has usually followed and often after a clear lag.[30]

It is not easy for a manufacturer to prove the novelty and uniqueness of a compound because many scientists are often working on the same plateau and possess the same information and the same techniques. Simultaneity of invention is common. To avoid that dilemma and to avoid embarrassing suits, companies with some claim to having created a new chemical entity or significant modification will license other companies to produce and market products on which a patent has been obtained under other names.

One of the more interesting case histories showing the means by which patents and cross-licensing are used against the public was provided during and after the Kefauver hearings. Tetracycline was a leading broad-spectrum antibiotic refined from Aureomycin by a Harvard professor, Dr. L. H. Conover, in 1952. A patent for the drug was awarded three years later to Charles Pfizer & Co. The patent, conservatively estimated to be worth at least a billion to the company during its 17-year life, was contested by the Lederle Laboratories Division of American Cyanamid and by Bristol-Myers. Later Squibb and Upjohn protested that they, too, had a right to manufacture the drug. They seem to have been aware, as the U. S. Patent Office was not, that the product's claim to being a new invention could be disputed.[31] Hoping to avoid what later became a public scandal, Pfizer agreed to license American Cyanamid and Bristol to produce and sell the antibiotic under their own names. Squibb and Upjohn were then licensed to sell under their names tetracycline purchased in bulk from Bristol. The five companies thus had formed a monopoly on the product, which was marketed as Tetracyn, Acromycin, Polycycline, Steclin, and Panmycin, and other brand names. All were sold to the public at "substantially identical prices."[32] The druggist paid 30 cents a capsule; the prescription holder paid about 50 cents. At the time the companies were charging the government 17 cents a capsule and the public 50 cents, manufacturing costs of one company were estimated to be less than 2 cents a capsule.[33]

A Federal Trade Commission study later revealed that the five companies had acted in concert in pricing tetracycline; that of 15,700 transactions the Commission studied that were made in eight major cities during a seven-year period, all but ten sales were closed at identical prices. When Squibb won a coveted contract with a Los Angeles hospital, a company official expressed alarm about a possible violation of the price agreement: "I was disturbed to learn that we were the successful bidder to Los Angeles County," he told an associate. An Upjohn salesman who took the competitive spirit seriously received an admonition from a superior: "It has been brought to our attention that you are inferring or directly stating to the physician that the Upjohn Company is going to reduce, lower, or bring the price down on Panmycin. This, I am sure, is the fartherest [sic] point in our minds."[34]

Government buyers got a reduction in price after they turned to foreign countries for supplies in 1961. Thus Pfizer reduced its price from 17 to 6 cents a capsule after an Italian company won an earlier order with a low bid of 8 cents. The public had to wait. But the abuse had become so widespread, and so much attention had been focused on it as the result of a suit brought by states, cities, and other groups that in 1969 the five companies agreed to make a $100,000,000 settlement for overcharges. Ads in papers across the country instructed people how to collect refunds for purchases of the drugs between 1954 and 1966. Dissatisfied with that settlement, the Justice Department filed an additional suit against Pfizer and American Cyanamid to cancel the patent for tetracycline and to obtain a $25,000,000 restitution for overcharges.[35] Five other large drug firms were also named in the suit, charged with conspiracy. In the summer of 1974, 9,500,-000 households in California, Utah, Washington, Oregon, and Hawaii received forms for making claims for refunds; no documentation was required for those up to $150. The mailing constituted one of the biggest experiments in legal history—the first large-scale attempt ever made to distribute to consumers money awarded to them in an antitrust settlement.

Further indication of the fact that drug companies overcharge was provided in a study made in 1972 by two HEW researchers, which indicated that companies in the United States were selling drugs to other countries for far lower prices than they were charging domestic consumers.[36] In the United Kingdom, for example, where the government does exercise some control over health care and exhibits equal concern about patient exploitation, prices of drugs made in the United States are often only a fraction of what is charged here. Lilly charges $7.02 in the United States for 100 tablets of an analgesic marketed under the name of Darvon but only $1.92 for the same product in the United Kingdom, sold under the name Doloxene. Abbott charges $26.12 in the United States for Trythrocin, $10.02 in the United Kingdom; Pfizer charges $20.48 here for Terramycin; $9.06 in the United Kingdom. The price for 100 tablets of Valium, produced by Roche, is $8.03 here, $2.88 there. Searle's Ovulen 21 oral contraceptives cost

$7.38 for a hundred tablets here; $4.10 in the United Kingdom.

In 1973, a U. S. District Judge in New York City acquitted five persons charged by the U. S. government in a mail-fraud case. Claiming to be foreign buyers, they had bought drugs for sale in this country at favorable prices. In dismissing the case, the judge charged that culpability lay with the major manufacturers who sell drugs for higher prices here than abroad. It is they, he pointed out, who are engaged in "a violation of the antitrust laws."[37]

The ultimate retail price of prescription drugs here has been a guesswork affair since druggists and the drug industry have lobbied through laws and regulations in 37 states forbidding price advertising. Just why it should be detrimental to public health and patient safety, as trade spokesmen claim, has certainly not been made clear to any disinterested observer looking into the matter of price advertising.

A number of retail drug outlets have courageously risked prosecution to make the point that price secrecy exploits consumers. Recently, the Dart chain challenged Maryland and Virginia price advertising laws by running full-page ads for the 40 "most wanted" prescriptions, as did the Osco drug chain. According to a report in Con$umer New$week, prices were estimated to be one-third lower than the national average.[38]

Efforts have been made and are being intensified on the state and national level to do away with laws against price advertising. California and some other states have since introduced laws making it mandatory to display prices and also to identify drugs by their generic names. Assemblyman Harvey Johnson, author of one bill, said that if consumers in California alone exercised comparison shopping, they could save at least $100,000,000. He cited a study in Los Angeles showing that buyers were paying anything from $13.95 to $33.60 for the same amount of Polycillin.[39] New York Congressman Rosenthal also conducted an investigation in 1972 before introducing a similar bill to make price-posting mandatory nationally. His investigators found that price secrecy had resulted in markups as high as 6000 percent, which is particularly cruel to persons sixty-five and older since they spend more than three times the amount younger people spend on drugs. He compared prescription prices in Washington, D.C., and New York City, where advertising is prohibited, with prices in Philadelphia and Miami, where it is not. For example, *100* capsules of a broad-range antibiotic cost $2.87 in Philadelphia and $1.93 in Miami; the price for only *30* capsules of the same drug was $4.31 in Washington and $3.44 in New York.[40]

Spurred on by the Consumer Federation of America, a number of activist groups in the 25 states that have prohibited price advertising have taken their claims to court to overturn laws and regulations. In 1974, the Virginia Citizen's Consumer Council won a substantial victory in Richmond Federal Court when a three-judge panel reversed a prohibitive state statute. The group's legal counsel, Raymond Bonner, an attorney with Ralph Nader's Public Citizen organization, called it "a tremendous victory for the consumer."[41] Since then, consumers in California and other states have been filing suits against pharmacy boards to challenge state codes.

Some consumers have been sensible enough to seek out mail-order drug firms offering quality products at prices far below those prevailing in their own communities. Concerned about the growth of these firms, the trade associations have been seeking to put them out of business.

Not the least reason for the high cost of drugs is the use of brand or trade names rather than generic (official) names. Thus tetracycline was produced by one manufacturer, and sold under its generic name to institutional buyers for a very low price; however, it was marketed at retail under a company brand name for a high price. So it is in other cases. In the summer of 1973, Senator Nelson pointed out that prices for the same product may range up to 30 times higher, according to the name under which it is sold. The confusion generated is almost total. For instance, he said, the City of New York bought 1000 50 mg capsules of Benadryl from Parke-Davis for $15.63; on another occasion it bought precisely the same quantity of the same drug from Parke-Davis, under its generic name of diphenhydramine for only $3.[42] Why should organized medicine go along with the absurdity that brand name drugs are better than their generic equivalents? The

179

answer is simple. It is because the drug industry makes it profitable for the AMA to do so. The battle of brand names, the only kind of competition that really exists in the industry, is waged in the pages of the medical journals every month. And that means millions of dollars of advertising for the AMA and the owners of other journals. (As a nonprofit corporation, of course, the AMA does not have to pay taxes on the income.)

The AMA was once opposed to the use of trade names. Indeed, its *Official Rules*, promulgated in 1955, specifically required that in the interests of diminishing "confusion" and to encourage the use of generic names, those names not be subordinated unduly to brand names in labels, labeling, and advertising. And Dr. Austin Smith, former editor of the *JAMA* and a vigorous opponent of what he had called the "absurd practice" of prescribing trade names instead of cheaper generic equivalents, found himself during the Kefauver hearings in the bizarre position of challenging his former statements. By that time, however, as Senator Kefauver reminded him, he was working for the manufacturers. The senator wondered audibly if Dr. Smith's new position as president of the Pharmaceutical Manufacturers Association had something to do with his change of mind.[43]

Forsaking its former position, the AMA was no less enthusiastic about trade names than Dr. Smith and has continued to push for them, advancing arguments it earlier considered specious—such as insisting that if the physician prescribes without mentioning the brand name he will have "no way of knowing that his patient will receive the drug in the form of highest quality and expected potency."[44]

Knowledgeable persons in and out of the AMA have been blunt about the reasons. Dr. A. Dale Console, former medical director of E. R. Squibb and Sons, said some years later that in his opinion: "Those who publish a journal and derive income from drug advertising are probably even more captive than the average practitioner."[45]

Commenting in an exchange with Senator Gaylord Nelson about the AMA's late enthusiasm for brand as opposed to generic names, Dr. Console said:

> The American Medical Association's contention that it is not a party in a tacit conspiracy with the drug industry is not convincing. Its denial fails to explain the astonishing, unscientific, pro-drug industry positions it has taken. It has given shelter to the drug industry under the cloak of immunity given to physicians, and the drug industry has been more than willing to accept the shelter since it gives the industry an ethical image while it uses the same profit-oriented tactics of any big business. It pays well for the shelter by buying advertising pages. . . .[46]

As late as 1973, some of the AMA's top advisers on drugs—the last two chairmen and the vice-chairman of its own Council on Drugs—were accusing the organization of being "a captive of and beholden to the pharmaceutical industry." Speaking for the group, Dr. John Adriani, former chairman of the Council on Drugs of the AMA, Clinical Professor at Louisiana State University of Medicine, and department director at Charity Hospital in New Orleans, said: "Until legislation is adopted that *one drug have one name*, namely, its generic name, and trademark names for drugs are abolished, this chaos will continue."[47]

A number of legislative reforms advocated by Congressman Rosenthal in that year could do much to prevent exploitation of the sick by the drug industry. He urged that all prohibitions on advertising prices be ended; that it be mandatory for druggists to post prices of the hundred most commonly prescribed drugs; that all perishable prescription drugs be dated; that the generic name be used in labeling and advertising: that licensing of new prescription drugs be compulsory. If a company manufacturing a new drug was found to charge more than five times the cost of production, the Federal Trade Commission would be given power to grant other companies an unrestricted license to make the drug.[48]

The likelihood of speedy implementation of the measures is not great, for the drug industry exerts a lot of influence on the nation's representatives, the regulatory agencies, and the medical establishment. Indeed, so much that aside from allowing its members to fleece the American people with impunity, it makes it possible for them to endanger American lives in the process.

11 Doctors, Dollars, and Dangerous Drugs

The notion is widespread that here in America, where things are *different*, drugs are safe. Surely, the drug industry can be relied on, that extension of all the Arrowsmiths who have toiled selflessly in their laboratories to defeat disease and hold back death. Surely, the government agencies are carrying out their mission of public protection. Surely, the AMA and its individual members, whose primary concern is the welfare of patients, would not allow us to be exposed to dangers and deceits. Had not the AMA been founded largely to protect Americans from being preyed upon by the makers of dangerous nostrums and useless quacksalver brews? Had not Sir William Osler spoken for the profession in 1902 when he branded the large pharmaceutical houses medicine's "insidious foe," which threatened to become "a huge parasite, eating the vitals of the body medical"?[1]

The situation had not changed, however, as was made clear during the Senate hearings more than a decade ago. In response to a nationwide demand for "something" to protect the American people from the profit-hungry drug and medical industries, Senator Estes Kefauver submitted the bill S. 1522 to Congress. It seemed to most sophisticated persons just what the doctors should have ordered long ago. Not only would costs be reduced, but patients would finally have some real defense against dangerous drugs. New standards would be set to ensure the quality, purity, effectiveness, and safety of all drugs; the Department of Health, Education, and Welfare would have power to enforce them. It seemed impossible to believe that any responsible person or organization could oppose such vital safeguards. HEW testified on its behalf; so did the Department of Justice, the Patent Office, the National Consumers League, the AFL-CIO, health-insurance groups, organizations of retired persons, many private physicians of distinguished reputation. Dr. A. Dale Console, former medical director of the Squibb drug corporation, appealed for enactment of the bill. Even the board chairman of the PMA, president of Eli Lilly, expressed approval of a large portion of it. Was it possible that the AMA . . . ? It was, indeed. In the face of incontrovertible evidence, over the opposition of its own Council on Drugs, with total disregard for public interest, the American Medical Association announced its implacable opposition to everything in the bill.[2]

In the decade that followed, the consequences of AMA opposition have been spelled out in considerable magnitude.

Iatrogenic diseases, which are induced in a patient by a physician's treatment and particularly by drug therapy, have become both endemic and epidemic. By 1965, at least 1,500,000 hospital admissions a year were held due to adverse drug reactions; and those reactions were of such severity that the hospital stay of those patients was about 40 percent greater than the average stay of all patients.[3] No improvement occurred during the next decade. In mid-1974, Dr. Milton Silverman, research pharmacologist at the University of California, and Dr. Philip R. Lee, former U.S. assistant secretary for health and scientific affairs, estimated that "unnecessary and irrational" use of prescription drugs is killing at least 100,000 Americans a year and making millions sick.[4] The researchers pointed out that the number of fatalities is actually much higher—between 130,000 and 140,000; however, they said, about 20 percent of those can be considered unpredictable, "acts of God," involving terminal illnesses or emergencies in which doctors use drug combinations they would not use if it were not a life and death matter.[5]

Their estimate is—despite AMA and pharmaceutical industry protests—conservative since they included only those hospitalized.

"We know nothing of those who are sick at home, or even die at home," Dr. Silverman pointed out; "Drug reaction is not a reportable disease." (Other researchers have pointed out that adverse drug reactions are frequently misdiagnosed as asthma, flu, infections, anemia, gastrointestinal, and kidney disorders.)

Once in the hospital, for any reason, the chances of succumbing to drug therapy are also pretty high. This is not surprising because patients often receive between 10 and 20 different medications daily during their hospital stay. Also, the number of medications that are given in error is thought to be pretty high. In a study of 900 patients at the Johns Hopkins Hospital several years ago, Dr. L. E. Cluff and his associates found the incidence of adverse drug reactions to be 10.8 percent, excluding "mild gastrointestinal side effects."[6] (Johns Hopkins, it should be pointed out, is one of the country's outstanding hospitals.) Other studies are even grimmer. A Canadian research team detected adverse reactions to drugs in 15 percent of the patients they studied; when combined with "errors in the administration of drugs," the figure rose to 30 percent. Thus, three of every ten persons admitted to hospitals studied (the better hospitals) become victims of drug-induced diseases.[7] Those diseases prolong the hospitalization of some patients by an average stay of nine days. They also increase the costs to the patient. A study was made of the direct and indirect costs incurred by 41 patients admitted to a Midwestern university teaching hospital. Because of adverse drug reactions, researchers estimated them to be at least $116,835.[8] How to measure the emotional, physical, and psychological costs to the victims? How to calculate the suffering involved for the victims' families?

Rational persons do not quarrel with the idea that in order to achieve major gains it may be necessary to accept some losses. And no rational person would deny the major gains that have resulted from drugs developed during recent decades that have surely played an important role in the dramatic decline in death rates from some diseases since "wonder drug therapy" was introduced in the 1940s. However, as specialists have been pointing out, antibiotics produce allergic responses: some mild, some fatal. Some are inherently toxic, damaging ears, kidney, liver, and blood.

184

Some cure one infection and provoke the development of another, which may be more dangerous. According to Dr. Louis Weinstein, chief of the infectious disease service of New England Medical Center Hospitals, they "must always" be used with circumspection and discrimination. They should be administered "only" in situations where they are known to be useful. "To do otherwise is to expose patients to the risk of reactions that may be more deadly than the infections from which they suffer."[9]

In 1972 Dr. Harry E. Simmons, director of the Bureau of Drugs in the FDA, estimated before a Senate subcommittee that "superinfections" may be killing tens of thousands of persons yearly in this country. He indicated that each year as many as 300,000 cases of superinfections may be caused by antibiotic therapy that kills one set of microorganisms and allows another group to flourish.[10] Between 30 and 50 percent of the cases of superinfections are fatal. Evidence also was submitted to Senator Gaylord Nelson's subcommittee which showed the overuse and misuse of antibiotics. Researchers studying a 500-bed community hospital found that antibiotic therapy was justified in only 12.9 percent of the cases; it was "questionable" in 21.5 percent; and "irrational" in 65.6 percent.[11] Is this circumspection and discrimination?

Of the 400,000,000 prescriptions for antibiotics written annually, many are for colds and minor viral infections, for which they are of not the slightest use. The same kind of casualness applies to other commonly prescribed medications, no less dangerous.

For years, doctors and scientific researchers on both sides of the Atlantic have been issuing warning notes about the indiscriminate vaccination practices in this country. England and other countries abandoned compulsory vaccination some years ago. Not only was there a general news blackout in this country about the matter, but government agencies were used to prevent information from reaching the public. For example, after writing a book called *Polio Control* in 1946, Dr. Eleanor McBean of Los Angeles received a memorable reminder of the power of the medical establishment. Performing what she considered a public service in alerting people to the dangers of vaccines and making every effort

185

to keep the book factual and legal, she had it checked twice before printing: with a lawyer and with officials at the Los Angeles Post Office. The Better Business Bureau, she reported, instructed newspapers not to sell advertising space. When the book continued to sell, the Post Office issued a fraud order against the book and her publishing company and refused mail delivery to her, entirely, as she pointed out recently, "without due process of law or proof of guilt."[12]

To be opposed to indiscriminate vaccinations was equated with being against the public good. Between 14,000,000 and 17,000,000 smallpox vaccinations have been administered annually in the country, although there has not been one case of smallpox since 1949. Adverse reactions have ranged from minor ailments to fatal encephalitis. In 1968 alone, nine deaths were linked to smallpox vaccination.[13]

In 1971, private warnings gave way to public concern after a research microbiologist in the Division of Biologics Standards reported that tests performed on vaccines against measles, mumps, and others that are commonly used "caused apprehensions of such grave nature that they might well serve as a basis for condemnation."[14] The U.S. Public Health Service followed up with a recommendation that states take action to halt or to curb vaccination programs.[15]

Risks all out of proportion to possible benefits have been accepted by unsuspecting patients so that the drug industry and the medical establishment could pursue profits. Senator Kefauver cited MER/29 as "a classic" instance.[16] By the end of 1963, only three years after its introduction, the Richardson-Merrell corporation had been indicted by a grand jury for having falsified reports about the toxic effects of MER/29 to the government, and the company was a defendant in more than 400 damage suits brought by injured persons. One of the plaintiffs won a $675,000 judgment.[17] The drug had appeared on the market in the summer of 1960, glowingly advertised in the *JAMA* as "the first cholesterol-lowering agent to inhibit the formation of excess cholesterol within the body. . . . [The] absence of toxicity [has been] established by two years of clinical investigation."[18] Soon after, warnings of danger came: another company discovered that cataracts developed in rats and dogs treated with the drug; the Mayo Clinic reported in January 1961, that skin disorders and loss of hair were associated with use of the drug and in October gave extensive information on side effects, including the development of cataracts. Yet the ads continued to appear in the *JAMA*. In the November 4, 1961, issue, it was claimed: "After three years' clinical experience . . . after use in more than 300,000 patients, few toxic or serious side effects have been reported."[19] The drug was formally removed from the market a few months later. Two years after that, the company and three scientists pleaded *nolo contendere* to criminal charges of suppressing and altering test results.[20]

Cortisone offers another striking example of the dangers of using a drug indiscriminately. Adrenal cortical hormones, cortisone, or corticosteroids can be valuable drugs to help patients suffering from Addison's or Cushing's diseases, in which there is an over- or under-production of hormones. However, as Col. Robert H. Moser of the U. S. Army Medical Corps pointed out recently, cortisone was introduced on the market with "fanfare." Newspapers carried "wild tales" of hospital patients who had been long crippled with arthritis dancing in the corridors. In short order, doctors were enthusiastically writing prescriptions for the stuff for almost anyone with an ache or pain.[21] But the dangers the patients faced covered an almost incredible range. The symptoms of Cushing's disease are most obvious: moon face, fat on abdomen and hips, purple streaks due to stretching of the skin, growth of a soft tissue lump on the upper spine, acne, and wasting of the muscles of the extremities. Less obvious symptoms often became apparent. Adverse reactions ran the whole gamut of psychiatric disorders, ranging from the wildest elation to suicidal depression. Blood pressure increased. The normal production of protein tissue was interrupted. The healing of surgical wounds was impaired. Patients suffered from cataracts. They developed large ulcers of the stomach. Still later, more subtle dangers came to light. Patients taking the substances for arthritis, asthma, or nephrotic syndrome might develop an acute appendicitis or pneumonia which could easily go undetected for some time since the drugs masked normal signs of infection. At the same time, it was found that the corticosteroids could facilitate the spread and propagation of tuberculosis, blood stream bacterial infections, virus and fungus infections. Some patients who had received a high dosage of corticosteroids for a long time might suffer irreversible shock while undergoing surgery.

It is not surprising that Dr. Moser warned his colleagues that:

> We must create an atmosphere of rational caution and critical evaluation, where each physician will pause before putting pen to prescription pad and ask himself, "Do I know enough about this drug to prescribe it? Does the possible benefit I hope to derive from this drug outweigh its potential hazard?"[22]

There is, sadly, no indication that physicians are likely to ask those uncomfortable questions as long as they continue to be propagandized by the drug industry.

With the exception of Thalidomide, there exists no more revealing example of the madness of the policy of administering drugs recklessly than the use of chloramphenicol.

During the 1940s, Parke Davis scientists discovered the substance in some Venezuelan soil samples of molds. It was found to be effective in treating Rocky Mountain spotted fever, scrub typhus, and several other diseases relatively rare in this country, but difficult to treat. Within a short time, researchers managed to synthesize it commercially at a low cost of less than 10 cents a capsule. The company named the antibiotic Chloromycetin, obtained a patent, and began production in the United States and Britain. Parke Davis was understandably confident it had struck gold. During 1949, its first year on the market, sales exceeded $9,000,000. A year later, they passed the $28,000,000 total; in 1951, they reached $52,000,000.

Shortly after Chloromycetin was licensed, however, "unexpected" clinical reports began to associate it with aplastic anemia, a blood disease with a fatality rate of about 50 percent. The Food and Drug Administration and the AMA's Council on Drugs both investigated the drug and took action in June 1952. An editorial in the *JAMA* warned doctors about possible reactions, and the FDA refused to approve further shipments of the drug until a National Research Council committee submitted its findings. Two months later, it revealed that 177 of the 410 cases of serious blood disorders studied were "definitely known" to have been associated with Chloromycetin.[23] Parke Davis was ordered to change the drug's label to warn that the drug should not be used "indiscriminately or for minor infections." However, the opinion was that: "It should continue to be available for careful use by the medical profession in those serious and sometimes fatal diseases in which its use is necessary."[24] Those cases, as has been noted, are rare in this country.

Sales plummeted. Parke Davis, which had soared to first place because of Chloromycetin, dropped to fifth place in sales in 1954. The sure cure for that, officials decided, was to pressure the company's 980 salesmen to persuade doctors that Chloromycetin was the safe answer for everything from acne to mild urinary infections. Memos and instructions from the president and sales director advised them to tell doctors that all was well, that the FDA had officially cleared the drug. Physicians looked at the ads, listened to the salesmen, and, despite continuing reports in medical journals, were persuaded. Among them was Dr. Albe M. Watkins, a general practitioner from southern California. In 1952, confident of its safety, he and a urologist had given the drug to his ten-year-old son James, who had suffered a urinary infection. Dr. Watkins first realized his son was in danger when the child kneeled on the living room floor to retrieve a toy that had fallen under a sofa. After he had stood up again, his knees were black and blue. The drug had presumably caused the depression of the production of platelets in the bone marrow. If the platelets are sufficiently decreased in number, bleeding may result. "From then on," Dr. Watkins said later, "there was no stopping the bleeding." After James's death, the Watkins family, the doctor, his wife (a graduate nurse), and two other sons, got in their car and headed east. His goal was to alert other doctors and government officials about the drug. Stopping at small towns and large, he called on other physicians to ask about their experiences with the drug. By the time he reached the Food and Drug Administration offices in Washington, he had recorded 294 other cases of adverse side effects and fatal reactions to the drug.[25]

His efforts to have the drug restricted were supported by others, also profoundly concerned about the dangers, and sales began to plummet, down $15,000,000 by 1963.[26] In that year, a California State Senate Fact-finding Committee launched an investigation. (It had intended at first to look into the entire antibiotics matter, but pressures from the drug lobby forced the committee to retrench.) The hearings were called ". . . *Particularly Chloromycetin,*" and the committee finally proposed that the use of the drug be limited to hospitals so that constant blood checks could be made on the patients.

Among the procession of victims testifying in favor of the proposal was another southern California physician, another bereaved parent. Dr. Franklin Farman, a diplomate of the American Board of Urology, told the committee that his five-year-old daughter had also died in 1952 following the administration of Chloromycetin. "In my opinion," he said, "there is hardly one case or one sick person in this state today that of his own free will would choose to take Chloromycetin knowing the full risk he runs in its causing either temporary or permanent bone marrow depression."[27] Another witness was Edgar F. Elfstrom, a California newspaper publisher. His nineteen-year-old daughter had died several years before after having taken the drug for a sore throat and mild urinary infection. Still another man told the committee that his mother had also died of aplastic anemia after taking Chloromycetin, which her physician had prescribed for a cold.

Parke Davis, has been forced to defend itself against a number of victims. The first settlement was made in 1961 on behalf of a woman whose doctor had prescribed Chloromycetin first for a sore gum and then for a bronchial infection. She died of the treatment. In making the judgment against the manufacturer, the court noted that Parke Davis had been "aware" that the warning label on the drug at the time it was prescribed was "ambiguous, inadequate and incomplete."[28] Twelve years later, the California State Supreme Court upheld a $400,000 award made by a lower court, agreeing with a jury finding that the drug firm "negligently failed to provide an adequate warning as to the dangers of Chloromycetin by so 'watering down' its warnings and so overpromoting the drug that members of the medical profession were caused to prescribe it when it was not justified."[29] Parke Davis has been successful using these measures and Chloromycetin has continued to sell well.

During the Nelson subcommittee hearings in 1968, Dr. Henry Dowling singled out the drug as "perhaps the most flagrant example of bad therapeutic judgment" on the part of some doctors.[30] It was pointed out that between 90 and 99 percent of prescriptions handed to patients should never have been written. The Food and Drug Commissioner had earlier confessed himself at his "wit's end" about the matter. "What it comes down to in bald terms is: What can be done to protect you from your doctors?"[31] Nothing, nothing at all. In 1970, an estimated 790,000 people in the United States were receiving the drug, sales topped $82,000,000, and new markets had been opened. The United States government was sending South Vietnam enough Chloromycetin to treat between 150,000 and 200,000 patients, *with no restrictions imposed on its use.* The government's position was summed up for reporters by Navy Captain J. William Cox, a physician who advises the Defense Medical Materials Board. Asserting that the South Vietnam rate of consumption of the drug "is not indicated by our standard or practice," he brushed off the drug shipments pragmatically: "But neither are leeches and lots of other things they use."[32]

Parke Davis has been making enormous profits on foreign sales of Chloromycetin in a way scarcely calculated to win friends for this country when facts are known. The drug has been marketed in Italy wtih the inducement that it is "remarkably without secondary reaction." In Japan, Chloromycetin has been touted as "a remarkably ideal antibiotic which increases the resistive power of bodies under stress and accelerates the recuperative process."[33] In Mexico, where it is sold over the counter, a doctor recommended it several years ago to me and my husband as a cure for our child's sore throat. He was positive of that, even without examining her throat or making any kind of tests. When I told him what I had learned about the drug from the legislative investigation in California, he looked at me pityingly and shrugged: "Well, aspirin is dangerous, too."

If the AMA had acted, who knows how many lives might have been spared, how much suffering averted. And the AMA could have acted, as its own Council on Drugs had urged. It could have insisted that the ads point out the dangers of the drug prominently as it did point out that the *only* disease for which it has continued to be a drug of choice is typhoid fever.

That kind of service for both doctors and patients had been provided in 1905, when the AMA had set up its Council on Pharmacy and Chemistry to provide members with reliable information about the safety and value of drugs in order to defend doctors from "the bastard literature which floods the mail" and to "protect the public and the medical profession against fraud, undesirable secrecy, and objectionable advertising."

Of paramount importance was the *New and Unofficial Remedies*, which the AMA began to publish in 1907. Every medication the Council considered might have merit was listed and described. In 1913 that was supplemented with a handbook, *Useful Drugs,* and in 1929, the Council adopted an insigne. Manufacturers whose drugs were approved received the AMA "Seal of Acceptance," which they were permitted to use on their packages and in their advertisements. No drug could be advertised which had not been evaluated by the Council and found acceptable.[34] The doctors relied on *Useful Drugs* and on the seal. A survey made by the AMA in 1953 showed that 71 percent of the physicians interviewed felt the seal had great value; more than half said they considered it more important than a company's reputation.[35]

The drug industry was less than enthusiastic about the control measures the AMA was imposing. It found a way to counter them in the 1950s, when the AMA was seeking new sources of revenue to fight compulsory insurance programs. The business staff invited Ben Gaffin and Associates, Inc., to discover how the sale of advertising space in the *JAMA* and other AMA publications could be increased. That was quickly and conveniently determined: The drug industry would step up its advertising in return for a number of "policy changes."

Changes included jettisoning the Seal of Acceptance and abandoning the publication of *Useful Drugs.* Instead, the drug industry would publish and distribute to doctors its own guide and index to prescriptions, the *Physician's Desk Reference.* Most doctors seemed unaware of the fact that it was an advertising tract. In it, all the material about every drug listed was prepared, edited, approved, and paid for by the manufacturer. As an indication of its objectivity and completeness, in the 1962 edition Parke Davis deleted from the Chloromycetin entry all references to hazards, and inserted a statement that doctors could get all necessary information from the package insert and from the salesmen.[36]

In return, the drug industry advertised. And what advertising drug advertising is. Ethical drug ads are as weighted with the cant of quacks and hucksters as pitches can be. Medical journals, which should confine advertisers to facts and scientific information, carry the same emotional appeals that characterize the ads for over-the-counter drugs in slick magazines and on radio and TV. The old familiar ills of insomnia, tension, obesity, constipation, coughs and wheezes, aches and pains are garishly portrayed and prescribed for. Smiling beauties and high-powered athletes suggest that depression, whether caused by stacks of dirty dishes or driving in freeway traffic, can be overcome and that "the active girl can stay active every day of the month."

Although the Kefauver-Harris drug law attempted to correct some of the advertising abuses by demanding that precautions and side effects be specified in detail, the advertising has found a way to overcome that important reform. For instance, in a recent full-page ad in full color for premarin, a hormone product, only one-fifteenth of the page is devoted to a cautionary note.[37] An ad for Haldol (haloperidol) that regularly appeared in the *JAMA* in 1972 is representative of the sales approach. The first page shows a framed picture of a smiling gray-haired woman. Above her head appears the quote: "We don't want to put Mother in a home, but . . ." The second page, in very large type, urges use of the drug "when disturbed behavior complicates caring for the elderly." On the third page, in small type, are warnings against the drug which is held useful in some cases of agitation and psychotic behavior. Mother might be better off in a home, judging from the fine print, although, of course, she might be dosed with it there. Adverse effects include: neuromuscular reactions, insomnia, restlessness, anxiety, euphoria, agitation, drowziness, vertigo, seizures of an epileptic type, impaired heart, liver, skin, and blood, loss of appetite, nausea, dry mouth, blurred vision, and urinary retention.[38]

Most distressing, perhaps, and certainly most popular are the ads for psychoactive drugs. The advertising in almost any medical journal being published offers clear explanation for America's having become "a nation of middle class junkies." Doctors have become drug pushers, writing nearly 100,000,000 prescriptions a year for uppers and downers and flattener-outers. Two of the most widely advertised tension relievers, Valium and Librium, were recently held so dangerous they were almost ordered off the market. For years, glowing ads had so deluded doctors and patients about their mildness and safety that they were widely prescribed for even the most minor display of tension.

Responsible professionals have protested such advertising abuses to no avail. Dr. Robert Seidenberg, a practicing psychiatrist and clinical professor of psychiatry at the State University of New York, said of the *JAMA's* ad policy: "Even *Good Housekeeping* and *Parents' Magazine* do better in protecting their reader-consumers. Is the AMA guilty of drug abuse?"[39]

Censorship charges were also made before the subcommittee by Dr. Edward Pinckney, a former editor of the *JAMA*. He listed a whole series of false and misleading claims that were made in the *JAMA* ads in a single 1969 edition, including Serc, which the FDA had started withdrawal proceedings against one year earlier. He said that an editorial protesting such advertising that he had written for the *JAMA* had been rejected by an AMA official on the grounds that drug advertising was the journal's "principal source of revenue."[40]

As dangerous as the education by media advertising can be, even more so is that provided doctors by mail and by the industry's

15,000 or so salesmen. In *The Doctors' Dilemma,* Dr. Louis Lasagna of Johns Hopkins, one of the most distinguished pharmacologists in the country, described the material sent out to doctors (whose names are on the lists that the AMA rents to the drug companies) as "a numbers racket, with its never-ending barrage of new products, confusing names, conflicting dosage schedules and indications, claims and counter claims." By 1969, the industry was spending at least $22,500,000 on direct-mail advertising to persuade doctors to write prescriptions for their brands.[41] The drug industry woos the men of medicine with inducements of all kinds: office equipment, "samples" (some of which are passed along to patients), golf needs, tickets, trips, food and drink. In order to influence doctors to prescribe their products, the drug industry has even invaded the medical schools. Among the gratuities provided students at most schools are textbooks and monographs, pocket notebooks and calendars, slide rules, black leather bags, with examining instruments, anatomical models. Additionally, it arranges trips to pharmaceutical plants and to scientific meetings, including board, room, and entertainment. Students are provided free drugs for themselves and their families; those with children are given baby food and other baby supplies.[42] The detail salesmen come to be their friends and benefactors.

The huge sales of Chloromycetin certainly prove the almost incredible influence the salesmen exert over the prescription pads. The popularity of Merck Sharpe & Dohme's Indocin also proves that the salesmen are effective. An antiinflammatory drug used for some arthritic problems, Indocin was so briskly promoted that within two years it had become one of the 200 most-frequently prescribed agents in the country. Despite hazards associated with its use, including asthma, aplastic anemia, hepatitis, jaundice (including some fatal cases), ulcerations, and sometimes fatal hemorrhaging, the drug was being improperly prescribed for such conditions as minor sprains and bursitis. Distressingly, it was also given to children, with fatal results in some cases, despite specific cautions against it.[43] In response to an FDA order to correct the misrepresentations and misleading claims, Merck modified its ads and the package inserts to convey the warning that the drug "must be used cautiously, if at all, and with the expectation that serious side effects may occur." However, bulletins to salesmen instructed them to convince doctors that "therapy with Indocin is safer"— presumably, safer even than aspirin.

To make sure that the story was told, financial encouragement was provided. "Now every extra bottle of 1,000 Indocin that you sell is worth an extra $2.80 in incentive payments. Go get it. Pile it on!!!"[44]

Doctors did have some partial defense against that kind of "education." But the AMA had disarmed the Council on Drugs in order to oblige the drug makers and to stimulate their financial support.

Several years ago, some insurgents in the AMA, particularly doctors working with the Council on Drugs, determined to launch a resistance movement—to revive the Seal of Acceptance and to provide doctors with a handbook of drug evaluations based on scientific evidence rather than the puffery that characterizes the *Physician's Desk Reference.*

The story of the killing power of the drug industry, as told in 1973 by Dr. John Adriani, a former chairman of the AMA Council on Drugs, director of the Department of Anesthesia of Charity Hospital in New Orleans, and a university professor, makes instructive reading for all who object to American citizens being used as guinea pigs and as gulls to be exploited.[45] Dr. Adriani determined to administer some life-saving aid to the AMA before it deteriorated completely. The AMA's image in the 1960s was badly tarnished, and its membership was dropping seriously. Finally what he calls the "paid bureaucracy" at 535 North Dearborn Street in Chicago agreed, after the Kefauver hearings, to do something. Three million dollars were appropriated and a staff hired to prepare an official book on drug evaluations, a replacement for the drug industry's *Reference.* However, when Dr. Adriani became chairman of the Council on Drugs in 1968, he found that the staff had written only one chapter of the proposed volume; it had managed to spend $2,000,000 in the process. Dr. Adriani had himself appointed chairman of a special ad hoc committee of three *volunteers.* He then enlisted the aid of other reputable specialists, and within a year the committee had prepared 89 of the 90 chapters.

In January of 1971, just as the first edition of *AMA Drug Evaluations* was about to be sent to the bindery, the chairman of the AMA Board of Trustees, Dr. Max Parrott, told the Council: "We want to hold the book up for a couple of months." The reason? So that "our friends" the Pharmaceutical Manufacturers Association could see it. Over the Council's objection, page proofs were sent. They came back three months later, accompanied by "three or four crates full of changes [the PMA] wanted to make." The PMA generously volunteered to pay for all the "changes," which actually amounted to revising the whole book. The Council agreed to some minor changes, but stood fast on substantive points. It condemned a number of heavily advertised drug combinations as "irrational." And it offended the drug industry in other ways.

AMA Drug Evaluations received excellent reviews when it appeared in 1971; doctors called it a "wonderful" prescribing manual since it categorized by disease rather than by drug; it specified the drug of first, second, and third choice; it recommended quantities for use; and it gave other vital information. Even so, Dr. Adriani and his colleagues were not satisfied. He noticed that without his consent or knowledge, the paid staff had made changes in ten of the chapters that he had written. Other unauthorized changes had also been made. Even before the book was circulated, he and Dr. Harry C. Shirkey, his successor as Council chairman, and Dr. Daniel L. Azarnoff voted to move ahead with a second edition.

Others were upset with the manual for a different reason, not the least of which were officials of the PMA. They were in a position to make their displeasure felt and they did. As a result, drug advertising in the *JAMA* dropped sharply after Dr. Adriani and his colleagues took on the job of preparing the book. Between 1968 and 1972, the page count fell from 4227 to 2558. That made the Board of Trustees unhappy, too. The feeling was enhanced, Dr. Adriani believes, because the PMA president was such a "good friend of the Board of Trustees." C. Joseph Stetler, former AMA legal counsel, took on that job as successor to Dr. Austin

Smith, who had become PMA president after a number of years as editor of the *JAMA*

In September 1972, a delegation of the Board of Trustees appeared before the Council and said that the statement "The Council does not recommend this drug" could not be used in the new edition. Dr. Adriani and his colleagues objected strenuously. Why not? The trustees answered with a lame explanation that the statement did not "mean" anything by itself. The Council countered with an offer to specify reasons. Understandably feeling trapped, the delegation agreed to "buy that." However, after leaving they apparently realized that they had left with a far worse bargain than they had originally gone to the Council for. The error was remedied a month later when the Board of Trustees summarily abolished the Council and thus halted all work on the new book.

The AMA denied charges of a "sellout" made by Dr. Adriani, Dr. Shirkey, and other Council members. PMA President Stetler also denied that pressure had been applied on the editors to conform with the wishes of the drug manufacturers. But, to date no convincing reason has been given for the action; no convincing defense has been made to the charge that the AMA and the PMA were "in cahoots" against American patients.

What can be done to halt the irrational and dangerous practices? The answer to that question is not easy, but a number of proposals that would be helpful were made to the Nelson subcommittee. For one thing, far more rigid restrictions should be placed on drug advertising; and the Federal Trade Commission and the Food and Drug Administration should be forced to move vigorously against makers of false and misleading claims. Disinterested experts like Dr. Adriani and his colleagues on the former AMA Council on Drugs, with the aid of other groups like the American Public Health Association, should be asked to prepare a compendium of prescription drugs. That committee should be charged with notifying physicians of adverse reactions. Drug dispensing should be monitored more carefully; recently hospitals have been employing pharmacists to improve drug-use practices. Computers should be used more widely, to store in memory banks and produce on demand the drug histories of patients.

The formulary system, which has been used in hospitals in this country since 1816, should be put into practice generally. Under that, drugs are screened, approved, prescribed, and dispensed usually by generic names, and drug quality is maintained, drug costs and drug inventories are minimal, and patient welfare is the objective of the hospital. State, regional, and even national drug councils could monitor the prescribing habits of doctors through computer systems, and either caution doctors who prescribe improperly or have them prosecuted for going beyond reasonable bounds.

Ultimately, of course, medical schools will have to do more to educate doctors more completely. Recently, Dr. Donald C. Brodie, associate dean of the School of Pharmacy at the University of California in San Francisco, demanded that an answer be provided to why the physician should be "the dupe of the detail man [salesman]." If a doctor cannot "hold his own" in a five-minute conference with a salesman, he said, "it is certainly an indictment of his profession and of the educational system that produced him."[46]

12 Do-Gooders, Keep Out

The greatness of America—its affluence, its genius, its compassion—has not been symbolized more dramatically than by the *S.S. Hope*, the nation's first peacetime hospital ship, which sailed out of San Francisco harbor in 1960 bent on carrying *H*ealth *O*pportunity to *P*eople *E*verywhere. The ship was supplied through donations from business and industrial firms, public tax money and by millions of individual contributors. It was staffed by doctors and dentists, nurses, and other health workers, most of whom were volunteers. Bent neither on conquest nor commerce, it had as its purpose to carry the light of modern medical science to the darker shores of Asia, Latin America, the Pacific Islands, and Africa.

Dr. William B. Walsh, the imaginative Washington, D.C., internist who conceived the idea, has described some of the needs it has met in *A Ship Called Hope*, an account of its initial trip. At Sumbawa in the Indonesian archipelago, he and his colleagues found that there were only two local doctors to care for 250,000 islanders. Bali was "Paradise Lost" to the voyagers, who entered wards packed with adults "destroyed" by leprosy and yaws, with tiny typhoid patients "gasping with pneumonia, their small bellies swollen from protein deficiencies, legs spidery from lack of vitamins."[1] In a filthy and overcrowded Vietnam hospital, one surgeon had the toe of his rubber boot eaten by a rat before it could be broomed out of the operating room. During a seven-month period, the *Hope's* staff treated more than 17,000 persons, performed more than 700 major operations, held more than 800 teaching sessions, X-rayed 10,000, mostly children, distributed 80,000 pounds of powdered milk, 86,000 pounds of medical equipment, 2000 artificial limbs.

In spite of the workload, the heat, the failures, the filth, the corruption, and even military attack the voyage was so successful that it was decided to continue the missions of Project HOPE. Although the ship was recently scrapped, the 13-year voyage will be remembered around the world. It gave new life to about 200,000 people condemned to death by diseases and deficiencies that modern medicine can cure or alleviate; it gave to 9000 poorly trained doctors and the untrained the knowledge of how to support life. It gave a new concept of American values. When civilian and military resources were called on to save a *Hope* nurse, Dr. Walsh noted, "it proclaimed around the world how precious is a single life to all Americans."[2]

That is the irony of the *S.S. Hope*. While it was projecting an image of engagement and benevolence abroad, the American medical establishment was exhibiting at home an attitude of noninvolvement. It continued to make sure that every applicant for medical care, whatever his need, drop money in the slot before any service would be given. This was the case even though medical conditions in many parts of the United States are no better than they are abroad. As Dr. Caldwell B. Esselstyn, president of the Group Health Association of America, pointed out to a Congressional committee at the very time the *Hope* was being given headline attention around the world, "The level of health in our country is directly related to the socioeconomic status."[3] As a result of the double standard, the "unlucky" Americans, chiefly nonwhite persons in depressed rural areas, on Indian reservations, and in urban slums, have been cut off from health opportunity as cruelly as the Indonesians who inspired such compassionate concern.

The policy of noninvolvement has been a major threat to the quality of public health in the United States. Many physicians still refuse to render aid even in emergency situations. To encourage doctors to help accident victims, at least, "Good Samaritan" statutes have been enacted, the first by the California legislature in 1959. It provided that:

> No person licensed under this chapter, who in good faith renders emergency care at the scene of the emergency, shall be liable for any civil damages as a result of acts or omissions by such persons in rendering the emergency care.

Maine, Nebraska, Oklahoma, South Dakota, Texas, Utah, Wyoming, and other states quickly moved to enact similar measures over the serious objections of attorneys that the laws might be unconstitutional since they set aside the common-law cause of action that has existed for injured persons.

By the end of 1972, the statutes had proved their workability; and no court decisions have been reported in which an injured person had successfully sued a physician for rendering emergency aid.[4] Nevertheless, many doctors were continuing to withhold aid, explaining that they feared they would become victims of a malpractice suit. Actually, a survey made by the AMA ten years earlier had established that exactly 50 percent of the physicians had declared that they would *not* render aid whether or not a Good Samaritan law was in effect.[5]

An almost incredible illustration of the noninvolvement policy was given in 1965, when the AMA proposed a statute that would weaken recently enacted laws making the abuse of children by parents or guardians a crime. "The battered-child syndrome" is one of the most serious health problems in the country today. About 60,000 cases are reported each year, but experts agree that there actually are many times that number. Savage, sadistic, and deranged parents and guardians have long been getting away with every brutality up to and including murder because no one intervened in time. Some of the injuries defy belief: fractured skulls, arms, legs, and ribs; damaged organs from punches; burns, bruises. And characteristic of the syndrome is that brutal treatment was repeated, often over a period of years.[6]

More than humanitarian considerations are involved in protecting children; they become carriers of the disease of savagery and violence. According to Dr. Gisela Meloy, a member of the staff of the National Institutes of Mental Health, children who are beaten may grow up to become parents who beat children; or they may vent their rage on outsiders. A recent study of six murderers, she said, showed that only two had had fairly decent childhoods: "The others had been kicked around by their parents and beaten unmercifully. It becomes a vicious cycle."[7]

Although doctors have had the moral responsibility to protect children from such assault by reporting suspicious injuries and conditions, many of them ignored it. Some failed to act because they held that the "confidential" nature of the physician-patient relationship outweighed all other considerations. Some were reluctant to *offend* patients, for not only poor and disreputable parents victimize children; torture and torment are also practiced in middle- and upper-income homes. Not a few doctors failed to act because they did not wish to risk a libel or slander suit.

A meaningful effort to protect battered children was made in 1963, when the Children's Bureau and the American Humane Society drafted guidelines to assist states in writing laws that would make it mandatory for doctors to report suspected cases. Doctors, it was believed, were best equipped to detect the battered-child syndrome. Physicians would no longer have to worry about irate parents suing; the model law guaranteed them immunity against liability. Few legislative proposals in the country's history have been so widely adopted in so short a time. Within three years, only three states were without protective statutes.

Meanwhile, the AMA came forward with a counterproposal. Doctors would be allowed to use their discretion about reporting "for professional reasons." The AMA also urged that other professionals who see children regularly be required to make reports, too. That would have seriously impaired the effectiveness of the laws, as Monrad G. Paulsen, Dean of Law at the University of Virginia, pointed out. If responsibility to report were widely spread, he said: *"Everybody's duty easily becomes nobody's duty."* Moreover, the chief aim of the legislation was to reveal cases which only medical skill can detect.[8]

The AMA has desperately maneuvered to maintain control of

medical services in the United States, against the efforts of a large number of groups and individuals who seek to provide care outside the approved entrepreneurial pattern, from the American Cancer Society to the American Legion.

Voluntary health agencies have long been regarded with suspicion by the leaders of organized medicine. But they have been necessary, if only to combat government intervention. As early as 1908, President Theodore Roosevelt's Committee of One Hundred on National Health was warning that public-health efforts should not be surrendered "to the weak and spasmodic efforts of charity, or to the philanthropy of physicians." Rather, it was a state responsibility.[9]

The AMA was not enthusiastic about voluntary agencies. Many that had come into existence during the reform fervor at the turn of the century had "dangerous" notions. They openly insisted that health is a social concern, and they placed an uncomfortable emphasis on preventive medicine. Lay persons on the boards frequently outnumbered physicians and thereby could determine the scope and direction of health programs. Not finally, some of the voluntary agencies were hiring doctors to work on salary.

The uneasy mutual need–mutual distrust relationship that existed between organized medicine and the voluntary agencies collapsed publicly for the first time in 1904. At that time delegates at a meeting of the College of Physicians found themselves forced by public demand to vote to establish a society to curb tuberculosis. (European doctors had acted 22 years earlier, when Koch announced his discovery that tuberculosis was caused by a bacillus; they had pressured governments to construct sanitoriums and to establish effective educational programs.) Although the delegates capitulated and voted to establish the National Association for the Study and Prevention of Tuberculosis, they were not happy. They resented lay interference in health care; they also resented the exposure of their failure to curb the disease and the expenditure of public money on a "private" medical matter.

An experiment, launched by the National Association and subsidized by the Metropolitan Life Insurance Company, revealed how successful a public program to control tuberculosis could be, if it was fully implemented. Framingham, Massachusetts, was selected as the site for the experiment because of its low economic status and high mortality rate from tuberculosis. Infant health clinics were set up; milk was pasteurized; infected persons were given medical care and proper nutrition. Within six years, the infant mortality rate dropped 35 percent; the tuberculosis death rate, 68 percent.[10] The Framingham experiment proved dramatically that the disease could be virtually eliminated if adequate medical and nursing care were provided, if high standards of sanitation were required, if economic support was given to house and feed the sick. However, those measures sounded so dangerously socialistic to the businesslike leaders of organized medicine that the experiment was not repeated.

Like the National Tuberculosis Association, the American Cancer Society has also learned on various occasions how formidable a foe the AMA can be. Richard Carter reported in 1961 that a physician working for the organization had told him: "It took us years to get the 'Pap smear' program going because we were afraid to antagonize the medical profession." In order to start an educational program to alert the public to the dangers of cancer of the colon, "We had to court the physicians first."[11] After it was learned that early diagnosis phenomenally increased the survival rate of cancer victims, the American Cancer Society decided to set up a network of free detection centers across the country. The centers were established, but thanks to organized medicine the service is not provided free. As a result, many who could have benefited by the service have not been able to "afford" to have their lives saved. (The AMA and the American Cancer Society also fought over the cigarette smoking issue which will be considered later.)

The most violent and widely publicized struggle that took place next was between organized medicine and organized "do-gooders" over the polio vaccine.

The AMA had been ready with thunderbolts in 1937, when President Franklin D. Roosevelt, who had been permanently maimed by polio, announced that a foundation had been created "to lead, direct, and unify the fight on every phase of this sickness." It was bad enough that he had attacked the inadequacies of medical practice. What was worse was the idea of using the money to pay for the treatment of those who needed it. "Until we learn more about it, any program which contemplates the prevention of infantile paralysis is a bogus campaign," declared an AMA spokesman.[12]

The National Foundation set about making the country conscious of the disease in a storm of publicity. And the dimes and dollars it collected as a result of "marches" were turned over to outstanding virologists. The Foundation supported the work of such Nobel Prize winners as Dr. Linus C. Pauling, Dr. John F. Enders, Dr. Thomas Weller, and Dr. Frederick C. Robbins. As a result of their work, scientists discovered that there were actually three kinds of polio viruses. They turned the drudgery of testing the theory and developing a vaccine over to Dr. Jonas Salk, who had been working on flu viruses. After three years of laboratory testing with a killed-virus vaccine, the Salk vaccine was tested with good results on more than 600 people in Pennsylvania. The National Foundation president, Basil O'Connor, then announced that it was going to pay $9,000,000 to drug companies to produce enough vaccine for a massive field trial during the summer of 1954 with more than 1,800,000 youngsters in 44 states. The money would also produce enough vaccine so that 9,000,000 school children could be immunized without charge if the field trials warranted that.

On April 12, 1955, confidence seemed justified. Dr. Thomas Francis, Jr., of the University of Michigan, reported in a "Hollywood atmosphere" that the tests indicated that the vaccine was a success.[13] But the reaction was mixed. Conservatives in and out of the AMA noted that the announcement had been made on the anniversary of Mr. Roosevelt's death. They charged that the announcement merely was a plot to glorify the late president. The AMA branded the program another milestone on the road to "creeping socialism." Most people, however, were ecstatic since polio had been made to seem Public Enemy Number One by sensational reporting.

Four days after Dr. Francis made his announcement, the Foundation launched its program in San Diego, California, for first and second graders. New York City announced plans to vaccinate free everyone under 20; and other local and state health departments across the country placed orders with the licensed manufacturers to get enough vaccine to immunize minors not included in the Foundation program.[14] Congress appropriated $30,000,000 for vaccine for pregnant women and for 30 percent of the nation's children.

Unfortunately, confidence in the vaccine was somewhat shaken after a number of persons were stricken with paralytic polio following vaccination with a product made by Cutter Laboratories.[15] AMA affiliates began to act to halt the free vaccination programs. New York and other communities that had established clinics were forced to postpone their opening. The AMA House of Delegates voted at a meeting in Boston to demand "immediate termination" of the free vaccination program, arguing that it was "a violation of principles of free enterprise." The House of Delegates held that only indigents could receive it free.[16]

The Department of Health, Education, and Welfare agreed to oblige the AMA resolution demanding the government get out of the vaccination program and return the vaccine it had purchased to "normal, commercial channels." The National Foundation was in a rage. So were millions of Americans who had given time and talent, money and effort to the campaign. They felt that the prize that had been won was in danger of being seized by the medical entrepreneurs. With the fury of Florence Nightingale confronting the British War Office, the foundation announced that unless the AMA modified its stand, it could expect an answering salvo. The foundation had won public loyalty and public support. It had also won some powerful allies.

The AMA had second thoughts. It issued warnings about "public apathy" and told member societies that they should encourage their patients to have children vaccinated. Even the requirement that vaccine be administered only in physicians' offices for the customary fee was modified. Dr. Dwight Murray, then AMA president, said: "Since medicine is a public service profession, we should and must do everything possible to inoculate every eligible person regardless of ability to pay."[17] However, the AMA continued to tout the superiority of the live-virus vaccine that had been developed by Dr. Albert B. Sabin.

In a carefully documented account of the "Salk versus Sabin" controversy, *Consumer Reports* raised serious questions about the AMA's having created hope about an unavailable product and doubt about the efficacy of the Salk vaccine, thus diverting attention and possibly delaying the eradication of polio.[18] The AMA's recommendation that doctors use the Sabin product had not made clear that a reason for the production delay was that manufacturers had been having safety problems with at least one of the vaccine's three components.

Thanks to skillful publicity by the National Association and vigorous action by many doctors and others who were bold enough to reject AMA policies and pronouncements, the controversy was resolved; people were immunized. Since then, polio has become relatively rare.

Oddly enough, one of the AMA's bitterest opponents on polio vaccine and other public health issues has been the American Legion. In many respects the Legion and the AMA are remarkably alike: cohesive, aggressive. They both fight actively for their special interests. They are politically sophisticated, politically conservative, and politically effective. Yet the two have attacked each other constantly over health issues with the anachronistic fury of a couple of saber-tooth tigers at a Cenozic water hole.

After World War I, the AMA began to have serious second thoughts about whether or not it was true that nothing was too good for the brave boys. What, doctors began to worry, would happen to their paying patients if the government extended its medical-care program beyond the sick and wounded among the 1,390,000 who had served on the battlefields to the other 4,000,000 who had been recruited, but who had not seen battle and were not eligible for government medical care? It was a delicate issue. Few wanted to go on record as opposing veterans' benefits, least of all an organization that was setting itself up as a benefactor to man. However, in 1924, the AMA decided to act to stop the expansion of "state medicine." This was done after Congress had approved a bill authorizing veterans of all military expeditions and occupations since 1897 to be given treatment in veterans' hospitals for disabilities that were not incurred from war, providing that the beds were not being used by those with service-connected ills.

The AMA branded the act intolerable since it denied the patient the "freedom" to choose his own doctor, it heavily burdened the taxpayer, and it tended "to pauperize an independent, self-supporting part of the citizenship" by providing them with free care even though they could afford to pay for it. Veterans were less concerned. In 1932 an AMA spokesman told Congressmen that the percentage of veterans treated for ailments that were not related to their military service in government hospitals had risen from 17 percent in 1925 to 77 percent in 1931.[19]

The struggle between the American Legion and the AMA intensified during and after World War II. The AMA increased its opposition after it saw that the British had integrated civilian and military medical services when invasion was threatened. The country had adopted totally nationalized medicine. The AMA visualized the same thing happening in the United States, with the Veterans Administration "empire" serving as the base.

The American Legion, which yields nothing to the AMA in its opposition to federal interference and encroachment, was unconcerned about the problems of medicine becoming socialized when it came to medical care for ex-GIs. Ironically, as Dr. James Howard Means pointed out, some of the staunchest fighters against socialized medicine were serving in veterans' hospitals with "the greatest equanimity." Yet, "if we have anything that amounts to socialized medicine, the veterans' medical services are it."[20] All during the 1950s the Legion carried on its defense against what it called "the AMA's campaign to destroy every facet of Federal care for nonservice-connected disabled veterans in VA hospitals.[21] Case histories were cited to show the need. For example, "Case 126" was a fifty-six-year-old fruit picker being treated in a veterans hospital for a compressed back fracture. He had been sent there from a private hospital because he could not pay. "Case 23" was a fifty-seven-year-old man with a service-connected heart condition. He was being treated for chronic rheumatoid arthritis after having spent $5000 of his own money for private care. Investigators claimed that the "Veteran spent his entire life savings before going to the VA for aid. Has had 19 operations since 1941 . . . has no income now except Part III pension."[22]

How did the AMA propose to "force" those men out of the veterans' hospital? the *American Legion Magazine* demanded rhetorically.

> The plan is beautifully simple. (1) Dig up, once more, every charge anyone has ever made against the VA (2) Raise a war chest (estimated to be $2,000,000) to finance the publicity campaign, speakers, and printing costs (3) Under the guise of economy, try to make the American people want them to be kicked out.[23]

The national commander of the American Legion made a speech in 1954: "If they [the AMA] want sick and disabled veterans removed from the hospitals, there's nothing in the world to keep them from saying so. But when they load their arguments with misinformation and half-truths, then somebody has got to stand up for the facts."[24] Dr. Charles W. Mayo of the Rochester Mayos, a former chairman of the American Legion Medical Advisory Board, denied that VA health care was socialized medicine. It is, he insisted, in the best American tradition. Moreover, he said that AMA arguments that government medical care would depress the quality were false. Veterans were getting treatment of quality "second to none."[25]

Legislators have been hard pressed by both groups. If the veterans' medical program was the equivalent of socialized medicine in the United States, it was also a sacred cow. Both organizations have plenty of political power. For example, when President Richard M. Nixon vetoed the Veterans Health Care Expansion Act of 1972, Congress overrode the veto with a resounding majority. Obviously, the AMA was opposed to Senator Alan Cranston's bill, for not only would it provide hospital and ambulatory care for 47,785 disabled veterans; it also made services available to 150,000 peacetime veterans unable to afford private care, and

282,000 wives, widows, and children of veterans who were permanently disabled or who had died as a result of service-related injury. In addition to expanding the quality of medical care, the bill sought to upgrade it.

In his appeal to colleagues, Senator Cranston revealed the havoc that has been wrought by the AMA, which had brought cutbacks in VA programs which, in turn, had caused deficiencies in the staff and facilities. In December of 1972, for example, there were 32,237 veterans on waiting lists or scheduled for admission to VA hospitals who had been determined to need care within 30 days. Senator Cranston pointed out that the ratio of the staff to patients in VA hospitals had dropped to about 1:5 as compared to about 2:7 for the average community hospital and more than 3:5 for the university medical center hospitals.[26]

The AMA also has been opposed to the opening of free clinics designed chiefly to treat veneral diseases (now epidemic in the country) and make efforts to protect millions of Americans from death or illness by blood transfusion. Despite the opposition of the medical establishment, the free clinics seem to have become permanent. Some of them were started by militants, like the Black Panthers and the Young Lords. Some of the centers were government sponsored; some were started by concerned doctors, dentists, nurses, and other health workers who were appalled by the toll exacted by some aspects of the counterculture. They volunteered their services to help the "flower children" sickened by drugs, malnutrition, and venereal diseases. As the young people learned to trust the clinics, the patient load zoomed. Without judgment, the youngsters have been helped with socially infectious problems: heroin and "speed" addiction, syphilis and gonorrhea, pregnancy and birth-control counseling. And they were helped, not by "freaks" in white coats as the medical establishment has frequently charged, but by some of the most outstanding doctors in the community. Recently, people of all ages have started to use the clinics, ranging from colicky babies to the arthritis-racked elderly.

Not long ago, a clinic was started in our neighborhood with the help of Dr. Donald Newman, a physician and "conservative" member of the Los Angeles School Board. It is housed in an abandoned store and kept going by donations from area residents and from groups like the Kiwanis Club. All professional services are volunteered, including those of Dr. Newman. During the first month, even with minimal publicity and much resistance from establishment doctors, more than 125 persons received treatment. That number has enormously increased, as word has spread and confidence has grown. Most of the patients are from the nearby high school and junior high; but others in the neighborhood have been coming for aid. They are mostly older people who are unable or too fearful to travel to county clinics.

When I asked Dr. Newman about the reaction of some of his medical colleagues, he said thoughtfully: "Well, the need is very great, and when any of them complain to me about care being given free, I remind them of the price of their office visits. That usually ends the discussion."

The problem of providing medical treatment for the poor has by no means been overcome by the volunteer free clinics. Nor have other important health problems, including the dangers threatening millions of Americans from contaminated blood. The American Red Cross and other voluntary agencies, as well as informed individuals, have been fighting for years to regulate the traffic in blood. Thanks to the AMA, the profiteers are still getting away with murder—literally.

The blood industry has been in existence since 1948, when "plasmapheresis" was introduced. In that process, whole blood is withdrawn from a donor and then separated into plasma and red cells. The red cells are injected back into the donor. The plasma is separated into its various fractions: fibrinogen, albumin, fibrin foam, thrombin. All these are needed for many types of surgery, hemophilia, anemia, obstetric cases in which much blood is lost after childbirth, accidents, injuries, wound shock, burns, and scalds. Another fraction, immunoglobulin, is used to prevent measles, rubella and infectious hepatitis.

One of the advantages of plasma and serum over whole blood is that they can be stored indefinitely. Moreover, they have no license restrictions because the commercial operators persuaded the legislators that plasma was also a commodity in "short supply" when license restrictions were lifted on rare blood types in 1948.

The profits that can be made selling both whole blood and its fractions are enormous. Even the nonprofit blood banks and the Red Cross levy fees for blood distributed to hospitals. Most of that blood comes from "volunteers," and usually no cost to the blood banks is incurred. The commercial banks, on the other hand, are interested in making high profits. They set up their blood banks among the poor and the desperate who are happy to accept $3 to $5 a pint for their blood. The donors include prisoners, narcotics addicts, skid row winos. A number of American-owned blood-bank companies operate in India, the Dominican Republic, and Haiti. Little or no protection is afforded the donors abroad or at home. In one southern prison, standards were so lax that as many as 1000 prisoners were afflicted with hepatitis, six of whom died.

No greater protection is offered to donors outside the walls. In England, persons are allowed to make two donations a year; only a few places in the United States have standards to protect the donor from being bled too frequently: the New York Blood Bank and the Central Blood Bank of Seattle both allow only five donations a year, well spaced. *Chicago Tribune* reporters investigating the commercial blood banks there found that the intervals of eight weeks that had been recommended were totally ignored; the reporters were readily accepted at banks one day after being bled; some banks made no effort to establish that they were not carriers of hepatitis or malaria or syphilis, all of which can be transmitted through blood transfusions. A similar investigation by *Washington Post* reporters revealed the same conditions there. (Ghetto donors there were being paid with $5 vouchers stamped "Cash at Moe's Liquor Store only.") [27]

The cost to the recipients of blood is high as well. Dr. J. Garrott Allen of Stanford University Medical Center has estimated that 50,000 patients who receive transfusions are injected with serum hepatitis every year, and 3500 die. Others set the figure higher. In an interview with *National Observer* reporter August Gribbin, officials of the Public Health Service's Center for Disease Control said that the real hepatitis rate could be as many as ten times Dr. Allen's estimate.[28]

There is no disagreement among experts however that the main way to prevent patients from being injected with hepatitis from a transfusion is to control the source of blood. Recent studies have shown that the risk of acquiring serum hepatitis was from ten to 70 times greater when blood was used that came from commercial blood banks. The incidence has been very low in the Boston teaching hospitals, where no blood was purchased from commercial firms. Another study in New Jersey showed an incidence 70 times greater when the blood was donated by convicted or suspected narcotics addicts. And still another, made by Dr. Paul Schmidt and colleagues at the National Institute of Health in Bethesda, considered two groups of patients undergoing cardiac surgery. One group received 94 percent of their blood from paid donors; 97 percent of the blood obtained for the second group was taken from volunteer donors. Although the second group received more units of blood and therefore could be considered to be taking a higher risk, the hepatitis attack rate of that group was *Zero*. The rate of the first group, which obtained blood from paid donors was 53 percent.[29]

Readers may be surprised to discover that the blood they donated to be held in store for themselves or given to another member of the family may be replaced with blood obtained from commercial sources.

Who will protect the public from the consequences of such profiteering? Congressman Victor V. Veysey wanted to provide some protection when he introduced a bill to establish a federal program that would encourage the voluntary donation of pure and safe blood. The measure would require the licensing and inspection of all blood banks and would establish a national registry of blood donors. The bill proposed that HEW be given authority over all blood banks in the country; presently, its Division of Biologics Standards has regulatory power over only 166 of the nation's blood banks, while the other nearly 5000 are "controlled" by state and local laws.[30]

Over the years, doing the research for this book, I have frequently been sickened and appalled at man's inhumanity. One of the best and brightest of times, however, occurred on the skid row in Los Angeles in the winter of 1973 at the Catholic Worker's Hospitality Kitchen, where a group of idealistic young people of all denominations from the Claremont Theological School were helping to organize a strike against commercial blood and plasma banks in the area.

I heard about the plan earlier, as I was pressed into service cutting and scraping carrots during an interview with Catherine Norris, then Sister Catherine, and Jeff Dietrich, who had left college to become coordinator of the program about a year earlier. Gracious and elegant in her corduroy slacks and torn sneakers. Sister Catherine, until recently the director of the Mayfield School for Girls in Pasadena, spoke movingly of the "awakening" she had witnessed on skid row. "It is a marvelous thing that these young people are doing," she said, "giving the men a sense of possible power to change things. The feeling here generally is that: 'Nobody cares about me, and I don't care about anybody—even myself.' "

Jeff Dietrich, too, marveled at what was going on. "The blood bank strike has given the men a feeling of pride and responsibility, a sense of commitment. It happens," he added, "when you demand the best of people."

And the theological students agreed—chief among them Ray Correio, the twenty-six-year-old strike leader, who had himself spent "time on the street." Anguished by family problems, as a child he had lived for some years in Boys Town in the Desert. In the Navy, he had begun to "put it all together" in 1966. Sickened by the war he was participating in, he went on a hunger strike that lasted 51 days before he was discharged "for medical reasons." Working his way through one of the California state colleges, he became involved in the peace movement and later the war on poverty. He moved from history into theology as the best way of helping others. Eventually, his concern led to the Catholic Worker's Hospitality Kitchen, where he envisioned a strike of the blood donors as a way of "helping the inhabitants break through the cycle of desperation and misery, to come together and work for the common good." He had recruited a contingent to help.

"Sure it means more money and better treatment," Ray said, his culminating experience on skid row having been the plasma donor center, which he described as "a human dairy." But it is more than that for the donors: "It means that they are helping to keep people from agonizing sickness and death."

Sister Catherine's appraisal of the "marvelous thing" seemed in no way an overstatement at the strike meeting. I had watched the men shuffle in for the midday meal a few hours before, apathetic, barely speaking, each with hands and arms protecting his own plate. Here they were, alert, eager to talk of their own experiences, obviously determined to make an effort. Not all of those who had been diners attended the meeting. The Hospitality Kitchen attaches no strings, hymns, sermons, or promises to reform.

Standing on East Fifth Street the next morning in a cold drizzle, I had a chance to check out the promises. It was reassuring: the Indian militant who pledged to be there "for my people"; the splendidly dressed gray-haired black man who wanted to "see this good idea through"; the young vacant-eyed veteran from Vietnam who refused to utter a word, but who somehow looked comforted; and a dozen others beneath seemingly incongruous banners that read: "Donor Dignity"; "Down with the Commercial Vampires"; "You Are Human."

A lot of the skid row inhabitants scoffed, including some who had admitted the day before that nurses in the banks told them, "If we see you on the picket line, no more money." Employees of the blood banks were grim about the affair. When I asked several if they would like to give their version of the conditions of the blood banks, they retorted: "Get out of here. You newspaper people are just trouble makers." "We have had orders not to talk with you." The off-duty policemen who were working as guards for several of the blood banks maintained a rigid silence. Those on duty were scarcely more communicative. When I asked several of them standing nearby, watching, what they thought the effect would be, it was not an encouraging answer: "Who'd pay attention to some winos and hippies?"

As it turned out, quite a few people did. Newspapers carried articles and editorials about the "disgraceful situation" and applauded the strikers' efforts; radio and television carried news items, features, and documentaries about the commercial blood banks. Where was the medical establishment? That is what two California legislators, Senator Anthony Beilenson and Assemblyman Alan Sieroty, wanted to know later that year after introducing bills to remedy the conditions of the blood banks. Rather bluntly, they held the California Medical Association responsible for "hundreds of unnecessary deaths" in the state each year caused by hepatitis that had been transmitted by blood transfusions.[31]

But blood banks are business, business that heavily involves drug companies and doctors. There is little likelihood that either the CMA or its parent organization would interfere with that.

13 The Medicinal Properties of Tars and Nicotines and Other Carcinogens

Perhaps the most startling evidence of the American Medical Association's willingness to defend economic interests at the expense of national well being was contained in *Smoking and Health: Report of the Advisory Committee to the Surgeon General of the Public Health Service.* The country was electrified when it was released on January 11, 1964. No longer could there be any reasonable doubt that cigarette smoking was a major health hazard. The unanimous verdict of guilty had been rendered after 14 months of study and deliberation by ten of the nation's outstanding scientists and physicians. No question could be raised about their authority to speak or their scientific objectivity. Few committees have ever been as carefully screened: the members had been chosen from an original list of 150, with nine organizations, including the tobacco industry's trade association, given the right to blackball any candidate for incompetence or bias.

Cigarette smoking was a major cause of lung cancer, the committee reported. It was "the most important cause" of chronic bronchitis in the country and increased the risk of dying from that disease and from emphysema. Moreover, although a causal relationship between cigarette smoking and heart and circulatory diseases had not been fully established, there was a strong association between them, strong enough to prompt the committee to note that it would be "more prudent to assume one" than to suspend judgment until no uncertainty remains.[1]

The reactions to the Surgeon General's report followed fast. Religious groups like the Mormons, Seventh Day Adventists, and many fundamentalist sects which had long been inveighing against the "evils" of tobacco were in the novel position of having their campaigns against the "noxious weed" deemed scientifically sound. Some of them established clinics to help smokers to quit. The American Cancer Society, which had played an important role in getting the investigation launched, joined with other voluntary health organizations and with the Federal Trade Commission in an attempt to have warning labels placed on cigarette packages and in ads, and to step up the educational campaign against smoking. They announced that one hundred Americans die every day from lung cancer caused by smoking and another 500 die daily from diseases linked to smoking.[2] It seemed as if everyone had something to say, making personal pledges, proposing legislation, advocating antismoking programs, preaching sermons.

Two groups said nothing. The tobacco industry, which had sold more than 500 billion cigarettes the year before and which had spent $250,000,000 to stimulate that sale, was momentarily silent. And so was the AMA. The silence of the AMA during the week after the report was published caused Drew Pearson to comment sharply on its "peculiar attitude" toward cigarettes as well as drugs. "Some senators," he noted, "are beginning to wonder whether the doctors are for health or against it."[3]

A month later, the wonder grew, along with indignation. The Tobacco Industry Research Committee, which had been formed by growers' and manufacturers' groups in 1953 to protect industry profits and bolster sliding stocks, announced that it was awarding $10,000,000 to the AMA's American Educational and Medical Research Foundation to conduct "further investigation" into smoking and health.

The AMA accepted. After all, cigarette companies had been

more than helpful in sponsoring programs like *Ben Casey* and *Doctor Kildare*, principal medical "image makers." Even before the Surgeon General's report was published, the AMA had attempted to minimize possible impact by announcing that more research was necessary. And the tobacco industry's spokesman, Dr. Clarence Cook Little, who, ironically, had been former director of the American Cancer Society, had issued a moving statement of appreciation: "We are gratified by reports of the AMA's recognition of the need for additional research on smoking and health."[4] The AMA needed money for that? Arrangements were made.

The AMA's first big opportunity to prove publicly what a loyal friend it could be came in March 1964, at hearings conducted by the Federal Trade Commission. The FTC had proposed within a week after the report was issued that as of January 1, 1965, all cigarette packages carry a clear and prominent warning that "cigarette smoking is dangerous to health and may cause cancer and other diseases." Failure to carry that warning would be considered "an unfair or deceptive act or practice," making companies liable to prosecution. The FTC also proposed that as of July 1, 1965, all cigarette advertising include that warning message.

On the first day of the hearings, the spokesman for the cigarette makers registered his objections with disarming frankness. "Every American smoker already has knowledge of the health danger from cigarettes as a result of the widespread publicity over the last ten years." Thus, he added, "there is no basis for requiring such recitals" on packages and in ads. The AMA supported his position fully. It asserted that "cautionary labeling cannot be anticipated to serve the public interest with much success." Moreover, "regulatory action in this matter should be instituted by the Congress rather than the FTC." News reports described the reaction of FTC members. "I really am perplexed," Commissioner A. Everette MacIntyre was quoted as saying. He described the AMA stand as "precisely" the position of the cigarette manufacturers.[5] Some Congressmen were furious, calling the AMA the "handmaiden" of the tobacco industry. So were some Senators. Maurine B. Neuberger of Oregon said bluntly: "The ostrich-like stand of the AMA on the labeling of cigarettes as a health hazard did little to improve that organization's already tarnished public image."[6]

When Dr. Wendell Scott, president of the American Cancer Society, appeared before the FTC members the next day, he urged the adoption of the labeling proposal. However, he added to the confusion when he was questioned about the stand of the AMA. Obviously determined to avoid open war (the AMA and the American Cancer Society had collided before, to the sorrow of the latter) he said that he did not think there was any conflict. Other society officials, however, were far more blunt. "For the AMA to be opposed to labeling is absolutely ridiculous," said Dr. Sol R. Baker, president of the California division of the ACS. In an interview with the medical editor of the *Los Angeles Times,* he charged: "Such a position is intolerable, unrealistic, and not representative of the feelings of the majority of individual doctors whom the AMA is supposed to be representing." His explanation for the AMA's stand? "I'd hate to think it was the $10,000,000 the tobacco industry gave the AMA to do research that is influencing them."[7] But the allegation that the AMA's opposition to cautionary labeling had been influenced by the multi-million dollar research fund gradually became more and more widespread. As a result, Congressman Harold D. Cooley of North Carolina, chairman of the House Agriculture Committee, felt himself impelled to comment after the FTC hearings: "I cautioned the Tobacco Institute against making this grant to the AMA." He added that he feared "some irresponsible people with axes to grind would charge that such a research arrangement was actually an attempt to bribe the AMA in its position on smoking and health." He denied the truth of the equally widespread allegation that the AMA and tobacco state legislators had worked out a *quid pro quo* so that in exchange for AMA opposition to cigarette labeling, Congressmen from tobacco-growing states would vote against pending Medicare legislation.[8]

The charge continued to be made, however, particularly in the summer of 1964 after the House Ways and Means Committee had shelved the Medicare bill. A number of writers were speaking pointedly of the "unholy alliance between the tobacco industry and the politically organized doctors in the American Medical Association."[9]

Before examining the intricate politicking concerning the publicity over the harmful effects of cigarettes, it is instructive to consider how the AMA came to allow itself to be the apologist for an industry whose existence and profits depend upon the creation and maintenance of a destructive habit. (*Addiction* is the word many prefer.) Very grave doubts about cigarettes had been expressed by medical scientists since 1921, when Dr. Moses Barron, a University of Minnesota pathologist, reported that lung cancer was becoming an increasingly significant cause of death. Medical journals also began to note an association between lung cancer and cigarette smoking. Two Chicago doctors reported in the *JAMA* in 1936 that 90 percent of the lung cancer victims they had examined were "chronic smokers."[10]

However, the medical profession generally did not exhibit concern. It tolerated the advertising claims of the tobacco industry that cigarettes not only tasted good, they were *good for you.* In the 1930s and 1940s, doctors were frequently used to hawk cigarettes: "More doctors smoke Camels than any other cigarette"; "Three out of four doctors smoke Philip Morris." Unlike medical organizations in other countries, the AMA did not demur publicly when male models were dressed in white coats to convey the impression that cigarettes were somehow actually *prescribed*, nor when the pages of the *JAMA* and other medical magazines were open to cigarette advertisers.

Individual doctors in this country and some medical groups, who were persuaded by the evidence in 1964, began to assail the choplogic propositions the AMA had offered at the hearings and the "educational" pamphlet it issued in May. "Smoking: Facts You Should Know" was ridiculed by doctors as the "don't-smoke-in-bed" tract. It made much of smoking as a threat to life only because "numerous deaths occur each year from burns and suffocation due to falling asleep while smoking." The cancer issue was carefully ignored.

Their indignation was further increased when the AMA announced in June that it had made the first awards of grants from the tobacco industry for studies on smoking and health. One of ten grants, to locate the "many gaps" in the case against cigarettes, was reported to have gone to a member of the awards committee and a member of the Tobacco Industry Research Committee's medical advisory group.[11]

The delegates to the AMA convention a few weeks later held a lively debate on cigarettes and cancer. By that time, at least 23 state societies had gone on record against cigarette smoking. Instead of making discreet criticism of the policy of the AMA during an executive session (as criticisms of the AMA are usually made), protesters made public statements during public sessions. Dr. Alton Ochsner of New Orleans, a leading authority on lung cancer, urged immediate action: "We must forthrightly say that this is a health hazard and not hide behind a cloak, saying we don't know the cause and must do more research."[12] Physicians from tobacco states countered with a claim that California vineyards and Iowa cornfields should be protested, as sources of alcohol. The delegates were calmed momentarily by the president of the AMA's research foundation, which had accepted the grant. While economic factors should not be "over-riding" in AMA decisions, he said, "they must be considered in any policy action."

The AMA House of Delegates did make concessions. It announced that changes would be made in the "don't-smoke-in-bed pamphlet" since there was a "significant relationship" between smoking and cancer. It also promised that all physicians would be urged to "engage more actively in intensive educational campaigns regarding smoking and health."[13] But within weeks, the AMA was cooperative again with the tobacco industry to insure that the warning notices would not have to be placed in ads, although they were to be carried on packages. This was acceptable to both the AMA and the tobacco industry; the package warning is generally seen by persons who are already hooked, whereas the ads have been designed to create new converts. Moreover, a note, of a properly vague and mild nature, would have the additional advantage of guarding the industry from suits by cancer victims. The number of suits had been growing. Now, they could be set aside on the grounds that: "We told you so."

A dozen leading health and educational organizations next joined with government agencies to form the National Interagency Council on Smoking and Health "to develop and implement effective plans and programs aimed at combating smoking as a health hazard." Its members included the American Cancer Society, the American Dental Association, the American Heart Association, the American Public Health Association, the National Congress of Parents and Teachers, the U.S. Public Health Service, the U.S. Office of Education, and others. The AMA had been invited to cooperate, but it maintained a silence that was to prove golden for the cigarette industry. The advertising Federation of America, the American Newspaper Publishers Association, the Magazine Publishers Association, the Radio Advertising Bureau, and the National Association of Broadcasters joined the industry, notifying legislators that warnings in cigarette advertising would be "detrimental." To their business, they meant. The cigarette industry is estimated to have spent $189,000,000 in 1965 on television commercials alone.

Legislators were properly impressed. Despite the brave words of the members of health groups bent on getting warnings published, they had not arranged even for legal counsel for the National Interagency Council on Smoking and Health. Its expenditures amounted to $450. As a result, the industry won its appeal. The role of the AMA was generally acclaimed. Not the least tribute came from the chairman of the board of a public relations firm, who applauded the AMA's having accepted the grant for research as "one of the most outstanding examples of social responsibility in American industry."[14] In dramatic circles, that would be described as king-sized irony.

In December 1974—almost 13 years after the Surgeon General's report had been issued—the *JAMA* took a decided stand on the matter, in an article and editorial holding Congress and other federal bodies responsible for the high death rates associated with smoking. Branding the tobacco subsidy "a national shame," Dr. Weldon J. Walker, a member of the editorial board and director of the cardiopulmonary laboratory of White Memorial Medical Center in Los Angeles, said that the 1964 report so bitterly contested by the AMA had had an effect: "The slight dip in tobacco consumption that followed the surgeon general's report has brought a drop in deaths from both these diseases" (coronary heart disease, which claims 600,000 lives a year, and peptic ulcer disease). "This dramatic breakthrough against coronary disease apparently has resulted chiefly from a modest reduction in tobacco consumption."[15]

The smoking drop, he acknowledged, had not had much effect on chronic bronchitis and emphysema, which has a toll of about 25,000 a year, or lung cancer, which claims 72,000 lives a year and has been linked with other cancer-causing substances by many researchers.

Oddly enough, the AMA's passion for "more facts" and "more research" on carcinogens seems to have been stimulated only by money from industries already threatened. That has been indicated by the attitude of the AMA toward other environmental dangers including smog, lead, mercury, hormones and antibiotics in animal feed, and pesticides, among the incredible list of hazardous chemicals to which people in this country have been wantonly exposed. Chemicals in the environment have recently been held responsible for at least 80 percent of cancer cases in the United States. Many of them have also been associated with other leading causes of death such as heart disease, diseases of the circulatory system, bronchopulmonic diseases, liver diseases, and vascular lesions affecting the central nervous system.

Demographers note the sharp upturn in mortality for men from 1952 to 1967 and since. In every age category over 15, male death rates have been rising steadily. The AMA, as the leading organization so far as health care in the country is concerned, should have played a leading role in conducting research or prompting research to identify the major chemical threats. Instead, it has remained aloof and allowed the slaughter to continue.

Consider the case of pesticides, which many sophisticated scientists regard as "potentially a much greater hazard than nuclear fallout."[16] No realistic laws prohibiting their overuse and misuse have been enacted, partly because, as one Congressman said of the tobacco problem, there is too much division of expert opinion.

225

That division of expert opinion has been brought about by ignorance or avarice or both. In the trade, the more than 45,000 registered synthetic commercial killers of weeds, bugs, funguses, rats, and other organisms considered pests are known as economic poisons. Lately, they have been called *biocides* because of their destructiveness to the web of life. A blunter but perhaps more meaningful label for them is *people poisons*. Pesticides came into extensive use only toward the end of World War II. But even then biologists and physicians were becoming troubled enough about them to speak out, protesting their effects on the human body. The *British Medical Journal* as early as 1945 began to carry reports of poisoning by DDT, the most notorious of the large family of chlorinated hydrocarbons that has occasioned such controversy. One researcher described reactions ranging from joint pains and irritability to a feeling of "incompetence in tackling the simplest mental task."[17] Another researcher said that after applying a solution of the chemical to his skin, he was bedded for three weeks and absent from work for ten.[18] Five years later, some doctors in the United States continued to question the unrestricted use of DDT. Not only did it induce the jitters, they said, but it was associated with hepatitis and other liver dysfunctions.[19] Still later, Dr. Wilhelm C. Hueper, former director of the National Cancer Institute, called it one of the chemical carcinogens. (For his concern, incidentally, his staff was immobilized and he was excluded from official meetings.)[20] By the 1970s, DDT was also known to be causing changes in sex hormones, reducing the effectiveness of a number of drugs, adversely affecting liver, spleen, and kidneys,[21] and, according to FDA scientists, damaging the hypothalamus, an important endocrine center, which helps to control emotional states, digestive processes, body temperatures, sex glands, sleep rhythms, and hunger and thirst.[22]

Other chlorinated hydrocarbons were far more poisonous. The former director of pharmacology for the Food and Drug Administration reported more than 20 years ago that chlordane causes depression of the bone marrow, reducing the number of red and white blood cells. So does lindane. Dr. M. M. Hargraves of the Mayo Clinic has also been warning the public and legislators about that for more than two decades. He has amassed more than a thousand cases implicating it in blood disorders. Among his patients was a young woman who had received 12 blood transfusions without success before going to Mayo. He determined the cause of her aplastic anemia, an often fatal disease, to be a lindane vaporizer that had been placed in her music room. where she practiced several hours a day. After it was removed, she improved and gradually recovered.[23] Heptachlor, endrin, dieldrin, and aldrin, all extremely toxic, induce muscle tremors, convulsions, and changes in the pattern of brain activity as well as occasional death. All are considered to be not only carcinogenic, but teratogenic (inducing birth defects) and mutagenic (affecting future generations).

England and other countries banned the use of chlorinated hydrocarbons for many purposes years ago. They have also exhibited concern about the other principal family of pesticides, the organophosphates. Closely related to "nerve gases," those substances affect the skin, eyes, and internal organs. Their effect is described in Army technical manuals. The first symptoms parallel those of relatively harmless irritants, running nose and blurred vision. Then nausea sets in, followed by vomiting, excessive sweating, uncontrolled salivation, and urinary incontinence. The heart, which beats rapidly in the early stages, slows. Convulsions follow; then coma and muscular paralysis. Breathing becomes increasingly difficult, finally impossible. Then death.

Physicians are rarely knowledgeable about pesticide poisoning. even in places where it is commonplace. A witness told Senator Walter F. Mondale's Subcommittee on Migratory Labor in 1969 that doctors often misdiagnose organophosphate poisoning as "flu." He held the chemicals largely responsible for the more than 100,000 cases of pesticide poisoning that occur each year.[24] That number may be even higher. Shortly afterward, Dr. Lee Mizrahi, with a rural health clinic in a California farm county, said that nearly half of the children he tested during the course of a nutrition study showed signs of organic phosphate poisoning. (The children, like their parents, were not in serious condition, and the discovery was made quite by accident.) To legislators, he indicated his dismay: "To me, it is tragically absurd that in 1969 such a study by an obscure rural doctor should be the first one ever done on children. We think this problem is widespread."[25] Other effects have come to light. Two British medical researchers noted that a number of persons who had been exposed to those pesticides for periods ranging up to two years had suffered "schizophrenic and depressive reactions, with severe impairment of memory and difficulty in concentration."[26]

Since all of us are exposed to pesticides all the time, in the food we eat, the clothes we wear, the surfaces we touch, the very air we breathe, surely it would have behooved the medical profession to research the relationship between pesticides and health. Instead, that was left up to concerned individuals and to independent researchers like Dr. J. L. Radomski and William B. Deichman, who revealed in 1967 the perils to which even people far removed from farms had been exposed. The study they made in Florida showed "highly significant elevations of pesticide concentrations" in cancer cases of all types of the lung, stomach, rectum, pancreas, prostate, and urinary bladder. The concentrations were particularly high among persons who used large quantities of pesticides in their homes.[27]

The medical establishment has continued a hands-off policy. And it will, until industry profits are seriously threatened. Lacking leadership and even cooperation, individuals and smaller organizations alone have been forced to persuade legislators to act before more destruction has been accomplished. Among those individuals is Dr. Samuel S. Epstein of Children's Cancer Research Foundation and the Harvard Medical School. Objecting to the inadequate testing methods now employed in order to get products on the market and pointing out that it often takes years for the dangers of weak carcinogens to reveal themselves, he pointed out that pesticides "could affect and catastrophically so, as many as 1/10,000 of the population and yet probably escape detection by conventional procedures."[28]

14 Insuring Sickness

The trouble with the kind of health insurance that prevails in the United States, thanks largely to the American Medical Association, is that the chief beneficiary is the multibillion dollar insurance industry. Next come the doctors and hospitals, while the policy holder trails in last across the finish line—if he makes it at all.

All insurance, of course, involves a kind of gambling, with the insured betting that he will need protection and the insurance carrier betting he will not. By creating an enormous demand and using both crude and sophisticated methods to minimize risks, the health insurance business has become one of the biggest businesses in the country today. And one of the most profitable. Although 80 percent of the people in the country under the age of sixty-five had some form of health insurance in 1970, benefits met only 40.3 percent of their expenditures for health. Yet the insurance companies were reaping a harvest, with some of them returning less than 50 cents of each premium dollar to the policy holders.[1] In some parts of the country, the averages were even lower. At least 90 percent of working Californians, for instance, had some form of health insurance in 1972; yet the average Californian was paid only 37 percent of his medical costs under health insurance policies.[2]

Reasons for the health insurance boom (for the insurers) and bust (for the insured) were summed up recently in a number of representative "case histories" presented to a United States Senate Health Subcommittee and other investigative agencies: the exclusionist devices, the deductibles, the inadequacies, the lack of control over costs and quality, the exploitation of the needy, the shady practices indulged in.

One of the witnesses before the Kennedy subcommittee was a Los Angeles insurance executive and attorney, Sumner Cotton. When he left the company he had been working for and applied for private insurance coverage, he was told that he could not have it for his wife who had been hospitalized the year before. "Wait a couple of years, old friend," they told him, "and if she has had no further claims and she is in good health, why, we will get her some insurance."

Before the wait was up, she was afflicted with an aneurysm in the anterior lobe section of the brain and hospitalized. Mr. Cotton's bill for his wife's illness was $13,000, bringing him, he said, to the verge of bankruptcy.[3]

Commenting on this kind of exclusionism before the Senate Judiciary Subcommittee on Antitrust and Monopoly in 1972, Leonard Woodcock, president of the United Auto Workers, said:

> The insurance companies do not assure universal access to health care. They are interested in profitability, not universality. They deal with people not as people, but as good risks, high risks and uninsurables, bad risks.[4]

The industry's actuarial "game plan," he said, has cut millions of Americans off from the possibility of obtaining coverage. Moreover, he added: "they do not sell health insurance at all." Rather, they sell "sickness insurance to healthy people."

And if those healthy people become ill, there are ways of insuring that they do not receive insurance benefits. One might think, as Senator Kennedy pointed out in his account of the hearings before his health subcommittee, "that for almost $500 a year a family could buy insurance that covered a problem with a newborn infant."[5] But the De Witt family of Denver offered evidence that this might not be so. The furniture repairman and his wife were making an insurance payment of $500 a year out of his $7000-a-year salary because they believed in protection. One of their twin babies was born with a ruptured bowel; that is when they learned they did not have all the protection they thought they did. According to the policy they had had with one of the most reputable insurance companies in the United States for seven years, no coverage is provided for newborns for the first 15 days, which is a common practice. When asked why the insurance companies did that, "It is," Mrs. De Witt told the Senators, "a pretty handy way to get the premiums and get out of the dangerous part of the new baby. This pretty well fixes them up, because if the baby is going to be sick when it's born this is the bill that's going to be big. . . ."[6]

Less prestigious companies, particularly the mail-order insurance companies, have found the "preexisting" clause a sure way to fatten company profits at the expense of the policy holders. Consider a few cases from the many compiled by the Senate Antitrust and Monopoly Subcommittee. They involved National Liberty Insurance Co., whose National Home policies were advertised from coast to coast on radio and television by Art Linkletter. A seventy-two-year-old man was hospitalized in 1972 for cataract extraction and heart disease. Although his doctor said that the ailments were first noticed in 1971, more than a year after he had bought the policy, his claim was denied because the hospital had told the company that the man had reported a gradual loss of vision for two years. Also denied was the claim of a fifty-year-old woman hospitalized for a month in 1972 for obesity and congestive heart failure. The doctor said the heart condition was new, but the company rejected the claim on the grounds that the patient's obesity preexisted the policy.[7]

Atypical? Not according to many expert opinions about the mail-order policies that have become big sellers, although not unique to them. As *Consumer Reports* pointed out, the wide power that such companies give themselves to determine whether a condition did exist before coverage was purchased makes it very difficult to collect benefits. "It is not surprising that some mail-order companies expect 50 percent of policyholders to drop their policies in discouragement before two years are out."[8] And the Council of Better Business Bureaus agrees: ". . . you may be sure that some insurance companies will try very hard to find some evidence to prove a policyholder is not entitled to benefits, if he makes a claim within the two-year period."[9] Some insurance companies have not even bothered to go through that formality. During Senate hearings in the 1960s, a California Congressman who is an expert in health insurance, Ronald Brooks Cameron, reported that in many cases persons who had paid for insurance for many years were notified that their policies would be canceled on the next renewal date when they reported an illness.[10] Another witness before that subcommittee told Senate investigators that when a number of persons had sent in claims to some of the more exploitive companies, they received by return mail a band-aid![11]

In contrast, a good many of those whose insurance policies *work* have found themselves with more health-care service than they have wanted or needed. Insurance is sometimes a *cause* for medical and hospital care.

A brief description of how the "Diagnosis: Blue Cross" game works was given a few years ago by an anonymous doctor in his revealing book, *The Healers*. The diagnostician called a specialist friend, with word that a woman had been in to see him with a sort of pain and he had referred her to the specialist.

"A sort of pain?" the specialist asked tentatively.

The diagnostician elucidated: "I mean it, two kinds [of pain]. She's got Blue Cross and Blue Shield at her office and her husband's got John Hancock Major Medical at his."[12] It was up to the specialist to take it from there, turning over a portion of the insurance payment to the diagnostician.

Since Medicare and Medicaid were enacted, the game has been expanded to take them in as "most popular" diagnoses in medicine in the 1970s. Perhaps most of the 2,000,000 and more unnecessary operations each year are due to the desire of physicians to take as much insurance money as possible; most of the unnecessary hospital and nursing home admissions are made for the same reason.

Bad as it is, not even the kind of protection currently provided would be in existence if the AMA had its way. The growth of the nonprofit (a word only loosely defined) Blue Cross and Blue

Shield plans as well as the frankly commercial health-insurance plans was countenanced by organized medicine only because of the "threat" of prepayment, group-practice plans, which are discussed in detail in a later chapter. After all, any kind of health insurance involves intrusion into the financial relationship between a doctor and a patient of "The Third Party," and the imposition of some kind of a fee schedule, which interferes with the doctors' free-wheeling determination of what the traffic will bear.

Basically, there are three types of voluntary health insurance. The service plans provide subscribers with most of the care they need for a fixed annual rate. The indemnity insurance programs pay specified dollar allowances for hospital and medical services. The major medical, or "catastrophe," insurance pays a large part of the cost of serious illnesses only, nothing toward minor episodes.[13] The AMA has chiefly resisted the service plans, particularly the prepaid, group-practice plans, since the latter aim at insuring health rather than sickness. Doctors are rewarded when subscribers are in good health, because they emphasize preventive care and early treatment in contrast to the ordinary insurance principle that rewards doctors when subscribers fall ill.

The idea of service plans is not new. They were a natural corollary of the industrial expansion in the nineteenth century, when lumber, oil, mining, and railroad enterprises isolated large groups of workers from urban doctors and hospitals. Companies found themselves forced to set up hospitals near mines and mills and to hire doctors. Frugally, they usually passed the cost along to the workers, who were asked to pay for the benefits through salary "check-offs." Some of the medical care was excellent. The Mayo brothers were at one time railroad "contract" doctors, and the outstanding health-insurance program carried on by the Southern Pacific Railroad Company dates back to 1868. Some of them were deplorable. William Faulkner gives a chilling, factually accurate picture of these in his novel *The Wild Palms*. The only concern of the company was protection from lawsuits.[14]

Prototypes of the various kinds of service plans evolved in 1929, when Dr. Michael Shadid began his remarkable experiment to provide both medical and hospital coverage, when Ross-Loos set up a comprehensive plan in Los Angeles for some city workers, and when a group of Dallas public school teachers worked out an arrangement with officials of Baylor University Hospital to provide up to three weeks of care in semi-private rooms for those ordered hospitalized by a doctor. Teachers paid 50 cents a month; later, the plan was expanded to include children and spouses. About the only things not included for the modest fee were the services of the patient's private doctor and nurse.[15] The plan was such a success that within five years, 400 other groups of employees in Dallas, including firemen, policemen, nurses, and newspaper workers, were enrolled. And insurance companies in a number of states began to work out contract plans between hospitals and employee groups.

The leaders of the AMA began to worry in print, especially because there also was great agitation in England to expand the national health legislation to include hospital coverage in addition to doctors' bills. The AMA feared that, as a result, there first would be hospitalization insurance, then medical, in the United States. Under the editorial direction of Dr. Morris Fishbein, the *JAMA* set about discrediting the plans. If the plans were allowed to continue, the *JAMA* warned, lay influence would "defile" standards; medicine would be commercialized; local medical societies would lose control; and hospitals, not doctors, would become the "preferred creditors." Moreover, the plans would probably lead to compulsory health insurance.[16] The leaders of the AMA sought legislation to block both hospital and medical-service plans, while working overtime to minimize the need for them. Contradictory to the findings of the Committee on the Costs of Medical Care, the AMA's Council on Medical Education and Hospitals came up with a glowing account of the quality of medical care in the country. Even in the state of Mississippi, where annual per capita income at the time was a little over $200, the AMA claimed medical care was adequate. To be sure, there were fewer doctors than in other places (1 to 1353 in contrast to the national ratio of 1 to 762); few hospitals accepted blacks, and all hospitals suffered from a shortage of highly trained workers. Nevertheless, the Council said blandly, "there is practically no one in Mississippi who cannot secure medical care regardless of his ability to pay."[17]

That statement was so ludicrously at odds with the facts that even traditionally docile legislators threatened that the government would act to provide decent hospital and medical care for the nation. In 1936 the AMA Board of Trustees reacted. They denied that they had ever been opposed to insurance and particularly to group hospitalization plans, designed for low-income groups, which had local doctors on their administrative boards.[18]

Plans that met American Hospital Association standards were allowed to use the official symbol and became known as "Blue Cross" plans. Organized as "public service," nonprofit insurance groups, they flourished. In 1937, only a million belonged; by 1972 there were more than 70,000,000 members. (Private insurance companies were offering a similar service to others so that 115,-000,000 had hospital expense insurance.) A few years after acknowledging the right of the Blue Cross hospital plans to operate, the AMA gave in on the Blue Shield plans. People had long been clamoring for protection against disastrous medical as well as hospital bills; as were some groups of physicians, for example, the American College of Surgeons. In 1934, the Michigan State Medical Society proposed a "mutual health insurance" plan that would cover doctors' fees; soon after, the California State Medical Society endorsed compulsory health insurance for certain groups. Both combined the indemnity and service principles for persons with a low income; the Blue Shield allowance for a particular service had to be accepted as full payment. If the patient's income was higher, doctors had the right to impose a surcharge! Thus, a doctor would have to accept $100 from the insurance plan if a patient's yearly earnings were below $2000; he could charge another $50 or $75 or more if the patient earned more.

For a time, the AMA would have none of such plans. Then, in 1939, Senator Robert Wagner of New York had introduced the first series of bills giving the federal government responsibility for creating a national system of prepaid medical care. To stem the tide, the AMA suddenly announced its approval of the Michigan and California medical society plans it had earlier opposed.

It favored chiefly plans that incorporated the cash indemnity principle; it insisted that doctors be in absolute charge. To win approval, medical insurance plans had to be sanctioned by the local medical societies, had to allow for free choice of physician, and had to observe the fee-for-service idea. Almost as much response was generated, and by 1962 the 74 certified Blue Shield plans had almost 50,000,000 members.[19]

By that time, more than 700 commercial companies had gotten into the act, selling some kind of health insurance. Aggressive sales campaigns, the application of shrewd business methods to "rating" prospective buyers and calculating possible benefits made them vigorous competitors of the Blues. Quickly, they took over a lion's share of the market.

The growth of commercial insurance plans—and by 1972 more than 1200 were in operation—had some unhappy consequences on the Blues. "A kind of Gresham's law operates here," is the way Seymour Harris has phrased it in *The Economics of American Medicine*; "the poor insurance drives out the good."[20] Blue Cross, for example, received its nonprofit tax exemption status largely because of its system of "community rating"; that is, the plan accepted the risky business as well as the safe, so that people who have few health problems subsidize those who have many. The commercial insurance companies have become highly selective, and as a result, Blue Cross is left with an undue share of the poor risks. Also, because of the many deductions, the emphasis on indemnity rather than service, the high rate of claims denials, the commercial companies could offer policies at lower rates than the Blues. In order to cut their high loss rates, the Blues began to adopt "experience" rather than community ratings, but they also reduced benefits and jeopardized national health.

Although Blue Cross and Blue Shield are technically nonprofit groups, that does not mean that they serve the public interest as well as they might. Blue Cross is dominated by the hospital interests; Blue Shield by the doctors. Neither they nor the commercial companies, which offer health insurance solely to make money, concern themselves with preventive medicine, with quality care, with efficient and economical distribution of services.

As early as 1932, the Committee on the Costs of Medical Care recommended that the least expensive and best way to assure that a person could receive quality medical care was to offer him pre-paid group-practice plans, with medical and paramedical workers "centered largely around a hospital." Over the decades, such plans have proved themselves time and again, as Professor Paul E. Hanchett, Chicago economist, has determined. He made a detailed study of the medical benefits offered the city's public school teachers under a comprehensive certificate of the Blues. He compared benefits with those offered by the Union Health Service group-practice plan, for which many organized employees in Chicago were eligible, including the school janitors. The Union health plan covered all surgical and medical costs the patient incurred in a hospital. Blue Cross-Blue Shield paid only stated dollar allowances toward charges; the teachers had to pay considerable expenses themselves. In addition, the Union Health Service covered office calls to the doctor, house calls (for an additional $3 fee), eye care, periodic examinations, and outpatient diagnostic tests, none of which was covered by the Blues. The price differential was startling: a three-person family paid $402 for the "comprehensive" certificate from the Blue; subscribers to the UHS plan paid only $314. "Evidently the families in Janitors Local #25 get a better deal than the teachers," Dr. Hanchett concluded his summary.[21]

More important than price, the UHS plan included quality service (the Blues have done almost nothing to guarantee that). It guarded members against unnecessary surgery and hospitalization. It encouraged health by urging early diagnosis and providing preventive medical care. The record of the commercial companies, by contrast with the Blues, was appalling.

Yet so great was the pressure of the insurance lobby that the enactment of Medicare and Medicaid in 1965 handed the Blues and the commercial companies a multibillion-dollar bonanza. Within two years, medical costs had reached crisis proportions. They have continued to soar since then; and the government's only answer has been more money. In 1972, Medicare patients were paying far more of the medical expenses than they were the year the program began. In addition to Medicare premiums of about $70 a year, average out-of-pocket expenses for an individual were $225; for an average couple medical costs would be almost $600—about 15 percent of their total income.[22] The insurance companies were doing very well; and if a government proposal to expand and extend the chaotic system had been enacted, it would have increased the premium income of the private health insurance companies from $23,000,000,000 to $30,000,000,000.[23]

In the *Report of the National Conference on Medical Costs*, Dr. Ray E. Brown, director of the graduate program in hospital administration at Duke University's Medical Center, described what could be expected from this country's effort to pursue its "crosspurposes" approach to solving the problem of providing medical care and selecting the "third-party scheme" for financing it.[24] The first is the extraordinarily high cost of administration. That has been running as high as 50 percent for some of the underwriters and averages 10 percent of the total premiums for all. Even the Blues, which as nonprofit enterprises return a far higher percent of the premium dollar than the commercial companies, have not been above padding the administrative costs.

Consider the case of the Virginia Blues. Blue Cross, the Medicare "intermediary," and Blue Shield, the Medicaid "fiscal agent," were charged with deciding how much should be paid to providers on a "reasonable cost" basis and were entrusted to disburse money for "reasonable" services. According to a Social Security Administration study, the Blues regarded the appointment as a chance to expand their power base. They hired a staff "about 23 percent in excess of requirements." Although the workload increased by only 22.3 percent, they upped their expenses for data-processing 1409.8 percent.

The Virginia Blues built a new office building soon after getting the Medicare-Medicaid contract and spent more than $1,000,000 on new furniture purchased without competitive bidding (much of it was bought from a furniture company whose sales manager was chairman of the building committee of the state Blue Cross board of trustees). Among other administrative expenses charged to Medicare was a company picnic, including 1050 buffet dinners, wages for two bartenders, bingo prizes, and the rental of six ponies. Medicare was also charged for one-third of the cost of 13 dozen golf balls imprinted with the Blue Cross-Blue Shield emblems, costing $2138.50.[25]

As Dr. Brown pointed out, the lack of any central control of standards allows underwriters to set up business in the states that best suit their purposes. Also, they can even bypass state regulations through newspaper, radio, and TV ads and direct-mail selling. That has certainly been the case with the mail-order insurance plans that make glorious promises in ads and deliver little in fact.

There were rich rewards in the mail-order insurance business for the entertainers and other celebrities who plugged the policies. According to the findings of the Ohio Insurance Department, Art Linkletter received $50,000 a year for his services, six days in personal appearances and ads, and six as a director of the National Home plan. The rewards were somewhat less for the policy holders, who, according to the Nevada Insurance Commissioner, got back between 35 and 37 percent of their premium dollar. Insurance commissioners in Washington, Pennsylvania, and Ohio have stopped the ads and similar ads by Paul Harvey for Banker's Life & Casualty of Chicago. (Reasons given by the Washington commissioner were that "their knowledge of insurance is unknown, they are not licensed agents, and the ads had the effect of deceiving the public.") [26]

Unfortunately, as Dr. Brown pointed out, *"In a real sense, the actuaries have been the architects of the medical care system."*[27] Emphasis has been placed on crisis medicine and on hospital coverage rather than on preventive medicine and emphasizing outpatient treatment. In 1972, an official of the Aetna Life & Casualty insurance company told Senate investigators that one of the studies it had made showed that the American people could save $100,000,-000 a year if minor surgery were performed "on a walk-in, walk-out basis."[28] But neither his company nor others have made any major effort to bring about a realization of that possibility. Since that kind of innovation would only lower the premium dollar, why bother with it? An indication of how the efficiencies of quality prepaid group-practice plans affect consumer pocketbooks was given by Dr. Milton I. Roemer of the school of public health of the University of California in a 1973 study of the real costs of three basic types of plan. The average premium paid to commercial insurers was relatively low compared with the "Blues" and group-practice plans: $208 as compared with $257 and $271. But the out-of-pocket expenses of those insured with both commercial plans and the "Blues" were very high as compared with those in group-practice plans: $156 and $190 as compared with only $52.[29]

Other new services that could be provided are the inexpensive homemaker, meals-on-wheels, and similar programs that would make it possible for millions of the elderly to live at home rather than occupying costly hospital and nursing home beds. But what insurance company is offering them under their plans?

The insurance system penalizes legitimate policyholders, yet makes it possible, as Dr. Brown pointed out, for some persons "to actually take cash out of the medical care system."[30] Chiseling has become a big business, with windfall benefits amounting to $1,000,000,000 a year paid to multiple policy holders bent on plunder. Investigators from the Health Insurance Institute have documented histories showing how people steal from the plan. A forty-nine-year-old Florida furniture dealer was hospitalized 23 times in an eight-year period because of back and hip pains, neck aches, and groin injuries. Records showed that for each two-week stay, he collected benefits from eight different companies. On one policy alone, he made a tax-free profit of $6400 after paying his hospital bills. Another, a sixty-two-year-old Arkansas carpenter, cashed in from back and head injuries. Three times in one year, he told hospital authorities that he had fallen, striking his head against a door. The days he spent in the hospital for observation were profitably spent; he collected seven times the amount of his bill from the various companies he was insured with.[31]

Chiseling by policyholders is deplorable; but it is small stuff compared with the even more deplorable chiseling that goes on among many physicians. The commercial insurers have been notoriously lax in checking on claims. A few have, with dismaying results. For example, when the Occidental Life Insurance company made a study of 6000 claims several years ago, it found that physicians charge on the average 20 percent more when coverage permits them to set their own fees for a service. In one case of gross overcharges, an insurance company intervened on the part of a family, although the policy had not gone into effect. A surgeon had submitted a bill for $3500 for operating on an eleven-year-old boy for a hernia and undescended testicle. As a result of that intervention, the company managed to get the bill reduced by $3000.[32]

Blue Cross and Blue Shield also have failed to protect the patients' financial interests. Pennsylvania Insurance Commissioner Herbert S. Denenberg decided to use his authority to insist on some basic reforms by Blue Cross such as an advance review of hospital budgets, public disclosure of hospital data, and protection of patients from being charged for unnecessary hospitalization. The consequences were dramatic. The rate of increase in hospital costs dropped from 18.4 percent in 1971 to 7 percent in 1973; the annual rate of increase of claims dropped from 14.8 percent in 1971 to 2.5 percent a year later. Other hospital statistics also improved: the admission rate per thousand subscribers dropped 7 percent, although the national figure showed no decrease; the number of days a patient usually was hospitalized dropped 11 percent, compared with a drop of 4 percent nationally. "As a result of our reforms and economies, Blue Cross of Philadelphia will not ask for a rate increase in 1973," Denenberg said, "it's first no-increase year within recent memory."[33]

Similar results were obtained when pressure was put on the Pennsylvania Blue Shield plan. It was the largest of these plans in the nation, covering nearly 6,000,000 people and paying some $170,000,000 in claims each year. After five days of public hearings, Denenberg and his commission proposed 44 guidelines. Among the most significant was greater consumer representation on the board that had been dominated by doctors and had "failed to protect the interest of the public as well as it protects the interests of participating doctors." According to Commissioner Denenberg: "We told Blue Shield we would not give it a nickel's worth of premium increases [it had asked for an $18,800,000 rate increase] today, tomorrow, or ever *until* it put into effect some

241

of the reforms and economies we were talking about."[34] Unhappy though it was, he added, Blue Shield has been responding to pressure.

Actually, the performance of the Blues is so superior to that of private commercial insurers that Commissioner Denenberg urged that they be allowed to provide all of the medical insurance in the state. As he phrased it, "As bad as the 'Blues' are, compared with commercial insurance companies, they look like angels."[35] Noting that one commercial insurer in Pennsylvania had returned only seven cents on the premium dollar in 1971, he told Senate investigators: "You could do better in the Pennsylvania lottery." However, neither the Blues nor the commercial carriers have observed any standardized or realistic guidelines for keeping costs at a reasonable level or maintaining quality.

The General Accounting Office recently reviewed the policies that seven paying agents in five states used to detect those instances when a doctor was possibly prescribing unnecessary services. The policies varied widely. One, for example, did question the need for more than four office visits a month; another had not questioned the need for visits unless they exceed ten.[36] Moreover, although the paying agents had identified many physicians who possibly were providing unnecessary services, they had not followed up to find out if the services actually were necessary. One paying agent, for example, identified 539 doctors whose services had exceeded established norms in 1970. It investigated only 12 of them.[37]

The insurance industry is very much involved in the political struggle for a national health plan. There are *billions* at stake. When HEW Secretary Elliot Richardson appeared before a Congressional committee a few years ago, he acknowledged that if the plan that the administration favored was enacted, it would increase the premium income of private health-insurance companies from $23,000,000,000 to $30,000,000,000 in the first year! Other experts regard that as an underestimate. Dr. Rashi Fine of the Harvard Medical School said that the plan would have produced a $12,000,000,000 windfall for the insurance companies and Blue Cross and Blue Shield. This would be more than a 50 percent increase over their current premium income.[38]

Most people, even AMA officials, have accepted the idea that some form of national health insurance is imperative. The principal issue is whether the plan shall benefit chiefly the insurance and health industries or the people of the country. The former have tremendous power and have no intention of surrendering the mine which has yielded such rich ore; for that reason, most of the bills proposed contain the flaws that now exist, erecting barriers between people and health care by expensive deductibles, making no allowance for preventive medicine, imposing no meaningful controls over the profiteers in either industry. Most promising was the bill drafted several years ago by Senator Edward Kennedy and Representative Martha Griffiths, advocating government financing. Senator Kennedy pointed out then that all Americans could receive comprehensive coverage if everyone contributed to a common fund according to their ability to pay. By spreading the risk among the entire population, premiums could be kept at a reasonable level; moreover, no one would be excluded from receiving health care. Public representation would help to insure quality of health care. In his original proposal, he warned:

> Only the government can operate such an insurance program in the best interests of all people. We can no longer afford the health insurance industry in America, and we should not waste public funds bailing it out.
>
> There is no place for profit-making and competition for profits and high salaries in health insurance. These motives are at the root of the failure of the health insurance industry to offer adequate protection to Americans and to assure that the health care system is responsive to America's needs.
>
> Even if we provide comprehensive government programs for the insurance industry's biggest problem cases —such as the poor, the disabled, the elderly, those with chronic diseases—and even if we wrote and enforced complex government regulations to reduce the gaps, the exclusions, and other traps in private insurance, the insurance industry still could not bring about change in the health care system to control costs, improve quality, and

offer health care services in a way most acceptable to the people. The industry would remain a moneychanger taking a percentage of our dollars for a dubious service.

The health insurance industry in its day has brought America a long way toward affording the cost of health care. But its day is past. I believe we should recruit the talented Americans who have operated this industry into the public service to staff a national health security program.[39]

Senator Kennedy was forced to modify his original position, to retreat. But the blueprint offered in the Kennedy-Griffiths Health Security Bill holds out promise of a more effective remedy of the health system's sickness than insurance companies have been able to provide.

15 Group Therapy
for a Sick System

The most dramatic development in Western-style medicine in the last half century was not the introduction of antibiotics, the procedures to transplant hearts and other organs, nor any of the other widely touted "miracles." It was, rather, that doctors began to render health care more effectively and economically by working cooperatively with each other and their patients to keep them well.

The terrible years of the Depression made it possible for many new concepts to be tested to answer social problems. Appropriately enough, the first experiment in prepaid, group-practice medical and hospital programs was launched in a small town in the center of the Dust Bowl by a Syrian immigrant physician. He was aided by the Oklahoma Farmers' Union and some concerned residents, among them a local bank president who had seen "too many farmers wiped out by a doctor's bill" not to encourage insurance against such disasters, however revolutionary the step appeared.[1]

In many respects, Dr. Michael A. Shadid was an unlikely revolutionary leader. He was, in 1929, the very model of a modern American success story. A charity student at the American University of Beirut's preparatory school, he had come to the United States in 1898 on borrowed steerage fare. His goal was to earn his family's fare to the land of opportunity and his own way through college and medical school. He fulfilled both objectives, over almost incredible hardships. While at the School of Medicine of Washington University, he had to scrape and skimp to such extent that one of his professors diagnosed him as "starving."[2] Nevertheless, he obtained his diploma in 1906; and without benefit of internship (he couldn't afford that luxury), he became a solo practitioner, first in Missouri and then in Oklahoma.

Dedicated, intelligent, ambitious, he shaped for himself a life and a career that fulfilled his dreams about the land of opportunity. He married the Syrian girl to whom he had been betrothed at the age of ten, and they had six thoroughly Americanized children, two of whom also became doctors. Although he often took payless leaves to do postgraduate study in Chicago, Philadelphia, even Vienna, the "foreign doctor" prospered. In the late 1920s, when doctors were averaging less than $4000 a year, his income was $20,000. By 1928, he was worth $100,000 and had a financially dazzling future, with a small hospital that enabled him to begin a new career as general surgeon in addition to his lucrative medical practice.

He was troubled about the fee-for-service "philosophy" of organized medicine, and the fee splitting and racketeering it encouraged among the greedy. He had seen doctors at their best, dedicated and competent like the Pennsylvanian who acted as chief surgeon at the university in Beirut. He had also seen, among his classmates and in practice, doctors at their worst. The fee-for-service type of medical care would have to go, he decided. He felt that he would work better and get greatest pleasure if he could forget about money. So could his patients.

Dr. Shadid reasoned that if farmers were willing to pay $100 to become members of the Cooperative Cotton Gin for the financial benefits, they should be willing to invest half that sum in a health cooperative for the medical benefits. The co-op could buy the two existing hospitals in Elk City with the first dues received. Thus, in return for annual dues of $25 for a family or $12 for an individual, members would be entitled to free examinations, medical and surgical care, X-ray and radium treatments, physiotherapy, and all laboratory work carried out at the hospital. Greatly reduced hospital rates could be offered. In 1944, it was only $3 a day for room, board, and general nursing service and 50 cents a day for new-born babies.

He unfolded his plan for the Community Health Association just nine days before the stock market crash of 1929 to an audience of union farmers in the basement of the Elk City Library. When he had finished, the chairman announced, "I'm with you, Doc." Others agreed to join, and a charter for a cooperative hospital capitalized at $100,000 was taken out. Within a few months, 700 had subscribed. They were asked to pay only $10 of the membership share, with the other $40 due in the fall of 1930 when operations would begin. But at that point organized medicine began the attack; 12 local doctors proclaimed in the Elk City *News* that the enterprise was "unethical"; they would never take a patient to the hospital.

Dr. Shadid had no intention of backing down in his crusade. He had a cause he "knew" to be right, a profound belief in himself as a man destined to realize dreams, a genius for attracting loyal followers, a superb talent for public relations. He also had financial resources.

The hospital committee had $10,000 on hand, and Shadid lent $10,000. A $15,000 bank loan was arranged from the Oklahoma Farmers' Union and secured by an insurance policy on Shadid's life. Building went ahead, and on opening day the committee held a barbecue on the hospital grounds for 3000 guests. The climax of the day was the announcement that Dr. Shadid and his assistant would perform free operations for all who needed them over the next four days; the only fees charged were for room, board, nursing care, and anesthesia.

The response provided awesome evidence of the need for the plan. "Most of the cases that came to us seeking relief were of many years' standing," he later reported. Among them were several persons suffering cancer in advanced states: a woman with incurable cancer of the womb who had mortgaged her farm to pay $600 to a couple of "skin disease specialists" for worthless treatments; a woman with cancer of the uterus who had almost bled to death; a man with cancer of the mouth who for some years had been using dentures he had carved out of wood with a jacknife.[3]

Not all in Elk City were delighted with the opening of the new cooperative hospital and health plan. A physician who was a friend of Dr. Shadid and sympathetic to the project arrived at Shadid's house after the hospital had been opened. He brought a notice of a special meeting of the Beckham County Medical Society, "called for the purpose of deciding what to do about the Community Hospital." No notice had been sent directly to Dr. Shadid, although he had been a member in good standing for twenty years.

Though Beckham County Medical Society meetings were often poorly attended, not a member was absent from this meeting. One member urged immediate expulsion: "I'm not going to tolerate foreigners coming over here and telling us how to practice medicine." Another denounced Shadid as an "alien slanderer"; he called the project: "socialism, communism, inciting to revolution, as Dr. Fishbein has correctly stated." Cooler heads warned that if Dr. Shadid were expelled without trial, he would have the right to appeal to the state authority. There was also the possibility of a suit for damages.

The Beckham County Medical Society decided to pursue another course. It was, Dr. James Howard Means of Harvard wrote later, a maneuver of "such fantastic indirection that it is difficult to believe that any members of a reputedly noble profession could bring themselves to perpetrate it upon brother physicians."[4] Members of the society disbanded and reorganized without Dr. Shadid. The next step was to intimidate Dr. Shadid and his assistant by threatening that they were petitioning the State Board of Medical Examiners to revoke their licenses for soliciting patients. But officials of the Farmers' Union obtained the support of Governor "Alfalfa Bill" Murray, who warned that:

> any organization of more than three persons having for its purpose the destruction of the hospital, or its injury, or the taking away of the license of any physician in such hospital will, under the criminal laws, be guilty of conspiracy, and will be prosecuted by direction of the governor by appointment of a special attorney.[5]

Group Therapy for a Sick System

The frontal attacks halted briefly, but the Medical Society continued to exert pressure from other directions. Dr. Shadid could not get malpractice insurance; he found prospective doctors and nurses reluctant to join his staff after they learned from the county medical association that the hospital was "in disrepute" with the medical profession in the state. The *Journal of the American Medical Association* refused for years to list the cooperative's ads for physicians; nor would it list the hospital until threatened with violation of antitrust laws.[6] The state boards joined the opposition: the Board of Nurses, the Board of Dental Examiners, the Board of Medical Examiners. The secretary of the nursing board, Dr. Shadid said, "made a point of warning all nurses taking state board examinations to shy away from us." After a number of doctors and dentists were denied license to practice because they indicated that they wanted to work with Dr. Shadid, the doctor began to instruct professionals who wished to become staff members to state on the examination form that they intended to practice anywhere but in Elk City.[7]

The variety as well as the vindictiveness of the harassment by organized medicine was genuinely astonishing. When Dr. Shadid went to Chicago to take a two-week course on fractures at the Cook County graduate medical school, an institution supported by tax money, he was denied admittance. "These courses are given for 'ethical physicians' only," the registrar told him. By that, of course, he meant duly accredited members of the AMA or local affiliates.

The federal government complied with the doctors representing organized medicine. The Resettlement Administration decided to make loans to people so that they could become members of Dr. Shadid's cooperative. Both the AMA and the Beckham County Medical Society passed resolutions condemning the plan, and sent copies of the protest to the President, Vice-President, and assorted Washington officials. Soon after, the 500 applications that had been approved were cancelled. A substitute plan was put forward under which the families were to pay $25 a year to a common fund for medical care. Each family was to have a "free choice" in selecting his doctor, providing the doctor belonged to the AMA. Doctors would submit monthly bills for their services and be paid out of the common fund. After the common fund was exhausted, Shadid noted, the hospitals turned away clients. In the meantime, however, they and the doctors had been "raiding it as though it were a private gold mine."[8]

Meantime, back in the ranch country where the cooperative was flourishing, the local medical society was working on other plans to ruin the project. The Beckham County doctors persuaded the State Board of Medical Examiners to revoke Dr. Shadid's license because of "unprofessional conduct."

This could have been a major threat to him since no doctor had ever defended himself successfully against the board. Dr. Shadid did, although it took four years. Next, the medical society tried to persuade the state legislature to do away with the cooperative hospital by amending the Medical Practices Act, making it illegal to provide medical care under any name other than a doctor's own name. By way of insuring its passage, the Oklahoma medical societies assessed members $10 each to build up a sizable fund. Fortunately, the cooperative, the Farmers' Union, and Veterans of Industry managed to get a substitute bill on the ballot, which was passed by the voters in 1940.

Still the attacks continued. A state senate investigating committee was set up to investigate the "subversive activities" of Dr. Shadid. During World War II, the medical committee of Beckham County's Procurement and Assignment Service declared every man of military age on the staff of the cooperative hospital "available" for the draft. One son, Dr. Alex Shadid, two dentists, a lab technician, and the hospital's only druggist promptly volunteered for military service. Another son, Dr. Fred Shadid, the only man of military age left, was kept at his hospital post only because a petition signed by 13,000 residents in the area was presented to the President.[9]

After the war the National Foundation for Infantile Paralysis asked Dr. Fred Shadid, then medical director of the hospital, to set up a unit for polio cases. The Beckham County Medical Society announced it would boycott the hospital and persuaded the State Commission for Crippled Children not to recognize the hospital. At that point, the National Foundation sent its regrets that it would not be able to grant money to treat polio victims at the hospital. After newspapers in the area exposed the situation, the Foundation withdrew the regrets and sent support. That was a fortunate decision since a serious polio outbreak occurred soon after, and youngsters from all over southern and western Oklahoma were sent to the cooperative hospital, which was the only one in the area equipped to care for polio victims.

By the summer of 1950, the hospital association decided that the situation had become so "intolerable" that it and 11 individuals filed a $300,000 antitrust suit against the Beckham County Medical Association. The case was finally settled out of court in 1952—ending a struggle of more than 20 years. The Beckham County Medical Society agreed to allow hospital staff doctors to become members and to end its boycott of the hospital. It was, as Dr. Means said later, "clearly a victory for the co-operative";[10] more important, it was a victory for quality medical care in the United States.

Dr. Shadid died in the summer of 1965 at the age of 94. Death came, his son Alex wrote to me later, "while he was playing poker with some cronies." But his idea has been felt far beyond Elk City and the courage he inspired has enabled thousands of doctors to brave the same attacks that his health cooperative experienced.

Despite the vehemence of the AMA's attack on Dr. Shadid, the principle of group practice was not a novel medical idea in the United States. The Mayo, Hitchcock, and Lahey clinics, for example, as well as large teaching hospitals had demonstrated that doctors working together provided care of far higher quality than solo practitioners. Dr. Will Mayo held group practice "a scientific cooperation for the welfare of the sick," emphasizing its role in lengthening "by many years the span of human life" and in improving ethics in the profession by "overcoming some of the evils of competitive medicine."[11]

Why had the AMA concentrated its opposition to group practice against the little Elk City hospital of Michael Shadid rather than the clinic of Will and Charlie Mayo?

The answer is partly that he was an easier target. The AMA was too skilled in the uses of power to oppose a couple of its former presidents who had captured the loyalty of the country and who had given American surgery an international reputation. Also, though the Mayos has violated a number of cardinal principles of organized medicine—patients were treated by doctors of the clinic's choice; physicians were hired and fired like ordinary men and worked for wages—the Mayos did not tamper with the "sacred" doctor-patient financial relationship; charges were what the Mayos deemed proper.[12] Nor did the Mayos practice preventive medicine. Therefore, on the occasions when charges of "unethical conduct" were brought against the Mayos by local medical societies, the brothers were "always exonerated" by the judicial councils of the Minnesota State Medical Society and the AMA.

The Elk City cooperative was not a wild idea either. In 1932 one of the most distinguished committees ever appointed to scrutinize medical care in the United States had approved its manner of operating. The committee was headed by a former AMA president and included some of the nation's most distinguished private practitioners, public health experts, economists, and laymen. It was financed by the Carnegie Corporation, the Julius Rosenwald Fund, the Russell Sage Foundation, and the Twentieth Century Fund. The committee studied the medical experience of 8700 families and other aspects of health care in the United States over a period of five years. It recommended:

---

1. That medical services, both preventive and therapeutic, should be furnished largely by organized groups of physicians, dentists, nurses, pharmacists, and other associated personnel, organized preferably around a hospital, for rendering complete home, office, and hospital care;

2. That the costs of medical care be placed on a group

prepayment basis through the use of insurance, through the use of taxation or both of those methods;

3. That the study, evaluation, and coordination of medical services be considered important functions of every state and local community; that agencies be formed to exercise those functions; and that coordination of rural and urban services receive special attention.[13]

The AMA rushed to defend the minority of the committee who dissented. Dr. Morris Fishbein, then editor of the *JAMA* and the organization's chief spokesman, denounced the majority report as "incitement to revolution" and branded group practice prepayment plans as "medical soviets."[14]

In spite of the warning, the plans continued to spread, often with many variations. Among them have been group plans set up by participating doctors. One of the earliest was founded by a Scottish physician, Dr. Donald Ross, and Dr. H. Clifford Loos, the gifted and socially concerned doctor-brother of the author of *Gentlemen Prefer Blondes*. While Anita Loos was making stage history, her brother and Dr. Ross were making medical history with a plan to provide prepaid medical and surgical care to 400 employees of the Los Angeles Water and Power Department in 1929. That two-man partnership has grown into one of the most prestigious group health plans in the country.

Another was the industry-sponsored Kaiser Foundation–Permanente Medical Group program. It was begun in 1933 by Dr. Sidney Garfield, a young surgeon who had recently completed his residency at the Los Angeles County Hospital, and a few colleagues. They went into the southern California desert to provide medical service for construction crews building the Colorado River aqueduct, 200 miles away from the nearest doctor. The physicians started work on the orthodox fee-for-service basis; but within a few months, the 15-bed hospital they had built on borrowed funds was facing financial collapse. When the contractors heard that the hospital might have to be closed, they joined the doctors in persuading insurance carriers to change the method of paying for industrial injuries to a prepayment plan. The seemingly modest sum of $1.50 was set as the monthly charge for each worker, but it was enough to alter the doctors' financial condition so dramatically that they soon could offer to cover nonindustrial illness and injury for a similar fee. Before the aqueduct was completed, the medical group had increased staff and services and had built two more small hospitals.

Equally dramatic was the change in the doctors' attitude toward patients. Dr. Garfield reported later:

> When we were on a fee-for-service basis, we had been anxious to have injured cases admitted to the hospital since that meant income and continued existence. Under this prepaid arrangement, we received the same amount of funds regardless, and we became anxious to keep those men uninjured.[15]

The experience was repeated several years later, when Edgar Kaiser asked Dr. Garfield to provide medical service for the 5000 men working on the Grand Coulee Dam. There, a plan for caring for workers' families was added, at a cost of 50 cents a week for adults and 25 cents for each child. In the early stages, the plan threatened to be a loss; people found it hard to shake off fears of "company doctors," a breed as disreputable as company storekeepers. But confidence grew so rapidly that by the time the Grand Coulee project was completed 90 percent of the families had enrolled. Again, Dr. Garfield was impressed by the "noticeable change" in the severity of illness: "We no longer saw seriously ill women and children. Terminal pneumonias became early pneumonias, ruptured appendices became simple appendices; mastoiditis and diphtheria practically disappeared." The reason was simple, as he pointed out: patients go to doctors sooner when there is no cost barrier.

By 1973, the Kaiser–Permanente program was offering service to more than 2,000,000 subscribers in the western states and Hawaii, offering them what *Fortune* and *Time*, along with other journals, has called more complete protection than is available from most other forms of U.S. medical insurance.[16]

Other rural and farm health cooperatives were organized, after the pattern set in Elk City. The first urban cooperative was established in Washington, D.C., in 1937, when a group of Home Owners Loan Corporation employees formed the Group Health Association. Other cities began to sponsor health plans, including New York. The Health Insurance Plan of Greater New York (HIP) was begun because of the interest of Mayor LaGuardia. Originally underwritten by loans from private foundations, that has become one of the largest groups in the country. In 1945, the Labor Health Institute of St. Louis was organized to provide quality care for workers and their families, with emphasis on preventive medicine and early treatment. And in 1946, the United Mine Workers organized a health-care program after a survey revealed that health services in an eight-county area were "so poor that their tolerance is a disgrace to a nation to which the world looks for pattern and guidance."[17] Even that plan was fought by the AMA.

The largest and most impressive of the health plans modeled after Dr. Shadid's is the Group Health Cooperative of Puget Sound. In his excellent study, *Group Practice & Prepayment of Medical Care*, one of the founders, Dr. William A. MacColl, describes the history of that and other groups along with the successes and problems.

Sparked by a speech given by Dr. Shadid, in 1945 a group of people interested in establishing a cooperative health program group joined with a group of physicians to take over a hospital and set up a clinic, and begin operation as a prepayment group-practice plan. Under the joint direction of laymen and physicians, the goal was to make coverage as comprehensive as possible. The Puget Sound cooperative became the first of the plans to cover all laboratory and X-ray charges, the cost of prescribed drugs, and the fees customarily added for anesthesia and other hospital services. Patients benefited to such extent that within a year the staff and facilities were becoming hard-pressed to handle new members. The doctors also benefited, personally and professionally, since the contract also recognized "that the physician apt to practice the best medicine was one who had time for relaxation, study, his family, post-graduate courses and participation in community affairs."[18]

What the Group Health Cooperative of Puget Sound means in human terms is best illustrated by the recent three-year ordeal of Leif E. Grefsrud, a thirty-six-year-old engineer at Boeing who suffered burns over 75 percent of his body after gasoline in a car on which he had been working ignited, enveloping him in flames. Grefsrud spent six months in the handsome new hospital of the cooperative attended by special nurses constantly for two and a half of those months. In addition to his regular doctor's treatment, surgeons performed eight skin grafts; specialists provided physical therapy; he was given drugs, intravenous feedings, and much laboratory work. For several years after leaving the hospital, he had to return at intervals for plastic surgery on his fingers, arms, and ears.[19]

The price? Experts estimate the treatment might have cost Grefsrud at least $25,000 to $50,000. But it cost him only the $40-a-month premium that all members paid at the time for themselves and their families.

Every one of the prepayment, group-practice plans encountered the kind of attack that was directed by the AMA and its affiliates against the Elk City cooperative. Participating professionals were harassed and the AMA had laws passed to prohibit their practice. Most of them had to take legal action to survive.

The first of what has been characterized as "some of the most bitter legal battles of recent medical history"[20] occurred in the nation's capital after the District of Columbia Medical Society, with the backing of the AMA, denounced GHA as a socialistically inspired plot to introduce European compulsory health insurance into America. The Department of Justice intervened on behalf of the HOLC employees, warning the medical society that legal action would be instituted if the attacks were not stopped. They were not; and on December 20, 1938, a federal grand jury indicted the AMA, three affiliates, and 21 individual physicians, including Dr. Fishbein, for violating the Sherman Antitrust Act. The AMA protested in the *JAMA* about the "persecution of the medical profession."[21] The evidence submitted by the Department of Justice, however, was highly damaging to AMA claims. An example of the way in which the local society had undertaken to restrain trade was the expulsion of a doctor who had been working with GHA. In another case, a specialist had been threatened with expulsion merely for consulting with a GHA doctor. Assistant Attorney General Thurman Arnold reported that doctors who had joined the cooperative had been barred from local hospitals, even in emergency cases. The "illegal activities" of organized medicine in the capital, he said, were "typical of what has occurred in other cities throughout the country whenever cooperative health groups have been formed."[22]

A verdict of guilty on the criminal charge of conspiracy was handed down in 1941 against the AMA and the District society. The former was fined $2500; the later, $1500. The case continued on through the U.S. Court of Appeals, where a unanimous decision was handed down against the appellants, in which it was pointed out that medicine's licensed monopoly enjoys severe restraints upon competition:

> But they are restraints which depend upon capacity and training, not special privilege. Neither do they justify concerted criminal action to prevent the people from developing new methods of serving their needs.[23]

The case was finally ended in 1943, when the U. S. Supreme Court affirmed the conviction of the lower court.[24]

Four years later the Complete Service Bureau of San Diego, a health cooperative, brought suit against the county medical society for its attempts to "poison the minds of the public against nonmembers of the society." A widespread rumor campaign had been organized: "The society members, nurses, employees, and members of their families frequently cause to circulate belittling and derogatory remarks about non-members, referring to them as quacks and their groups as 'outfits' and the prepaid medical plan as a 'scheme.' " That cooperative also won its case.[25] So did the Group Health Cooperative of Puget Sound against the King

County Medical Society and related defendants. In an appeal from a lower court decision, attorneys for members of the cooperative described the tactics and techniques employed by organized medicine. Aside from slandering the doctors and staff members of the cooperatives, the medical society refused to admit them to membership. It threatened to expel any member of the society "guilty" of consulting with doctors who worked in the cooperative. Members of the medical society threatened hospitals with ruin if they allowed the doctors who were members of cooperatives to use their facilities, often making the threats in the most direct and crude manner. Thus, during the trial of one of the King County Medical Society members, Dr. M. J. Schultz was questioned about threats that had been made to commissioners of the Renton hospital. He answered:

> Q. I suppose that you told the commissioners of the hospital that is what you would have to do if the hospital were opened up to non-members?

> A. We not only told them. I threatened that we would walk out and pull every patient out and leave them go broke.

> Q. You told that to Mr. Wright?

> A. I told him that we would just have to take our patients out; there wouldn't be enough in the hospital to keep it operating in the black, over the red mark, like we do now. . . . If seventeen Renton doctors, or twenty, would take our patients out and leave a matter of five or six patients . . . the hospital would go broke in a hurry. And the commissioners realized it. . . .[26]

Similar threats had been made successfully to the Seattle General Hospital, Children's Orthopedic Hospital, the Swedish Hospital, and others in the Seattle area. They accordingly had denied even emergency privileges to the cooperative's medical and surgical staff. Additionally, doctors are required by their professional code to seek consultation when a question arises about patient care. But the society's opposition to sharing knowledge and skill was so stiff that only a few members were willing to brave expulsion by consulting a qualified doctor who might be a member of the staff of a cooperative.

In its decision in 1951 in favor of the group health cooperative, the state supreme court said: "In our opinion, the Society may not, through the mere use of the term 'unethical,' clothe with immunity acts which would otherwise fall under the ban of the antimonopoly provision of our constitution."[27]

Other group-practice plans experienced the threats made to the Elk City cooperative during World War II. Since representatives of the AMA and its affiliates only could serve on the Procurement and Assignment Service's medical advisory group, they had the sole authority to determine which doctors were essential to civilian service and which were not. One doctor told a Senate subcommittee that he had been warned orally that if there was any attempt to make prepaid medical care available to Kaiser shipyard workers' families, doctors on his staff would be classified as "eligible" for armed service.[28]

Because of these tactics not all of the early prepayment group-practice plans survived the assaults of organized medicine. Those who did, as Jerry Voorhis, former president of the Cooperative League of the USA and one of the founders of the Group Health Association of America, said recently, had to survive "the hard way"—thanks to the courage of the doctors and the "earnest commitment" of members of the cooperatives, imaginative union leaders like Walter Reuther, and the integrity of those politicians at the state and federal level who refused to condone the program mapped out by the AMA.

Although the AMA officially did an about-face regarding prepaid group-practice plans in 1949, it still permitted local and state affiliates to harass them; and in more than half the states restrictive laws made it impossible to start one.[29]

Pressed to cope with rising welfare costs, in 1970 a number of states began to authorize contracts to Prepaid Health Plan organizations to provide care for the poor. A new stimulus to their establishment was given in December 1973, when ex-President Nixon signed into law the Health Maintenance Organizations legislation, offering them as an option to individuals and families because the experimental HMOs had demonstrated themselves so successful. (More than 60 were providing services to about 5,000,000 enrollees at the time the bill was signed; another 3,000,000 were served by plans less comprehensive than HMOs or more restricted in the field of membership.)

Unfortunately, many of those set up did not adhere to the standards set down by the Group Health Association of America, but were regarded as simply another means to loot the public purse. Many, masquerading as nonprofit operations, were boasting about the kinds of returns investors could reap—as much as 2500 or 3000 percent on their money.[30] Medical and lay hustlers alike joined the gold rush. In Southern California (where PHPs, as the HMOs are commonly called) widespread protest has been made about some of the profiteering plans, the methods of enrolling patients and the kind and quality of services provided. At a hearing I attended in 1973, it was revealed that some of the plans had commission salesmen and women—some of whom were dressed in hospital uniforms—canvassing low-income neighborhoods, telling householders that the law required all Medicare and Medicaid patients to sign up. Other salesmen and saleswomen were reported to be identifying themselves as welfare workers; more blatant types of promoters sent trucks through poor neighborhoods, offering fried chicken dinners and other inducements to anyone who would sign up.

Rewards were rich for the salespersons as well as the contractors, many of whom have been doctors. Services, although legally required to be comprehensive, were sometimes of the sketchiest sort. One large group provided no emergency care of any kind; clinic offices were not open after five or on weekends. Many, including one of the largest, had "inadequate numbers of physicians, on the whole inadequately prepared to provide a reasonable range of modern medical services, and hospitals that are generally inadequate," according to Dr. Lester Breslow, dean of the school of public health at the University of California at Los Angeles.[31] A number of the contractors were using the emergency rooms of public hospitals; a number of them were finding the plans a sure way to cash in on their own hospital investments. One doctor–contractor was sending patients to his own hospital—a hospital that had been denied accreditation by the Joint Commission on Accreditation of Hospitals because the structure was so flimsy that fire could consume it before bedridden patients could get out.

The price for the services provided by some of the profiteering plans was sometimes very high. Two of the largest in the state, each with about 100,000 members, were sending in bills well above those of the regular Medi-Cal program—a practice forbidden by state law.[32]

The shoddy HMOs are a far cry from plans like Kaiser–Permanente or the Group Health Association of Washington or the Group Health Cooperative of Puget Sound. All of those, as well as other members of the Group Health Association, provide a wide range of high-quality services at reasonable cost, placing emphasis on preventive medicine and early diagnosis. For instance, the Kaiser–Permanente plan provides comprehensive hospitalization benefits for illnesses and injuries in one of the Kaiser Foundation hospitals; unlimited visits to Permanente doctors for diagnosis and treatment, specialists' care, physical checkups, and physical therapy, as well as laboratory tests, and X-ray examinations. Drugs are provided at low cost. (The Puget Sound Cooperative provides them as part of the services.) Psychiatric care for mental illness or disorder is covered; so is emergency care 24 hours a day at any of the foundation's excellent hospitals. If illness occurs during a trip or temporary absence, reimbursement is provided by the plan.

Patients have almost complete freedom to choose the doctor they want. Some laymen may know how to select quality doctors; most of us have only the vaguest idea. At Kaiser standards are kept very high: the probation period for each doctor is relatively long, doctors who don't measure up are dropped, and the performance of those who do is constantly scrutinized. Decisions about serious surgery are made by several doctors, and even the diagnostic and prescribing practices of doctors in the group are reviewed. Nor are the doctors impersonal. As one of them explained his attitude: "I can become more personally involved in a patient's case when there isn't the problem of money between us."

Commenting on the quality of the outstanding group-practice plans, Dr. Alan Gregg of the Rockefeller Foundation, a medical philosopher as well as practitioner, observed some years ago:

> The service given a patient by group practice gains in quality by the criticism of the other members of the group whether the criticism be tacit or fully expressed. Whether we realize it or not the presence of merely a competent nurse tends to raise the doctor's level of performance. Reluctant as an anxious patient may be to think that his doctor above all people might ever need the stimulus of competent critics, the fact remains that doctors sometimes do need and usually respond well to the realization that their work is observable and observed.[33]

The economic benefits group medical practice can provide are impressive. The Twentieth Century Fund estimated a few years ago that *the application of group health economies to all medical practice would cut the costs of health care in the United States by almost 50 percent.*[34] In California, where about 20 percent of those eligible for Medi-Cal benefits were enrolled in prepaid health plans by 1973, it was estimated that a potential savings of $150,-000,000 to $300,000,000 a year could be effected if the other eligibles elected them instead of fee-for-service medicine.[35] Hospital admissions are much lower because doctors are not encouraged to indulge in and order them for personal gain. Most important, the mortality rates of those who belong to group-practice plans are much lower than among the general population. In 1963, a demographic analysis of the membership of Group Health Association of Washington, D.C., for a three-year period showed an annual death rate three times lower than that of the whole country.[36]

In summary, that most essential concern of any system of medical care was revealed years ago in an exchange between Senator Claude Pepper and Kaiser's Dr. Garfield during the hearings on procurement policies. Dr. Garfield said:

> The most amazing part of the whole thing was that when

we had the plan started and in operation, people stopped dying. That sounds funny, but actually what it meant was that they came to us. . . .

Senator Pepper provoked some bitter laughter in the hearing room when he interrupted to ask: "You don't mean that the American Medical Association opposed a plan which made it possible for the people to stop dying, do you?"[37]

Unfortunately, that was the way of things.

16 How Other Countries Manage Health Care

Residents of truly wonderful Copenhagen are proud of the city's Tivoli Gardens, zoo, Deer Park, Schumann Circus, museums, and the statue of the "Little Mermaid," but they are even prouder of their country's services for its people. Several summers ago, our family boarded a bus for a "life-seeing" trip, to find out about those services.

Before shifting into first gear, the driver gave us an introductory talk, explaining the significance of the schools, the child care centers, the apartments for elderly persons, the hospitals, playgrounds, and other public facilities we were to see. Those things, he said, do make for relatively high taxes; but they make it possible for Danes to pursue happiness wholeheartedly and lightheartedly. He said with enormous pride that no Dane has to worry that sickness in the family will not be treated or that the treatment will wipe out the family's life savings. For very small annual sums, the government guarantees that when need arises all health care bills will be paid: hospital, medical and surgical, drugs, and other items.

A young American sitting nearby, who had been frowning, spoke up sharply: "But that's socialized medicine." The driver looked at him thoughtfully for a few minutes before replying mildly: "You, sir, may call it *socialized*, if you will. In Denmark, we prefer to call it *civilized*."

Today, no advanced country in the world is without some type of what the AMA scathingly denounces as "socialized medicine." Many of the more backward—even feudal—nations have also come to regard government-sponsored medical and hospital programs as a mark of civilization in the twentieth century. Among them is the little oil-rich kingdom of Kuwait, which has perhaps the most socialized medical system in the world. In 1950 the country had only four doctors; by the middle of the 1960s it had one for every 700 inhabitants, a high ratio, and more hospital beds than it needed. The government pays all medical expenses for everyone, including transients. Even the animals are protected: a Bedouin nomad wandering into a populated center with a sick camel can obtain free veterinary service for the beast.[1]

Needless to say, persons detecting any resemblance between the Kuwait government and socialistic or communistic control can only be considered to be envisioning a mirage.

So many slanted reports have been circulated by the medical establishment about the health-care programs sponsored by governments in other countries that it is not surprising that Americans have been deluded into believing that they are no good. Those who do know have, for the most part, very different attitudes. Two episodes brought those differences to our attention some years ago.

One occurred at a party in Los Angeles, when the wife of an attorney told us of her difficulties in getting her citizenship papers. A New Zealander, she had met her husband during World War II. They married and came to the United States. A decade later, she decided that this country was "it" and that she wanted to make it her homeland. All went well during the citizenship examination until she was asked her opinion of the "socialistic" health-care system. When she said that she thought it was fine, the examiner terminated the interview with the recommendation that she "think things over and come back next year." She did; and although her opinion had not changed, she answered more evasively and was admitted to all rights and privileges.

The second episode took place some years later at Paestum, a coastal town in southern Italy near some glorious ruins left by the ancient Greeks during their expansionist movement centuries ago.

It was not a full-fledged tourist resort, although some of the shopkeepers and hotel and motel owners were hoping that it would become one "when people realize that you could have archaeology and wonderful bathing, too." Chief hopeful was the man who had the bathing house concession at the beach, a rather tacky operation in which he took great pride. After we became acquainted, we expressed some concern about his ability to weather out the waiting period until word about the place spread. "Oh, we make our living in England," he explained. He and his brother had a fish-and-chips place in Brighton; each of them and their families spent six months at home. "We will always keep that," he added. "The medical treatment in England is so fine that we will always have to have that."

If, like most Americans, our family had been misled about the British health-care system, it is small wonder. The American Medical Association has spent enormous sums to insure that our thinking was confused since the National Health Service plan in the United Kingdom has been its chief target.

Even before the passage of the National Health Service Act of 1946, the AMA was denouncing the proposed legislation as a plot to "enslave" the British medical profession and "make every one of its physicians a clock-watching civil servant."[2] The *JAMA* printed many articles and comments of doctors about the plan which the British Medical Association repeatedly protested as "misleading and inaccurate." The BMA held one account of an American doctor before a U.S. Senate Committee to be a "gross libel."[3] Other medical publications as well as general circulation magazines have given inordinate space to non-medical critics of the British program—principally John and Sylvia Jewkes and C. Northcote Parkinson, that delightful practitioner of Blimpmanship whose satirical attacks on bureaucracy are best sellers on both sides of the Iron Curtain.[4]

Those Americans who have had experience with British health care have generally expressed gratitude. Fairly typical was the reaction of William P. Keim, who spent a year as a visiting professor at Langside College in Glasgow in the 1960s. During that time his wife had to undergo major surgery for a lung tumor.

Commenting on the quality and cost of the care she received, Keim said: "I am convinced that the only freedom lost under National Health is the freedom of the doctors and dentists to charge all that the traffic will bear."[5] Nor is government medicine the impersonal, patronizing experience it is held to be. Another example —this one cited by Roul Tunley in *The American Health Scandal*—sheds some light on that aspect of British health care. When a retired journalism teacher and his wife landed in London as first stop on their first Grand Tour, he was stricken with a heart attack that kept him bedded in St. Thomas Hospital for three weeks—where the nurses said "Thank you" when they performed such services for him as changing his bed, bathing him, or even bringing him a cup of tea. When he was dismissed at the end of three weeks, he owed not a shilling for medical, hospital, nursing care, for X rays, tests, physical therapy. His comment to Tunley: "How is it possible to express gratitude [for help] given so graciously and freely to a stranger? There are no words for it."[6]

Nor are the British people confused about the value of the National Health Service, despite their grumblings about long waits, not enough service, and similar complaints. Since its inception, no serious aspirant for public office—Conservative, Liberal, or Labour—has remotely suggested abandoning it. In the 1960s, Dame Patricia Hornsby-Smith, one of the leading Conservative members of Parliament, startled American audiences prepared to hear the worst with the comment that: "If our health services, which are more comprehensive than Medicare, came up for a vote, 97 percent of the British people would vote to retain it."[7]

Nor do most British physicians have a desire to return to the old days. To be sure, many of them—an estimated 400 a year— are attracted to Canada and the United States by the rich rewards to be found in medical practice in those countries. (But since those countries attract many more from such underdeveloped countries as India and Mexico, where medicine is not socialized, that can scarcely be considered a condemnation of the *system.*) And many British doctors, chiefly the nation's General Practitioners, protest that they are underpaid and overworked in contrast to the hospital specialists who enjoy high salaries and regular hours and holidays.

However, in that situation they are the authors of their own woes since they insisted that their "professional integrity" could be maintained only if they were permitted to make private contracts as individuals to provide services for particular individuals in the traditional small-businessman pattern of medical practice.

The need for a comprehensive health-care program was brought home to Britain by World War II as a national security measure, since people were principal national "resources." A first step had been taken in 1601 with the enactment of the Poor Laws, which made it mandatory that local governments set up institutions to shelter the aged, the sick, the insane.

Before that, caring for the sick had been a religious and moral affair. Christianity imposed the moral obligation to care for the "blessed" sick, as Dr. Henry E. Sigerist has pointed out in *The Sociology of Medicine*.[8] Believers became hospital and health facility builders; religious orders evolved that were dedicated to nursing the sick; religious individuals devoted themselves to medical missionary work as a sure route to Heaven, since caring for the ill was an ultimate expression of charity, that highest of virtues.

Like other virtues, however, it was less easily practiced than preached. And when the pattern of feudal life—the castle, the church, the cluster of peasant huts—was obliterated by sprawling, lusty, and filthy cities, it became obvious that religion could not do the job of protecting public health; the economic and political consequences of bad health were too great to leave to individual consciences.

The Poor Law institutions were not much help, thanks to the frugality of prosperous Britishers who blessed the poor and the sick on Sunday with religious fervor, but rejected on all other days the idea that their "good" money be spent to improve the lot of the less fortunate.

During the nineteenth century, conditions became so bad in Britain as in other parts of western Europe that clergymen, writers, some medical experts, and the newly emerging trade unionists raised a clamor for reform. However, it was not until 1911 that the foundations of comprehensive national health care were laid with the Health Insurance Act. That authorized benefits in kind and cash for workers during periods of sickness; medical benefits included only the services of a general practitioner, not specialists or hospital care.

During World War II, the nation's health resources, along with all others, were mobilized to meet the threat of invasion and to cope with the devastation wrought by the bombing of Britain. In 1940, the Emergency Medical Service was set up to utilize all hospitals and medical services. The EMS worked so well that at war's end the government was called upon (partly because the country was in such bad financial shape) to operate the nation's hospitals and medical schools.[9]

Demand for an extension of coverage resulted in the National Health Service Act of 1946. That had as its goals: (1) to provide complete medical care for all people; (2) to promote health; (3) to prevent disease. Aneurin Bevan, its chief architect, hailed Parliamentary approval as "the greatest single health measure of our history."[10] Corresponding acts were approved in Scotland and Nothern Ireland, with slight variations in administrative structures. On July 5, 1948, when all municipal and voluntary hospitals were transferred to the various governments, the National Health Services began operating throughout the United Kingdom.

In scope and financing, the services are much like the public school system in the United States. Predicated on the notion that a democratic government has the obligation of providing all citizens with adequate health care, all who are able must pay to guarantee that right. The costs are met through taxes—just as all persons in the United States are taxed to support public schools, whether or not they have children and whether or not they elect to send their youngsters to private schools. Also, as with our public school system, no person is forced to use the public health and medical services. Harley Street doctors and private practitioners at other addresses are available for persons who prefer them. Private hospitals and nursing homes may be used by anyone wishing and willing to pay for them privately. Not finally, as with our public school system, the National Health Services represent cooperation between laymen and professionals and coordination of local and central agencies.

All aspects of health care are under the Ministry of Health; however, much responsibility has been delegated to the Regional Hospital Boards, Local Health Authorities, and the Executive Councils. The hospital boards were created so that the hospital and specialist services in each area would be associated with a university medical school—an association that has been demonstrated as vital to modern medical practice. The 148 local health authorities are in charge of providing such services as maternity and child welfare, midwifery, health visiting, home nursing, vaccination and immunization, ambulances, health centers, preventive medicine programs—including mental illness. They also provide domestic help when it is needed because of sickness. The 138 executive councils in England and Wales supervise the medical, dental, optical, and pharmaceutical services. They decide the number of professionals who may participate in an area (a help toward solving the problem of maldistribution); they also investigate complaints about the services provided by them and have the right to disqualify practitioners who do not meet the standards.[11]

Great freedom of choice obtains. Patients may choose any doctor they wish, provided that he is enrolled in the service and that he agrees to attend them. Patients may change doctors simply by filling out a new card with the new practitioner. Doctors have equal latitude; they are free to accept or reject patients at their own discretion (except in emergency cases). Their enrollment in the service does not prevent them from attending private, paying patients, and about 70 percent do. The fees thus collected supplement the money they receive from the government, a modest sum for each patient on their lists. To encourage equitable distribution, doctors may not have more than 3500 patients on their lists.

The British plan differs chiefly from those of other medically advanced western European nations in that doctors are not paid fees for particular services: the GPs are paid according to the number of patients on their lists, the hospital-based specialists are on salaries. Moreover, it has jettisoned the insurance principle on the grounds that health care is as much a public service as a post office or a fire department or a public school. Patients, however, are free to supplement government benefits with private insurance to cover special services.

But even where the insurance principle is maintained and where doctors technically charge a fee for a service rendered, the government maintains control over the insurance funds, insures that medical treatment is available to all, and operates the hospitals so that they are healing centers rather than doctors' "workshops."

Germany, which has one of the highest reputations in the world as regards the quality of medical care, is a case in point. The "oldest" government program began in Germany under Bismarck, who has long been regarded by the AMA as the author of its deepest woes, the "diabolical scheme" to foist socialized medicine upon an unsuspecting people. Actually, Bismarck's health insurance program was designed primarily to halt the socialist movement in Germany in the nineteenth century. Having deprived all political action groups of freedom of assembly and freedom of the press, he believed that he needed some kinds of social security to eliminate the threat to the state caused by workers' social insecurity. One of the measures to remedy that was the Sickness Insurance Act of 1883, providing benefits for medical care, maternity cases, and funerals; it also allowed workers to draw money in cases of sickness or accident for up to 13 weeks, at which point their disability insurance program was effective.[12]

German health care is largely funded by worker-employee money paid to about 2000 nonprofit "sickness funds" based on types of work: e.g., a taxi driver would pay into a taxi drivers' fund. Special government funds cover those who are not so classified; but about 85 percent of the people are. The financial burden is the hospital program, assumed chiefly by local governments.

In return for the nonprofit insurance premiums, workers have all doctors' bills completely paid, total hospital bills paid for up to a year, basic dentistry at no cost, free maternity benefits, prescriptions for only pennies whatever the cost of the drug, and even free rest cures when ordered by a doctor. In addition, they receive cash sickness benefits from the first day of illness.[13]

One of the interesting aspects of the program is that general practitioners do not make much lower sums than specialists—a cause of profound unrest in most other countries; and all German doctors are handsomely rewarded even though there is no shortage in that country since German medical schools turn out a very large number of graduates each year.

Sweden, too, which has had compulsory health insurance—"socialized medicine"—since 1955, has a high ratio of doctors. It has placed great emphasis on remedying the consequence of disease on living conditions rather than simply offering medical services. Thus, its primary concerns have been to offer cash benefits to the ill and their families, free hospitalization up to two years, reimbursement of doctors' fees up to three-quarters of a standard fee schedule; free lifesaving drugs, such as insulin and some hormones, and others largely subsidized by the government.[14]

It has focused much attention on early health care: free treatment is given to mothers and children at health centers in towns and stations in rural areas; the School Health Service, which begins where Child Welfare Service ends, works actively to maintain the health of school children and to implant hygienic habits in them. All beginning school children are medically examined; every child between six and fifteen is given a complete annual dental overhaul at no charge.[15]

The glory of the Swedish system is its hospitals, among the most coherently and carefully planned institutions of their kind in the world. Radiating out from the central general hospital in each county are other general hospitals of smaller size, an epidemic hospital, geriatric clinic or hospital, nursing homes for chronically ill, nursing homes for mentally ill, schools for mentally deficient persons, and homes for mentally deficient persons. Such gradations encourage economical use of appropriate facilities; they encourage quality since all are staffed by specialists working on salary full time.

Norway, which established a government plan to insure the entire population in 1956 not only for citizens but for all who have established residence in the country, also provides comprehensive health-care service and has also introduced innovations.

In Norway as in Sweden and many other countries, coverage is not total. The patient must pay 60 to 65 percent of the cost of the first and second visits to the doctor. For subsequent visits, the program pays full costs or close to that sum. And if the illness requires expensive examinations and treatments, the patient's part of the fee is reduced: "People should not be financially penalized because they become seriously sick," according to the program's philosophy. When a patient is hospitalized, the program pays all the bills. Maternity care is covered; physiotherapy, convalescent and rehabilitative care are provided—including occupational training and even school expenses. Because the vast sparsely populated areas create special problems, if a patient is too ill to make the journey to the nearest hospital or physician's office, the insurance program pays the doctor to go to him. If he can make the journey, he is reimbursed for necessary transportation expenses. If he must live away from home while receiving treatment, his insurance covers the cost of a stay in one of the "sick hotels" Norway has pioneered.

Other important protections are guaranteed. In addition to maternity benefits, cash allowances cover lying-in expenses and simple, but dignified funerals. Sick workers and their families are compensated for salary losses. "Essential" drugs are covered.

Financed by workers, their employers, local communities, and the national government, the Norwegian program has never been seriously opposed by any group. Unlike other forms of taxation, Dr. Karl Evang, a director-general of Norway's Health Services, pointed out recently, the health insurance premium "enjoys popularity." People do not object to buying medical security for themselves and their families at a very reasonable price.

"Socialized medicine" in Norway, as in Britain, Sweden, Germany, and other countries in western Europe, offers dramatic rebuttal to the typical objections to national medical programs that have been raised by the AMA: charges of lowered quality; destruction of the physicians' incentives to improve their skill; restriction of doctors' freedom; "bureaucratic" paper work; and breakdown of doctor-patient relationships. Have the sums Norway has invested in health-care services been a "sound" investment? Through Dr. Evang, the country has answered that:

> Money has, as we know, no value in itself. It is a con-
> venient yardstick for a large number of material values.
> But the health and life of an individual, as well as the
> health of the nation, cannot be measured by that yardstick.
> If we, entrusted with protecting and defending the health
> of the population, give in to a salesman's scale of values,
> we are lost.[16]

We have given in to that salesman's scale of values largely because the AMA has successfully persuaded us that to do otherwise would be to court socialism or communism. But politics and health services are very different things.

Anyone who imagines that Russia is medically unsophisticated simply hasn't been reading scientific journals, or even the conservative popular press. The Russians, too, are transplanting hearts and other organs and talking about brain transplants; they too, are using computers, electronic devices, nuclear medicine. They, too, have plastic bone banks and advanced drug therapy.

Perhaps more important, they have one of the finest systems of preventive medical care in the world, and certainly the most massive system of national health care. They have an ample supply of doctors—one of every five of the world's 2,500,000 physicians is a Russian. And these doctors are supplemented by another 500,000 paramedics, *feldshers*. According to an article in *Life* a few years ago, the feldshers constitute "a benevolent army of paramedics."[17] Most of them women, they study basic medicine for two to four years. Ranking between the nurse and the doctor on the professional scale, they serve as doctors' aides or on their own in rural areas; they watch over sanitation and hygiene, conduct routine physical examinations, administer mass immunization programs, give emergency care, and direct more serious cases to hospitals.

Other Communist countries have made use of paramedics and have stressed health education and other methods of preventive medicine to good effect. Among them notably is China. Members of the entourage that traveled to Peking with ex-President Nixon were astounded by the kind and quality of medical care they found there—delivered by highly trained physicians and "bare-foot doctors" alike.

Health care is highly politicized in China. For example, the fight against venereal disease has been waged with exhortations to workers that VD belongs "to the old" and that the new society "can't afford" to take up with such diseases.[18] The health care policy and goals are undoubtedly shaped in Peking; importantly, witnesses agree, they work. Indeed, as Dr. Leon Cooper, former director of health affairs for the Office of Economic Opportunity, told delegates to an International Health Conference in 1973, the "attitudinal fixation" has aided the organization of an efficient health-care delivery system in a relatively short period of time. One of ten physicians whose tour of China was sponsored by the National Medical Association, he prefaced his comments with the assertion that he had not been *brainwashed*: "It's just that the system was so impressive."[19]

Basically, the system contrasts with United States medicine in that in China it is not a "business." The sophisticated specialist and the barefoot doctor he has trained are alike "medical workers," who perform their duties as a state service. As United States-trained Dr. Huan-Chen Cheng, an associate professor of surgery at Peking Medical College Hospital, summed it up, the medical worker is not torn between personal gain and benefit to the sick "no matter what their motives were before." In China, he added, "Patients feel it is their right to be cured, but the relationship between medical worker and patient must be cordial and harmonious."[20]

No one is above service. Medical school professors have an obligation to spend two months a year treating patients in outlying areas and holding classes for health workers. No one is beyond criticism since the doctors—whether wearing western-style shoes or without any at all—are responsible to the patient.

Oddly enough the man who helped to shape China's health-care program and who has become one of the great heroes of the Chinese revolution is Dr. Norman Bethune, a Canadian physician, who had lived in Detroit and had achieved a highly successful career as thoracic surgeon and inventor of dozens of medical instruments before becoming a revolutionary medico.

In 1936, he went to Spain to join the Republican cause against Franco; there, among other things, he organized a mobile blood bank, an innovation which proved valuable to the partisans. In 1938, he went to China to provide medical help for the Eighth Route Army, then struggling against Japan. With doctors in short supply, he set about training health cadres—laymen and women who were given intensive instruction in all aspects of medical care, while caring for the dying and the ill. Teaching materials were so scarce that he had to write the training manuals himself. In the short time he was there, he organized mobile hospitals and a system of first-aid stations and clinics that have become a vast network of health facilities. Dr. Bethune established the idea of taking medicine to the people and of learning from them.

He contracted blood-poisoning as a result of having cut himself during an operation in 1939. His grave and a statue to honor him are in the North China Martyrs Cemetery in Shijiachuang; and a museum that honors him is at the center of the Norman Bethune International Peace Hospital there.

On one of the walls is a tribute to Bethune from Mao Tse-tung:

> A foreigner, without selfish motive whatsoever, taking the Chinese people's liberation movement upon himself as his own business, what moral character is this? It is the doctrine of internationalism and of communism also. So each and every one of our fellow communists in China must try to obtain this kind of moral character.[21]

Chinese doctors, as well as businessmen, scientists, athletes, actors, and diplomats have made pilgrimages over the years to Bethune's birthplace, to the School of Medicine of Toronto University, his alma mater, and to McGill University Medical School, where Bethune was a member of the faculty. The most recent visit in 1972 was headlined in papers in the People's Republic as "Chinese Doctors in Bethune's Land."

North Vietnam, that hapless, defoliated, devastated country of a million bomb craters, survived largely because it adopted from

China the idea of training large numbers of persons without formal medical schooling to carry out specific important health-care jobs. Recent American visitors to the country have expressed amazement at the efficacy and quality of care. The infant mortality rate, 400 per 1000 births a year in 1954, dropped so dramatically despite wartime conditions that in 1970 it was 23 per 1000 births. (By contrast, the United States figure was 26 per 1000.)

According to Dr. George Roth of the Medical Aid to Indochina Committee, mass vaccination has virtually eliminated smallpox, cholera, and plague "for the first time anywhere in Southeast Asia." Trachoma, which afflicted more than 60 percent of the people in 1954, "is now so rare that medical students must rely on photographs instead of clinical cases to study the disease."[22]

Despite round-the-clock bombings at the time of his visit, he and fellow doctors were asked to send advanced medical journals; and he found that at the central hospital in Hanoi research was being carried out in viral diseases and epidermiology, immunology, fundamentals of shock, and in child diseases and development. Dr. Roth said:

> The striking impression that one gets of North Vietnamese medical care is that it is humane, intelligent, and tightly-organized. Despite the ravages of war, it provides excellent care, both preventive and therapeutic, to all its citizens.

The first line of defense against illness, he pointed out, is carried on by the medical workers in the 6000 villages in which a small dispensary acts as center. That provides traditional herbal medicines—among them one identified as digitalis—which have been used for thousands of years and which Western doctors are now coming to value. The dispensary also provides immunization treatment, takes care of common medical complaints, and serves as a maternity hospital. (About 14,000 midwives are functioning in North Vietnam.)

At the next level are the province hospitals, which provide more complicated care and correspond generally to small community hospitals in the United States, with full medical staffs of nurses, X-ray technicians, laboratory technicians, and other paramedical workers. Those hospitals, Dr. Roth said, continued to function despite the American bombings, which curtailed activities in 32 of the 36 existing ones.

Other American doctors have contrasted the health-care system in North Vietnam with that in the south. Dr. John Champlin, who spent three and a half years as a physician there, said of that: "We are protecting a regime in South Vietnam that by its health care policy alone is responsible for more deaths than those caused by all military actions combined."[23]

There, according to figures given by the Walter Reed Army Research Institute, infant mortality is about 800 percent higher than in North Vietnam. There, another 25 percent of all children born alive die before the age of five.

The American-style doctors charge private patients, Dr. Champlin said, about $1.30 for an office visit, exclusive of treatment costs. That is one percent of the annual per capita income of a typical South Vietnamese, or the equivalent of a doctor charging a $10,000-a-year patient in the United States $100 for a single office visit. Also, according to his indictment, "in government health centers many nurses, doctors, and administrators steal large quantities of drugs, medical equipment, and even the patients' food to sell or use in private practice." The captain of the Helogoland Hospital Ship anchored in Da Nang officially reported that South Vietnamese Red Cross personnel secretly charged peasants a stiff fee for admission to the "free" floating ship. Although, as he told Dr. Champlin, he tried to put an end to it, the illicit profiteering continued—"as it does today in many other foreign-run hospitals in South Vietnam."

The American medical establishment has more to answer for than the Vietnam situation. During the 1960s, all over Western Europe, including Britain, strikes by physicians threatened health-care services. Their demand? To become as rich as American doctors. Their weapon? To emigrate. While fees in the United States skyrocketed after World War II, European governments kept doctors' fees in line with other prices.[24]

The first doctors' strike in European history was launched in Belgium on April 1, 1963, after the government decided to put an end to their patient exploitation and tax dodging. The way the system worked was that doctors could—and some did—charge patients stiff fees, enter only half the amount on their records, and pay taxes on the lesser amounts. The government had no way of knowing how much they were charging or the size of the income on which they paid taxes since patients gave cash to the doctor and were reimbursed up to 75 percent by the insurance societies to which they belonged. (The societies, in turn, were reimbursed by the National Medical Fund, which collected money through payroll deductions and which had been slipping deep into the red.) To curb doctors' income and to regulate tax returns, the Belgian government passed a law setting standard fees for medical services and requiring doctors to give patients receipts for payments on which were listed diagnosis and treatment as well as charge.

Likening themselves to the heroic *maquis* of anti-Nazi fame, many doctors were pledging opposition "to the death"—although, as some noted thoughtfully, the death was not theirs.

After 18 chaotic days, the strike was settled by mutual agreement, with the doctors winning higher fees. The people of Belgium felt less enthusiastic about the "triumph." One of them told reporter Pete Hamill that if anything had happened during the strike to one of his children, "I would shoot a doctor in retaliation. And I would keep shooting doctors until I found the one responsible." Another, whose wife had waited four hours for treatment of an asthma attack, said simply: "We have finally seen the true faces of our doctors. It will never be the same."[25]

Later, another uprising occurred in France, where the doctors —who received the highest fees in western Europe—were demanding huge increases. The two disturbances that brought greatest joy to the medical journals in the United States were the British GPs' strike threat in 1965 and that of the Canadian doctors a few years earlier.

The General Practitioners in Britain, as has been noted, exempted themselves from salaried government service—as the hospital-based specialists did not do—preferring to accept the fee-per-patient arrangement as the next best thing to fee-for-service. Their rewards lagged, far behind the specialists'. And the excessive demands they made in the mid-1960s did not fit in with the government program to curb inflation. Through their trade association, the British Medical Association, they were demanding a 15 percent hike "or else."

The strike was abandoned and the GPs won a whopping increase, but the episode indicated to many observers a need for more imaginative approaches to health care than the establishment has encouraged or even permitted.

Perhaps the best summing up was contained in an article in *The Observer*, which applauded the Minister of Health's rejection that patients should pay fees for attention from the General Practitioners. It stressed that even the report of their own College had pointed out that GPs are generally not overworked, nor beseiged by hordes of well patients interrupting their nights, prolonging their days. *The Observer* tartly noted that such a system of fees would "destroy the one great achievement of the Health Service: free access to the patient by the doctor."[26]

A somewhat similar situation occurred in the Canadian province of Saskatchewan in 1962, when 700 doctors struck against a medical program instituted in the prairie province by the government. A leader in government-financed health care, Saskatchewan had set up the first comprehensive hospitalization program in Canada in 1947. All provincials were required to pay a hospital tax, which, coupled with other revenues, covered most of their hospital bills. That was so successful that all other Canadian provinces adopted the plan.[27] (Persons unable to pay were also protected.)

The doctors did not revolt then or later when the Saskatchewan government pioneered medical care plans financed by taxes for residents of rural areas and small towns and for persons afflicted with cancer, mental illness, and some other diseases. But in 1962, when the legislature enacted a bill to pay nearly all doctor bills out of the provincial treasury, the doctors began to utter the familiar rebel yells: "Dictatorship," "Down with slavery," "Bureaucratic medicine is bad medicine."

Urged on by their professional organizations, which relied

heavily on the AMA arsenal of verbal and tactical weapons, the doctors acted on July 1. Their strike shut down two-thirds of the province's hospitals and cut off almost all medical care except for emergency services at some larger centers. The government was equally adamant. It encouraged other Canadian doctors to practice in Saskatchewan; it flew in physicians from England and Scotland to minister to the sick and injured. At the end of three weeks a compromise was reached: provincials would receive medical care financed by taxes; the doctors would be allowed to bill the nonprofit agencies operating the medical insurance plans instead of billing the government.[28]

Peace was restored, and the government's insurance program did not result in the threatened mass exodus of physicians. Quite the reverse. Within two years, 100 more doctors were practicing in Saskatchewan than before the strike. And why not? As reporters pointed out, the doctors had never made so much money in their lives. Unpaid bills were a thing of the past, and they could charge full fees for anyone they treated—including their own wives and children.[29]

Even before the strike had started, a massive investigation was under way by the Royal Commission on Health Services. The 914-page report issued in 1964—named to honor the Canadian Supreme Court Justice E. M. Hall who headed the Commission—emphasized the need for action by the national and provincial governments. Less than half the population had "some degree of reasonably adequate" health insurance coverage; and insurance programs covering mental illness, dental and optical care, drugs, retarded and crippled children were "hardly worth mentioning."[30] During recent years, Canada has been placing much emphasis on health promotion and disease prevention, as well as on the treatment of illness since the country's showing in life expectancy, maternal and infant mortality has been relatively poor—although not as low as this country's showing. Some of the primary goals and objectives were spelled out recently by the Science Council of Canada in a study prepared by Dr. H. Rocke Robertson, a distinguished surgeon who was until recently Vice-Chancellor of McGill University.[31]

281

First priority is to improve the quality of health of Canadians, while improving the quality of health care and of the system—insuring, meanwhile, that inefficiency and extravagance do not cheat people from getting their money's worth.

Canada has already embarked on expanding its medical schools for reasons summed up by Dr. John Evans, President of the University of Toronto:

> . . . it is doubly unjust to drain skilled manpower from other less well developed countries and at the same time deny the career opportunity in medicine to the abundant number of well-qualified young Canadians who currently seek entry to our programs of medical education.[32]

Medical education is being shortened in many cases; although quality is being enhanced by requirements for continuing post-graduate education and by the move to make mandatory periodical review of doctor competence. Moreover, liberalized admission policies may result in a new breed of health professional to alter the character of the "academically-oriented professional insensitive to the needs of the people." Again, as Dr. Evans pointed out, by opening the medical door wider, it serves to offset the forces of academic competition "which deny admission to highly committed individuals whose earlier formal educational opportunities have been handicapped by ethnic background, poverty, or inadequacies of the educational system in the remote geographic areas in which they have lived."[33]

To supplement the number of doctors and the imbalance created by the abundance—even over-supply of specialists in relation to family physicians—Canada has been placing increasing emphasis on the "nurse–practitioner." Now staffing the 60 stations in the north, they have had special training in midwifery and in general medicine. In contact with a doctor by radio or telephone, they have done an impressive job, judging from the improvement in the infant mortality and maternal mortality rates in the Territories. Nurses in Canada are also playing an important role in urban areas as full-fledged members of health teams. For example, the 40 nurses of a health team in a company with 40,000 employees presently carry out all preplacement examinations (referring 5 percent of the female and 10 percent of the male applicants to a doctor for an opinion) and most of the periodic health examinations. The first to see an employee reporting sick on the job, they are able to handle most of the problems. "The overall opinion of the medical staff and the employees of the quality of work performed by these nurses is unequivocally favourable," the Robertson report noted.

Like the United States, Canada has a long way to go. But at least it is taking big strides, hoping to reach soon to the condition where a person will have access, "without barriers of any sort, to a coordinated system of health care which embraces the full range of facilities of high quality, operated considerately and efficiently."[34]

Curiously enough, one of the most promising solutions for Canada as well as for all other western European countries concerned about the cost and the quality of health care is the system of prepaid group practice, pioneered in this country forty years ago and continually attacked by the AMA in its long-standing war with the people.

17 Rx for American Medicine

Even the most casual consideration of the American health-care system indicates that despite the remarkable gains in medical science and the billions spent to make those gains widely available, the American health-care system is gravely ill. The cure depends upon the willingness of physicians and laymen alike to substitute new values and new methods, to work cooperatively to realize the system's potential.

A first step is to replace the "single voice" of the AMA with a truly representative planning council and commission to set priorities and standards at the national level; similar councils and commissions should be set up on regional and local levels. The AMA and its affiliates should have representation on those councils, but it should not be allowed to dominate them. The AMA's power is waning; membership has plummeted by almost one-fourth in the last few years. It has recently modified some of its positions, including sanctioning the Professional Standards Review Organizations and allowing intern and resident members to elect their own committee members, but it will be hard pressed to modify others without outside help. That was dramatically illustrated late in 1974, when the Board of Trustees tried to free the organization from drug industry domination by proposing to drop nearly all advertising from its fourteen publications and make up part of the revenue by increasing members' dues from $110 to $200 a year. "No way," members said. And the proposal which could

284

have saved Americans billions of dollars and removed them from serious dangers, was rejected.

Those organizations of medical men—such as the Group Health Association of America, the American Public Health Association, the Association of American Medical Colleges, The Physicians Forum, and the Medical Committee on Human Rights—which have demonstrated themselves concerned about quality and cost and availability should be given representation equal to that of the AMA. Other health care professionals should be included: hospital administrators, nurses, paramedics, and directors of non-profit nursing homes. Importantly, consumer groups should have representation equal to that of the professionals. Like the professionals, the consumer representatives should be drawn from organizations that have demonstrated their concern about the cost and quality of health care and that have worked to achieve it: the Consumer Federation of America, the Cooperative League of the USA, Ralph Nader's Health Research Groups.

No representative of a profit-seeking group should be allowed to serve; if advice and counsel are needed from special-interest segments, such as the drug and insurance industries, they may be obtained on a temporary basis. A primary goal should be to remove medicine from the marketplace.

The councils would have multiple responsibilities, one of the first being to set national priorities. People all over the world have been excited and impressed by the dramatic gains made in the more esoteric aspects of medicine—like heart transplants; since persons and agencies of so many nations have contributed to the advances, here would be a splendid field for international cooperation. There is, however, something radically wrong with our priorities when, as Dr. Richard Nesson, Medical Director of the Harvard Community Health Plan, pointed out recently, we are presently spending about one-fourth of our health care budget on exploring the potentials of liver and lung transplantation.[1] In contrast, as has been pointed out earlier, we spend very little on preventive medicine and something less than 1 percent of the budget on health education. Both of those areas would pay immediate and long-range dividends. As the comprehensive report of the Comptroller General emphasized recently, the first order of business—if costs are to be cut and health improved—is to substitute for acute crisis care the strategy of preventive medicine, precluding illness or injury and intervening as early as possible in order to halt or delay the progress of disease toward a more critical state.[2]

Benefits would be even greater if people could be taught early enough the importance of adopting life styles that ward off, among other ills, the major chronic diseases in the country—heart disease, stroke, and cancer. Health education must be stepped up in the schools and carried beyond them to the public, using some of the "prime" time to inform and enlighten people that is now devoted to detergent- and analgesics-sponsored programs glorifying Young-Doctor-What's-His-Name. The education should also provide some training in semantics, to offer protection against the corrupt language of much advertising. It is not surprising that pill-popping has become one of the nation's favorite indoor sports. How could it be otherwise, with the constant bombardment of urgings to take this tablet or that to relieve any minor frustration or discomfort? Fine though it is to have school children given "Don't" instruction about dangerous drugs, few of those sessions compare in entertainment value and effectiveness with commercials that advocate "Do."

Some semantic training should also help people to distinguish between *socialized* and *socialism*. We do not recoil with horror at sending our children to socialized schools; we do not consider the American way threatened by our socialized protective services—police and fire departments, Coast Guard, Army, Navy. Much of our health-care system is already socialized, including the medical education given doctors, even in private medical colleges. What is needed here, as Dr. Caldwell B. Esselstyn pointed out a decade ago, is less antagonism to government intrusion into medicine and more "synergism," to bring about "an integrated program which alone can achieve the best in health and medical care for the American people."[3]

Care should be made available immediately when it is needed; and that is particularly important with children. The screening

programs in schools to detect health problems are not very
helpful if those in need are simply told to "see your family
doctor." Many have none; many cannot afford to follow up the
recommendations. As a consequence, lives are blighted, and social
costs are enormous. A recent study, for example, showed that
many youngsters are doomed to deafness and blindness for lack of
medical care. Even children with communicable diseases are
allowed to go without care. Sweden and other countries provide
necessary health care for school children; there is no reason why
we could not, since, among other things, it would be an investment in the future. Restrictions that prohibit doctors, dentists, and
nurses from rendering professional care should be eliminated;
their only purpose is to protect physicians' bank balances, certainly
not children's health. And they are now handicapped; the direc-
tive noted in *Up the Down Staircase,* in connection with the death
of one of the students, is common across the country: "The school
nurse may not touch wounds, give medication, remove foreign
particles from the eye. . . ."[4] What is a school nurse for?

By rendering care where need is, much professional time could
be saved. And, in this case, time means billions.

The councils should and could seek to alleviate the shortage
of physicians and provide for more comprehensive care by more
fully utilizing the services of nurses and by training paramedics,
rather than continuing to raid other countries, whose doctors have
established a flourishing underground here. Often ill-trained, unable to pass licensing examinations, they have been lured here—
most from Asia—by promises of rich rewards in American medicine. In ironic contrast many admirably trained American nurses
and paramedics have been barred in many cases from all but
minor duties. Yet in the instances in which they have been allowed to function up to the level of their training, their performance has rated high. In one case—reported, incidentally, in the
JAMA—a graduate nurse who had finished a year of preparation
as practitioner undertook the care of chronically ill patients in a
medical clinic. In addition to having a wide range of diseases, patients were also suffering from major social and psychological
problems. Patients were seen by a doctor only if they or the nurse

felt it was necessary, although their course of treatment was followed by a physician who was always available for consultation. At the end of six months, the nurse was following up 110 patients, all of whom were reported to be "pleased with their care."[5] And the care was satisfactory.

Paramedics trained to give emergency care have been performing as effectively on the homefront as in Vietnam, despite physicians' protests that they be allowed to function at all. The Los Angeles Board of Fire Commissioners, for example, felt that the only way of obtaining voter authorization for a $43,200,000 bond issue in 1975 was to add another $1,000,000 and tie it into the popular paramedic program. No immediate need for the money for paramedics had been established, but the Commission president declared that it was necessary to sell the issue to the voters: "He [the voter] wants to know lifesaving. He wants that magic word 'paramedic'—that's all he cares about when he goes into the booth."[6]

The paramedics or physicians' aides, or whatever their title, should be under the supervision of physicians, but that can be done best and most effectively in a group-practice plan or health-care center, where they have ready access to consultation and advice when needed and when their performance, like that of the doctors, can be constantly scrutinized. Other persons could also be used in such a situation—social workers, psychologists, family counselors, health educators; and more legitimate experimentation could also take place. As Dr. William A. MacColl, medical director of the Group Health Cooperation of Puget Sound for many years, has pointed out, there is a real need for that since an increasing amount of illness is related to stress, rather than to illness of a viral or bacteriologic origin. "Many of these persons," he said, "are better treated through some form of counselling and assistance than through the laying on of the stethoscope, and this can often be accomplished by nonphysician professionals."[7] Such a comprehensive health care center with various forms of aid available could also take care of the large number of patients passing through doctors' offices daily who require little more than what he called "high quality first aid."

Nationally and at regional levels, the councils should insist that the medical profession step up quality and cut costs. Comprehensive care of excellence can be best provided by salaried doctors working as teams either through government agencies or the prepaid group-practice organizations. Many of the Health Maintenance Organizations authorized in 1973 do not meet the standards set by the Group Health Association of America, although that should be a requirement for any contracting organization since they guarantee a wide range of services, careful review of performance, preventive care, and reasonable freedom for patients to choose their own physicians, in addition to offering economies. Some of the HMO contracts have demanded nothing in the way of quality; and several instances have occurred in which they offer nothing at all to patients. They have been merely a chance for get-rich-quick doctors and other promoters to make windfall profits on investments. In one case in California recently, three doctors and their accountant received a contract to provide care for a maximum of 10,000 poor persons for a maximum income of $2,600,000 a year. The doctors did nothing to implement the contract for almost a year. At that point, they sold their interest for $50,000 to another doctor who had been denied a contract by the state.[8]

Legislation providing for Professional Standards Review Organizations will not be of maximum benefit to consumers unless the review committees are required to open membership to outsiders. Laymen are presently serving as judges of medical care as jury members sitting on malpractice cases; with computerized auditing procedures they can make intelligent contributions to improve quality. And they could do a whole lot about costs. Insurance companies and government agencies have permitted the professionals to commit—unpunished—petty and grand theft. There is no valid reason at all why the prices of medical services should not be public knowledge rather than a confidential matter between the patient and the professional who demands the right to guess what the traffic will bear. A major blow to that kind of secrecy was struck by one of Ralph Nader's Health Research Groups in 1974, with the issuance of the nation's first directory of doctors' fees, office hours, training, education, and other data. Limited to one Maryland county, the pilot directory inspired other research groups in other areas to make such comparative guides and issue them free of charge. The director of the group in Springfield, Illinois, said of the work to provide a directory there: "The medical society has a vested interest in keeping consumers in the dark. They don't want consumers to be able to make easy comparisons of such things as fees."⁹ Because of the opposition of the society, the research group had been able to obtain the cooperation of only 54 of the city's 215 doctors, but that was enough to give people the idea. Similar directories rating the quality of care doctors provide would be even more valuable.

Governments at all levels have done little to upgrade standards and keep down costs. What organized medicine has wanted, organized medicine has gotten. Its role in the misuse and overuse of dangerous and expensive drugs has been a national scandal for several decades, thanks to the government's hands-off policy. Some relief is being obtained by recent court decisions overturning bans on price advertising and by the requirement that generic names be given. But those gains must be supported by agencies and by health care providers independent of the industry. An outstanding example, as indicated earlier, is the drug program of the Group Health Cooperative of Puget Sound, which has been functioning in a rational manner for years at very low cost. A committee of the medical staff and the chief pharmacist develop a formulary, including drugs by generic name whenever possible, for use by all the doctors. The formulary is reviewed continuously, so that new and effective drugs are added, unsafe and ineffective ones removed. And the doctors are educated by the committee, not by salesmen. A council could function nationally to do the same job, with its findings checked regularly against those of other legitimate groups.

Hospitals and nursing homes, which take the largest share of public and private health care dollars must be more rigorously controlled by the government. The nursing home situation is a continuing horror story, with only the feeblest efforts being made by government agencies to correct conditions in those pre-mortuaries. In California in 1975, an audit was finally demanded after authorities learned that courts had been releasing persons picked up as alcoholics to a man claiming to represent a senior citizens welfare group, but who was actually a commission patient-procurer for a chain of nursing homes. The men were kept in the homes as long as their Medicaid benefits lasted, drugged to prevent their leaving, and told they would go to prison if they objected to the treatment. A nurse testified that nursing home administrators opened and destroyed patients' mail and monitored telephone calls to prevent their seeking outside help.[10]

Substandard nursing homes should not be rewarded—as they are now; nor should hospitals. A 1974 HEW proposal to police hospitals and doctors treating Medicare and Medicaid patients was blocked when the AMA went to the White House, raising the threat of a doctors' boycott. Forced to acknowledge how much of the $20,000,000,000 spent that year on the two programs was being wasted, the proposal would have required doctors to get permission before putting patients in medical hospitals, mental hospitals, and nursing homes. What was substituted instead was a concurrent review within two days after patients are admitted, a review conducted the first day by nurses and technicians, the final decision to be made on the second day by groups of doctors. That is not much more than an agreement to allow the ineffectual self-policing to continue.

The savings would be enormous, if there were proper utilization. General Accounting Office investigators reported not long ago that a study showed that about $3,000,000,000 could have been saved in 1970 alone if patients' needs had been matched by appropriate facilities. It was their finding that about 25 percent of the patients in the country are treated in facilities that are excessive to their needs.[11] The haphazard building of hospitals and nursing homes has encouraged this; indeed, some areas are so "overbedded" that parts of hospitals have been transformed into luxury hotels. Like the nursing homes, the hospitals have been scouting the highways and byways for occupants, putting pressure on doctors to hospitalize patients and to keep them hospitalized in order to increase revenues. A friend of mine was needlessly incarcerated for nine days recently for a simple knee operation that could have been performed on an outpatient basis. After four days of enforced "resting up" for the operation, she insisted on returning home for the weekend; she returned Monday morning for the operation and was subsequently kept in the hospital—one of the largest and most respected in the Hollywood area—for five days. She and her husband could not believe the bill that was sent to them by the hospital and their insurance company. She had been charged the standard daily rate, plus meals and medications, for the two days she was "on leave" with her doctor's permission. Her husband, who becomes irate about such matters, finally obtained a refund for their share of the bill and also for the insurance company. Not expectedly, the insurance company told him to "forget it; it will just cause more paper work."

Much more use should be made of ambulatory facilities and other substitutes. One hospital recently estimated that on the basis of its own savings in performing surgical procedures in the clinic, the country could save well over $1,000,000,000 a year by that simple expedient. Homemaker programs, which provide help with cleaning and shopping, have demonstrated themselves remarkably effective in California in keeping people out of hospitals and nursing homes. Under those programs, a worker paid by the state performs basic household chores one or two days a week and does shopping for foodstuffs. Yet a good many doctors and hospital officials have objected effectively to those programs. Consider one case brought to my attention recently by a social worker involving the young mother of three children. The woman demanded release from the hospital; her broken leg simply needed time to heal, she was in need of only minimal medical attention, and she was worried about the tots. Instead of helping her and the Medicaid program by signing authorization for the Homemaker Service, the doctor told the social worker bitterly: "She can stay in the hospital until she is ready to walk around again; I'm not certifying any charity patient for the services of a maid." The cost differential would have amounted to thousands, since the children would have been placed in foster homes or state facilities for the duration. The social worker persuaded a voluntary organization to provide household help; the woman was able to stay at home comfortably with her children.

The government agencies administering health programs have long had an obligation to see that unnecessary surgery and hospitalization are averted. They have also had an obligation to act against those hospitals that endanger lives and health by unnecessary operations and to insure that the types of hospitals they were supporting were essential. That is another area of much needed reform. It is wanton for hospitals to continue their empire building at the expense of taxpayers and patients instead of sharing special facilities. For example, in 1971 an average of only about 40 percent of the newborn beds were occupied; labor and delivery rooms were also "underused" then. Other beds unused are those set aside for pediatric patients and open-heart surgery patients; of the 416 hospitals equipped to perform open-heart procedures in 1969, 97 percent used those facilities less than four times a week —much below the standards set by the Inter-Society Commission for Heart Disease Resources.[12]

Little attention has been given to costs, although a number of studies have indicated that virtually no economic competition exists in the hospital industry. And patients are not allowed to choose on the basis of cost and quality; they go where the doctor or the emergency service directs them.

The government should act promptly to halt the monopolistic situation that exists in all aspects of medical care. Some promise of that was given by former Attorney General William B. Saxbe shortly before he left office in 1974. In a speech to the National Association of Manufacturers, a kind of farewell speech, he raised the possibility of antitrust actions against doctors, dentists, pharmacists, along with funeral directors and veterinarians and other so-called professionals. State regulation, he said, and in some cases self-regulation have led to price fixing and monopoly behavior.[13]

The insurance industry should also be investigated since it has encouraged those things in our health-care system. Usually, benefits are limited to expenses incurred during hospitalization as well as in crisis medicine and surgery. It has discouraged early treatment and preventive medical care; it has discouraged out-patient treatment and the use of facilities appropriate to patients' needs.

The superior prepaid group-practice plans—like Kaiser-Permanente, Group Health Cooperative of Puget Sound, Group Health Association of Washington, D.C.—have a different objective since they are rewarded for keeping patients well and out of the hospital.

Beyond all those measures, however, what is needed is a kind of moral revolution within the medical profession. The possibility of that was first suggested in 1963, when the president of the Association of American Medical Colleges attacked the "entrepreneurial" philosophy of the AMA and declared that the time had come when "medical colleges can adapt themselves to the social and economic changes of the country."[14] A kind of declaration of independence from the AMA came several years later in a report bearing the name of Dr. Lowell T. Coggeshall, vice president of the University of Chicago and chairman of the AAMC committee drawing up what has been described as one of the most significant documents since the Flexner report. The Coggeshall report proposed to close the gap between practice and research, break down the barriers between physician and the society in which he lives, establish preventive and rehabilitative care as a national policy. It urged that consumers and other health groups join medical schools in seeking solutions to the country's health care needs.[15]

Consequences of the report have been evident in such things as an expansion in the number of medical schools and the size of entering classes, an increase from 8500 in 1965 to 13,500 in 1972. Many of the schools were going out of their way to attract minority students and women, who had traditionally been shut out from becoming MDs. More than tokenism was involved; schools like Northwestern established tutorial programs to help less qualified students bring their academic skills up to the mark, and Harvard started summer programs to give cram courses to academically disadvantaged Black, Puerto Rican, and Chicano undergraduates interested in becoming physicians. In 1969, it also replaced the Hippocratic Oath with the "Declaration of Geneva," with students pledging themselves to use their medical knowledge in conformity with the laws of humanity.

294

Curriculums have been expanded, and many schools have followed the example of Western Reserve by assigning each freshman to a pregnant patient to care for her and her family during his school years. Many of the medical schools are getting students through at a faster clip—an especially important innovation since it will help to ease the shortage. The activism characteristic of liberal arts students in the 1960s also touched medical school students: for example, in 1967 a hundred students strode into a meeting of the AMA in Chicago to accuse it of "plotting to silence the anguished cries of the poor." A year later, the Student Health Organization (SHO) financed and administered multidisciplinary health care projects in nine disadvantaged areas of the country.

I witnessed the rise of that activism at the University of Southern California School of Medicine, where SHO was founded during the years Dr. Roger O. Egeberg served as dean. He encouraged students to organize a revolt from mediocrity—setting up a speakers' forum featuring such outstanding "liberals" in the profession as Dr. Louis Lasagna, Dr. H. Jack Geiger, and Dr. Allan Butler, who helped them to establish the SHO in contrast to SAMA, the students' branch of the AMA. Within a few months, students at Harvard, Chicago, Tufts, Boston University, Stanford, and the University of California medical schools organized similar groups of students pledged to work in the slums of their own cities and wherever else they found suffering and need.

Some of the USC students worked in Los Angeles, testing the vision and hearing of slum children; some, along with some nursing students, set off for the migrant labor centers in the state's central farming valleys; some, with funds "dug up" by Dean Egeberg, went to Mississippi. Their reactions were enthusiastic. Peter Nash, who worked in Mississippi with the Medical Committee on Human Rights, described hardships calmly, including a bomb scare and a dynamite explosion. But he was enthusiastic about his fellow workers: "For the first time, I felt proud of the medical profession in areas other than medicine." Craig McMillan, a freckled, red-haired student with a desire to become a medical missionary, wrote to me of his experience with migrant farm families in California:

They have no hope, no expectations, no promising future. They have no education, no knowledge of basic hygiene, basic nutrition, basic sanitation. NOTHING. We can't expect to do much for them, but we can try to clear some of the obstacles out of their children's future. Our project is beginning to show promise.

Nearly a decade later, in the spring of 1973, I saw the social concerns of the Sixties generation translated into meaningful action at the clinic set up by Cesar Chavez's United Farm Workers Union on the desolate "Forty Acres" that is the central headquarters just outside Delano, California. The clinic is a handsome building, a long one-story rectangle made of adobe bricks, with a gallery extending along one side that provides a welcome respite from the blazing heat. The main door opens into an attractive waiting room, with toys for children and colorful signs in English and Spanish urging adults to support the boycott. A large poster reads:

> ESTA CLINICA ES SUYA. UTILIZE VD. TODOS LOS SERVICIOS
> PARA TODA SU FAMILIA.

Beyond are laboratories, examining rooms, cubicles where ambulatory treatment and surgery are given, a pharmacy, a storeroom, an office for a former priest who serves as counselor, and a kind of kitchen–meeting room where the staff holds informal sessions.

There I talked with four of the young doctors who had been working in the clinic for the past two years: Peter Cummings, Dan Murphy, Peter Rudd, and Caleb Foote—MDs of recent internship.

Peter Cummings, a Western Reserve graduate interested in general medicine, found the "whole spectrum" of problems at the clinic and was appalled by the needs: the "horrible" mortality rate among farm workers, the frequency of diseases among the young, the acute illnesses from pesticide poisoning and other hazards of field labor. He and his colleagues found patients so miseducated that it took almost a year before they could disabuse them of the notion that a shot of penicillin would cure a common cold. (For many of the poor in this country, as in others, medicine means a shot of antibiotics for whatever ails them.) He was disgusted by the quality of care they had been receiving. "Outrageous, outrageous," he kept repeating, citing case after case. One involved a man who had lost 22 pounds in a nearby hospital and who was discharged because "nothing seems to be wrong with him." Cummings intervened successfully.

Peter Rudd, who had come from an internship at Stanford, was understandably proud of the changes wrought in the year and a half he had been there. When the clinic opened in October 1971, only 40 a day came in search of medical care; by mid-1973, more than 140 were coming. Thanks to volunteer help from other California doctors, the patient load was only 20 a day—allowing 20 minutes for each patient. Like other prepaid group-practice plans, the UFWU's Kennedy Health Plan emphasizes early treatment and preventive measures—in contrast to more traditional workers' insurance plans, which doctors in the area had been exploiting, Rudd said. Among the examples he cited was a case he had encountered in the local hospital, "still a proprietary institution in its philosophy," when he saw a fifteen-year-old boy enter with abdominal pains. Without making tests of any kind, the physician in charge of the emergency service told the boy that he needed an appendectomy. "Where does your father work?" he asked. "Have you a medical card?" When Rudd asked the doctor what was going on, he shrugged: "These people are always wasting our time without proper insurance."

One of Rudd's greatest success stories reveals the kind of medical care the young doctors provided. A twelve-year-old boy who had been exhibiting a peculiar pallor was brought to the clinic by his parents after he failed to respond to an iron preparation a doctor in town had given to him. When all the usual tests proved negative, Rudd decided to seek help from the hemotology departments of Stanford and the University of California at Los Angeles. An analysis of the child's bone marrow indicated that he was suffering from a rare disease—one of only about 40 cases until then reported in the world—related to B-12 absorption. Proper treatment resulted in a dramatic response.

All agreed that the experience was important for them. They found the "team" experience, working with nurses and counselors as well as other doctors, stimulating. They broadened their skills: "Here we have all learned how to take X-rays, give tests, and do much else that was not taught in medical school." They learned some of the facts of social life in the agricultural center. Unlike the single doctors, Caleb Foote lived in a small house in Delano with his wife, who has a Ph.D. in history, and their three-year-old child. Their neighbor, an auto mechanic, would not allow his child to play with the Footes' child; only "suspect" people had dealings with the farm workers.

All four of them felt bitter about the medical establishment in Delano. In order to bring about change from within, they had decided to join the Kern County Medical Society; however, within a few months, they dropped their membership. Reasons? They said that the high fees medical society members charged farm workers had caused insurance premiums to increase sharply— more than the workers could afford. They were disturbed by the avariciousness of the members of the society; Rudd called them "money hungry, socially unconscious people." What precipitated their leaving the society was a meeting during which one of the officers announced that scientific discussions would be eliminated from future programs on the grounds that members were not interested in them and not attending such meetings. He drew a tremendous round of applause for that and for the announcement that the fee schedule the society had been instrumental in establishing in the county was "one of the highest in the country."

All were leaving at the end of two years, and they had some concerns that the great ferment in medical schools had died, that there would not be enough replacements. But boxes of books heaped in corners bearing the names of MDs who were on their way minimized that worry. So did comments of other people involved in the farm worker program.

We found the clinic at Salinas no less inspiring. A nondescript stucco had been converted into a modern medical center: the living room an attractive waiting room, the kitchen an examining room, the back porch a well-organized dispensary. Patients, many of them in family groups, sat quietly. For many patients, this was their first encounter with professional care; for all of them, it offered help with a whole range of ills that resulted from poverty and overwork. What was remarkable was the staff: volunteers clad in the "costume of the country"—blue jeans or simple cotton dresses—totally dedicated to their medical mission.

Chief among the volunteers was Dr. Jerome Lackner, an internist from nearby San Jose. He, his wife, and their five children had spent weekends and holidays for more than a year at the place. Why? "Well," he paused between gulps of milk from a carton that his fifteen-year-old daughter had brought him for lunch and said thoughtfully, "I like practicing medicine and enjoy giving medical care to people who need it. Here, I am also helping people to organize their own structure—to acquire power." He added: "The farm workers' union movement is about the only thing going in the United States I see any hope for."

Others found one of the most hopeful signs that the old order is changing the appointment of Dr. Lackner as director of the state health department by California's recently elected Governor Edmund G. Brown, Jr.—over the heads of the medical establishment.

There are other hopeful signs, however, in and out of the profession that American medicine may abandon its horse-and-buggy delivery service and find a vehicle more suitable for carrying to all people the gifts that science has made. The help of everyone is needed, patient as well as doctor, to cure the sickness of American medicine and American society.

Notes

Introduction

1. *Statistical Abstract of the United States, 1974* (Washington, D.C.: Government Printing Office, 1974), p. 69.

2. *United Nations Demographic Yearbook, 1973* (Canada: United Nations, 1974), pp. 336-55

3. Ibid., pp. 256-76.

4. *Scientific American* (September 1973), pp. 65-66.

5. *Congressional Record* (August 2, 1973), p. S 15532.

6. "Doctor Demands $30 Cash, Refuses Case," *Los Angeles Times,* April 18, 1974.

7. *Limitation of Activity Due to Chronic Conditions, United States 1969 and 1970*, Public Health Service, U.S. Department of Health, Education, and Welfare (Rockville, Md.: DHEW Publication No. (HSM) 73-1506, April, 1973), pp. 1-3.

8. *Barriers to Health Care for Older Americans*, Hearings Before the Subcommittee on Health of the Elderly of the Special Committee on Aging United States Senate (Washington, D.C.: Government Printing Office, 1973), Part 1, p. 15.

Chapter 1

1. Painting by Robert A. Thom, reproduced on the cover of *JAMA* (*The Journal of the American Medical Association*), May 8, 1972.

2. Anonymous, M.D., *The Healers* (New York: G. P. Putnam's Sons, 1967), pp. 195-96.

3. James Burrow, *AMA: Voice of American Medicine* (Baltimore: The Johns Hopkins Press, 1963), p. 37.

4. Ibid., p. 101.

5. *JAMA* (July 1, 1916), p. 41.

6. Elton Rayack, *Professional Power and American Medicine: The Economics of the American Medical Association* (Cleveland: World Publishing Company, 1967), p. 66.

7. Abraham Flexner, *Medical Education in the United States and Canada* (New York: Carnegie Foundation, 1910), pp. 28-51.

8. *JAMA* (September 3, 1949), pp. 27-93. [Slightly different figures are presented in *Historical Statistics of the United States, Colonial Times to 1957* (Washington, D.C.: Government Printing Office, 1957), p. 25—

which indicates that in 1915 there were 96 medical schools, and in 1920 only 85.]

9. *JAMA* (August 27, 1932), p. 765.

10. Walter L. Bierring, "The Family Doctor and the Changing Order," *JAMA* (June 16, 1934), p. 1997.

11. *Conditions and Problems in the Nation's Nursing Homes,* Hearings before the Subcommittee on Long-Term Care of the Special Committee on Aging, United States Senate, Eighty-Ninth Congress (Washington, D.C.: Government Printing Office, 1965), p. 615.

12. Robert J. Weiss, Joel Kleinman, Ursula C. Brandt, Jacob J. Feldman, and Aims C. McGinness, "Foreign Medical Graduates and the Foreign Underground," *New England Journal of Medicine* (June 20, 1974), pp. 1408-13.

13. Rayack, op. cit., p. 242.

14. *Los Angeles Times*, March 20, 1974.

15. Walter H. Tompkins, "Chiropractors Fight AMA's Charge of Alleged Quackery in Treatment," *Santa Barbara News-Press,* May 28, 1972.

16. Rayack, op. cit., p. 257.

17. Everett Forman, "Face It: We Can Learn From Chiropractors," *Medical Economics* (March 5, 1973), p. 201.

18. Louis Lasagna, *The Doctors' Dilemma* (New York: Harper and Brothers, 1962), p. 38.

19. Rayack, op. cit., p. 258.

20. Harry Nelson, "Medical Schools Asked to Halt Advanced Training for Nurses," *Los Angeles Times*, November 24, 1973.

21. "New Acupuncture Believer: Nixon's Doctor," *Medical World News* (April 7, 1972), pp. 17-19.

22. John J. Fried, "Biofeedback—Teaching Your Body to Heal Itself," *Family Health* (February 1974), pp. 18-20.

23. Carter L. Marshall, "Psychiatrists Question Two 'Social Myths,'" *JAMA* (February 28, 1972), pp. 1146-47.

24. Ida Honorof, "Public Education Bows to Business Pressure," *A Report to the Consumer* (Vol. III, No. 63), pp. 1-3.

25. Burrow, op. cit., p. 81.

26. Oliver Garceau, *The Political History of the American Medical Association* (Cambridge, Mass.: Harvard University Press, 1941), p. 101.

27. Odin W. Anderson, "Medical Care for Americans," *Annals of the American Academy of Political and Social Science*, ed. by Franz Goldman and Hugh R. Leavall (Philadelphia, 1951), p. 108.

28. Robert M. Cunningham, Jr., *Hospitals, Doctors, and Dollars* (New York: F. W. Dodge, 1961), pp. 208-9.

29. Caldwell B. Esselstyn, "The Professions Respond to the Challenge," Speech to the Southern District Branch of the American Public Health Association, May 3, 1962. (Typescript)

30. Richard Dudman, "Socialism in the Armed Forces," *The New Republic* (November 9, 1963), pp. 24-26.

31. James Howard Means, *Doctors, People, and Government* (Boston: Little Brown, 1953), pp. 145-49.

32. Ibid., pp. 152-53.

33. Richard Harris, "The Sacred Trust," *The New Yorker* (July 2, 1966), p. 29.

34. Rayack, op. cit., pp. 11-12.

35. Francis Ward, "Two Nixon Stalwarts in Indiana Will Test Watergate Backlash," *Los Angeles Times*, October 30, 1974.

36. "Horror Story," *Time* (December 10, 1973), p. 107; "Doctor, Hospital Ordered to Pay $3.7 Million in Malpractice Suit," *Los Angeles Times*, December 2, 1973.

37. Harry Nelson, "Many Pupils with Positive TB Tests Not Given Followup Check," *Los Angeles Times*, November 28, 1973.

38. Letter, March 12, 1973.

39. *Prism* (October 1973), p. 6.

Chapter 2

1. *San Francisco Examiner*, September 23, 1965; *Los Angeles Times*, September 24, 1965.

2. Seymour E. Harris, *The Economics of American Medicine* (New York: The Macmillan Company, 1964), pp. 143-49.

3. *Medicare and Medicaid Problems, Issues, and Alternatives*, Report of the Staff to the Committee on Finance United States Senate, February 9, 1970 (Washington, D.C.: Government Printing Office, 1970), pp. 163-98.

4. *Los Angeles Times*, July 3, 1969.

5. "A Doctor in Michigan Gives Back $169,000 in 'Medicaid' Payments," *Wall Street Journal*, August 4, 1969.

6. "AMA Leader Defends Doctors' Medicare Fees," *Los Angeles Times*, July 3, 1969.

7. Gilbert Cant, "An X-Ray Analysis of Doctors' Bills," *Money* (August 1973), p. 24.

8. Rudy Maxa, "What Can You Say About a Doctor Who Makes $75,000 a Year Treating Poor Patients," (*Potomac*), *Washington Post*, January 14, 1973, p. 11.

9. "Doctors Refuse to Deliver Baby," *Los Angeles Times*, February 21, 1975; "Eye for Sale—Price, $35,000," *Los Angeles Times*, February 1, 1975.

10. Edward M. Kennedy, *In Critical Condition: The Crisis in America's Health Care* (New York: Pocket Books, 1973), pp. 16-18.

11. "Too Poor to Aid Son; To Rich for Help," *Los Angeles Times*, November 1, 1972.

12. "Man Divorcing His Dying Wife," *Los Angeles Times*, January 19, 1973.

13. Dial Torgerson, "Popcorn Removed from Ear of Child, Bills Total $420," *Los Angeles Times*, January 20, 1970.

14. *Medical Economics* (May 30, 1966), p. 154.

15. *Annual Report on Medical School Income and Expenditures*, Continuing Survey of American Association of American Medical Colleges, 1970.

16. *Journal of the American Medical Association* (February 5, 1973), pp. 710-18. (Classified advertising section)

17. "Hahn Probes Outside Teaching by Doctors," *Los Angeles Herald-Examiner*, February 6, 1973.

18. *Los Angeles Times*, May 13, 1974.

19. $20,000-a-Year Pay for Part-Time Jail Doctor Reported," *Los Angeles Times*, August 18, 1973.

20. *Money* (August 1972), p. 26.

21. Roger Rapoport, "It's Enough to Make You Sick," *Playboy* (September 1973), p. 114.

22. *Medical Economics* (April 16, 1973), p. 88.

23. Paul W. Kellam, "Vacation in Vietnam?" *Medical Economics* (June 13, 1966), pp. 48-58.

24. "Diet Doctor Tells of $1 Million Annual Gross," *Los Angeles Times*, January 27, 1968.

25. Rudy Maxa, op. cit., p. 14.

26. Harry Nelson, "Doctors View Above $100,000 Incomes as Justified," *Los Angeles Times*, May 18, 1969.

27. "Drew Pearson Column," *Los Angeles Times*, October 8, 1965.

28. Harris, op. cit., p. 147.

29. Richard Carter, *The Doctor Business* (Garden City, N.Y.: Doubleday, 1958), pp. 55-56.

30. Edward R. Pinckney, *How to Make the Most of Your Doctor and Medicine* (Chicago: Follett Publishing Co., 1964), pp. 92-94.

31. *Money* (August 1973), p. 26.

32. *Medical Economics* (April 2, 1973), p. 142.

33. Laurent P. LaRoche, "How Medical Practice Can Change Overnight," *Medical Economics* (September 7, 1965), pp. 98-103.

34. Anonymous, M.D., *The Healers* (New York: G. P. Putnam's Sons, 1967), p. 302.

35. Helen Clapesattle, *The Doctors Mayo* (Minneapolis: University of Minnesota Press, 1963), pp. 197-99.

36. Abraham J. Heschel, "The Sisyphus Complex," *Ramparts* (October 1964), pp. 45-49.

37. Robert Mighell, "Why Some Doctors Charge Too Little," *Medical Economics* (January 11, 1965), pp. 191-204.

Chapter 3

1. Donald T. Atkinson, *Magic, Myth, and Medicine* (Cleveland: World Publishing Co., 1956), pp. 74-75.

2. Ibid., pp. 120-22.

3. Ritchie Calder, *Medicine and Man* (New York: New American Library, 1958), pp. 206-7.

4. Henry E. Sigerist, *A History of Medicine* (New York: Oxford University Press, 1951), Vol. 1, pp. 425-34.

5. Osler L. Peterson, "Medical Care in the U.S.," *Scientific American* (August 1963), p. 19.

6. Edward R. Pinckney, *How to Make the Most of Your Doctor and Medicine* (Chicago: Follett Publishing Company, 1964), p. 56.

7. W. Palmer Dearing, speech given at a seminar on medical care sponsored by the Institute of Industrial Relations of the University of California at Los Angeles, March 10, 1965.

8. *Scientific American* (September 1973), pp. 65-66.

9. *Violence in the City—an End or a Beginning*? Report by the Governor's Commission on the Los Angeles Riots, December 2, 1965, p. 74.

10. " 'Glob of Sand' Finally Gets Its Own Doctor," *Medical World News*, August 27, 1965.

11. "California Area in Search of a Doctor," *Los Angeles Times*, February 18, 1969.

12. Gregory S. Slater, "The Case of a National Fee Schedule," *Medical Economics* (March 5, 1973), p. 146.

13. "City Finds Fraud in Medicaid Cases," *New York Times*, June 20, 1969.

14. "Medical Scandals Point Out Need for HEW Watchdog," *Washington Post*, June 15, 1969; also *More Needs to Be Done to Assure That Physicians' Services—Paid for by Medicare and Medicaid—Are Necessary*, Report to the Congress by the Comptroller General of the U.S. (Washington, D.C.: General Accounting Office, 1973), pp. 37-39.

15. "2 Million Medicaid Fraud Uncovered, Paper Reports," *Los Angeles Times*, April 19, 1975; also, *Time* magazine (May 26, 1975), p. 55.

16. "Physician Fined $112,500 for Writing Illegal Prescriptions," *Los Angeles Times*, January 30, 1973.

17. Osler L. Peterson, *et al*, "An Analytical Study of North Carolina General Practice," *Journal of Medical Education* (December 1956), Part 2.

18. H. Rocke Robertson, *Health Care in Canada: A Commentary* (Ottawa: Science Council of Canada, 1973), p. 41.

19. *Annals of Internal Medicine of American College of Physicians*, January 1965, quoted in *Los Angeles Times*, January 7, 1965.

20. Pinckney, op. cit., p. 96.

21. *The Voice of ACSUP*, October 1973, pp. 2, 3.

22. *Medicare and Medicaid, Problems, Issues, and Alternatives*, Report of the Staff of the Senate Finance Committee (Washington, D.C.: Government Printing Office, 1970), p. 87.

23. Harry Nelson, "Cause of Death: Who Is Best Fitted to Tell?" *Los Angeles Times*, February 4, 1973.

24. "Santa Barbara Physician Under Investigation Quits County Job," *Los Angeles Times*, October 20, 1972.

25. *More Needs to Be Done to Assure that Physicians' Services—Paid for By Medicare and Medicaid—Are Necessary*, p. 9.

26. *Report on Medi-Cal Program by the California Department of Justice*, November 6, 1968, p. 37.

27. Morris N. Placere and Charles S. Marwick, "Is This Operation Really Necessary?" *Family Health* (October 1973), p. 20.

28. Peterson, op. cit., p. 165.

29. Donald McDonald, ed., *Medical Malpractice: A Center Occasional Paper* (Santa Barbara: Center for the Study of Democratic Institutions, 1971), p. 20.

30. Placere and Marwick, op. cit., p. 20.

31. *Meeting the Challenge of Health Care Today*, Teamsters Joint Council No. 16 and Management Hospitalization Trust Fund (265 West 14th Street, New York, N.Y.), p. 2.

32. Richard Shoemaker, "Evaluating Medical Care," *AFL-CIO American Federationist* (May 1966). (Reprint, no page number)

33. Eugene G. McCarthy and Geraldine W. Widmer, "Effects of Screening by Consultants on Recommended Elective Surgical Procedures," *New England Journal of Medicine* (December 19, 1974), pp. 1331-33.

34. *Los Angeles Times*, February 7, 1966.

35. Herbert S. Denenberg, Pennsylvania Insurance Commissioner's *Shopper's Guide to Surgery* (Reprinted by Consumer Insurance, 813 National Press Building, Washington, D.C. 20004.) no page number.

36. Talk given at a meeting of the California Public Health Association in Los Angeles, May 16, 1975.

37. *Group Health and Welfare News* (January 1970), p. 3.

38. Howard and Martha Lewis, *The Medical Offenders* (New York: Simon and Schuster, 1970), p. 222.

39. Morton K. Rubenstein, "The Outdated U.S. Doctor," *Los Angeles Times*, December 3, 1972.

40. "AMA Leadership Yields to Calls for Revision of Stance on PSROs," *The Nation's Health* (January 1974), p. 4.

Chapter 4

1. Morton Mintz, "AMA Denounces Doctor–Salesman Curb," *Washington Post*, March 2, 1967.

2. "AMA Official Denies Misuse of Bank Funds," *Los Angeles Times*, September 10, 1973.

3. "Penalty for Medic's Tax Evasion: $10,000 Fine or Public Service," *Long Beach Independent*, January 19, 1965.

4. Louis Nizer, *My Life in Court* (New York: Pyramid Books, 1961), p. 435.

5. James P. Gifford, "Why 9 M.D.s Were Jailed as Tax-Dodgers," *Medical Economics* (December 28, 1964), pp. 76-83.

6. *Medical Economics* (February 22, 1965), p. 64.

7. Philip Stern, *The Great Treasury Raid* (New York: The New American Library, 1965), pp. 154-56.

8. Robert Schram, "Will They Rob Your Office Next?" *Medical Economics* (September 7, 1964), pp. 135-50.

9. Raymond V. Martin, *Revolt in the Mafia: How the Gallo Gang Split the New York Underworld* (New York: Duell, Sloan & Pearce, 1963), p. 79.

10. "Tax Evasion by 1,500 Doctors Told Senators," *Los Angeles Times*, September 23, 1970.

11. Harry J. Anslinger with J. Dennis Gregory, *The Protectors* (New York: Farrar, Straus & Cudahy, 1964), pp. 141-48.

12. Ron Einstoss, "Doctor Made Her Addict, Writer Says," *Los Angeles Times*, December 1, 1965; also, "Doctor Gets Jail Term in Drug Case," *Los Angeles Times*, January 6, 1966.

13. Mickey Deans "Her Husband's Story of Judy Garland, Her Last Tragic Months," *Look* (October 7, 1969), pp. 84-90.

14. "Newsmakers," *Newsweek* (July 5, 1969), p. 44.

15. "Society Speed," *Time* (December 18, 1972), pp. 76-77.

16. Robert Rawitch, 'Surgeon-Actor Indicted in Dope Case," *Los Angeles Times,* January 6, 1975.

17. *Congressional Quarterly Almanac* (1964), pp. 253-54.

18. Jack Star, "The Growing Tragedy of Illegal Abortion," *Look* (October 19, 1965), p. 43.

19. Joseph Heller, *Catch-22* (New York: Dell, 1962), p. 52.

20. "Dr. X," *Intern* (New York: Harper & Row, 1965), p. 168.

21. *Los Angeles Times,* March 23, 1965.

22. William Michelfelder, *It's Cheaper to Die* (New York: Braziller, 1960), p. 89.

23. Selig Greenberg, *The Troubled Calling* (New York: The Macmillan Company, 1965), p. 208.

24. Carl Dyster, "Health Plans Rocked by Fee Frauds," *Medical Economics* (July 1952), pp. 97-108.

25. Mintz, op. cit.

26. *Medical Economics* (June 1953), p. 82.

27. Michelfelder, op. cit., p. 82.

28. Michael M. Davis, *Medical Care for Tomorrow* (New York: Harper & Brothers, 1955), p. 156.

29. "Attack on MD-Owned Pharmacies," *Medical World News* (September 11, 1964), pp. 111-14.

30. *Physician Ownership in Pharmacies and Drug Companies,* Hearings of the Subcommittee on Antitrust and Monopoly of the Senate Judiciary Committee, 1964 (Washington, D.C.: Government Printing Office, 1965), p. 122.

31. Ibid., p. 345.

32. Ibid., pp. 346-47.

33. Ibid., pp. 41, 376.

34. Morton Mintz, "The Merchant Doctors," *Progressive* (October 1967), p. 34.

35. "Making Spectacles," *New Republic* (December 25, 1965), p. 6.

36. "Negligent Lab Testing," The Wells News Service, May 15, 1967, p. 4.

37. Donald T. Atkinson, *Magic, Myth, and Medicine* (Cleveland: World Publishing, 1956).

Chapter 5

1. John Lear, "The Patient's Right to Know," *Saturday Review* (June 26, 1965), p. 20.

2. John Lear, *Saturday Review* (March 5, 1966), p. 65.

3. John Lear, "Human Guinea Pigs and the Law," *Saturday Review* (October 6, 1962), p. 55.

4. Irwin Feinberg, "Threats of Progress: Medicine and Liberty," *Civil Liberties* (July 1972), pp. 1-3.

5. Henry K. Beecher, *Experimentation in Man* (Springfield, Ill.: Charles C. Thomas, 1962).

6. "A Tempest on Human 'Martyrs'," *San Francisco Examiner*, April 4, 1965.

7. "Documenting the Abuses," *Saturday Review* (July 22, 1966), pp. 45-46.

8. Feinberg, op. cit., p. 6.

9. Thomas Thompson, "The Texas Tornado vs. Dr. Wonderful," *Life* (April 10, 1970), pp. 62B-62D.

10. "Battle Looms Over Definition of Death in Heart Transplant," *Los Angeles Times*, September 14, 1973.

11. *Quality of Health Care—Human Experimentation, 1973*, Hearings Before the Subcommittee on Health of the Committee on Labor and Public Welfare, United States Senate, Ninety-Third Congress, Part 2, p. 359.

12. Ibid., p. 442.

13. Ibid., p. 442-43.

14. Ibid., p. 445.

15. Ibid., Part 3, p. 794.

16. Ibid., p. 797.

17. Aileen Adams and Geoffrey Cowan, "The Human Guinea Pig: How We Test Drugs," *World* (December 5, 1972), pp. 20-21.

18. *Competitive Problems in the Drug Industry*, Hearings Before the Subcommittee on Monopoly of the Select Committee on Small Business of the United States Senate, Ninety-First Congress, (Washington, D.C.: Government Printing Office, 1973), Part 14, pp. 5755-64.

19. "28 in Study Died From Syphilis, Reports Say," *Los Angeles Times*, September 12, 1972.

20. "Doctor Tells of Order Not to Treat Syphilis," *Los Angeles Times*, August 8, 1972.

21. "Syphilis Suit Pact Reached," *Los Angeles Times*, December 17, 1974.

22. Adams and Cowan, op. cit. pp. 22-23.

23. Les Payne, "U.S. Sterilization Abuses Disclosed," *Los Angeles Times*, January 5, 1975.

24. Hubert H. Humphrey, "Myths About Federal Drug Policies," *New Republic* (May 16, 1964), p. 17.

25. "Quote Without Comment," *Consumer Reports* (January 1965), p. 6.

26. "Drug Regulation, Investigating the Investigator," *Time* (August 5, 1966), p. 65.

27. Leonard Gross, "Preview of a New German Horror Trial," *Look* (May 28, 1968), pp. 43-52.

28. "Thalidomide Case in Belgium: Doctor Disagrees with Verdict," *Los Angeles Times*, November 18, 1962.

29. John Lear, "The Unfinished Story of Thalidomide," *Saturday Review* (September 1, 1962), pp. 35-40.

30. Will Jonathan, "The Feminine Conscience of FDA: Dr. Frances Oldham Kelsey," *Saturday Review* (September 1, 1962), pp. 41-43.

31. Joe Alex Morris, Jr., "Thalidomide Trial Ends on Inconclusive Note," *Los Angeles Times*, December 19, 1970.

32. "Thalidomide Babies Awarded $50 Million," *Los Angeles Times*, July 31, 1973.

33. John Lister, *New England Journal of Medicine* (February 22, 1973), pp. 406-7.

Chapter 6

1. Morton K. Rubenstein, "The Outdated U.S. Doctor," *Los Angeles Times,* December 3, 1972.

2. Bryce Nelson, "Doctors Meet to Bring Problem of 'Deviate Physicians' Into Open," *Los Angeles Times,* February 11, 1973; also, Selig Greenberg, *The Troubled Calling* (New York: The Macmillan Company, 1965), p. 206.

3. *Medical Malpractice, Report of the Senate Factfinding Committee on Public Health and Safety* (February 1965), Senate of the State of California, p. 14.

4. *Meeting the Challenge of Health Care Today,* Teamsters Joint Council No. 16 and Management Hospitalization Trust Fund (265 West 14th Street, New York, N.Y. 10011), p. 1.

5. *Medical Malpractice, Report of the Secretary's Commission on Medical Malpractice,* DHEW Publication No. (OS) 73-89 (Washington, D.C.: Government Printing Office, 1973), Appendix, pp. 668-80.

6. "Principles of Medical Ethics," the American Medical Association, 1957.

7. "Dr. X," *Intern* (New York: Harper & Row, 1965), p. 220.

8. Ibid., p. 282.

9. Richard H. Blum, *Commonsense Guide to Doctors, Hospitals, and Medical Care* (New York: The Macmillan Company, 1964), p. 49.

10. Rubenstein, op. cit.

11. *Bulletin of the Los Angeles County Medical Association* (January 4, 1973), p. 20.

12. James Wechsler, with Nancy Wechsler and Holly W. Karpf, *In a Darkness* (New York: W. W. Norton, 1972), p. 14.

13. *Medical Malpractice, Report to the Secretary's Commission . . .* Appendix, pp. 594-95.

14. Howard and Martha Lewis, *The Medical Offenders* (New York: Simon & Schuster, 1970), p. 68.

15. Ibid., p. 62.

16. "Grievance Committees of Medical Societies Handle More Gripes," *Wall Street Journal,* October 17 1967.

17. *Report of the (California) Senate Factfinding Committee on Public Health and Safety,* p. 14.

18. "Grievance Committees of Medical Societies Handle More Gripes."

19. Lewis, op. cit., p. 62.

20. *Medical Malpractice, Report of the Secretary's Commission . . .,* Appendix, p. 295.

21. Lewis, op. cit., p. 37.

22. Ibid., p. 41.

23. *Society for Social Responsibility in Science Newsletter,* May 1964, p. 1.

24. Ibid.

25. *Report of the (California) Senate Factfinding Committee on Public Health and Safety,* p. 12.

26. Walter W. Stiern, "Explanation of Senate Bills 400 and 403," Statement by the Office of Senator Stiern, April 6, 1965.

27. Ibid.

28. Vincent J. Burke, "Nader Team Calls for Controls Over Doctors," *Los Angeles Times,* November 9, 1970.

29. Al Stump, "State Watchdog Agencies Crack Down on Professional Malpractice, Business Misconduct," *Los Angeles Herald-Examiner,* April 28, 1974.

30. Herbert S. Denenberg, "Dr. Strangelove Joins Alice-in-Wonderland in Quest of a National Health Plan." *Progressive* (May 1973), p. 20.

31. *More Needs to Be Done to Assure That Physicians' Services—Paid for by Medicare and Medicaid—Are Necessary,* Report to the Congress by the Comptroller General of the United States (Washington, D.C.: General Accounting Office, 1972), pp. 12-13.

32. Ibid., pp. 36-38.

33. *Medical Malpractice, Report of the Secretary's Commission . . .,* p. 85.

Chapter 7

1. *Medical Malpractice, Report of the Secretary's Commission on Medical Malpractice,* Department of Health, Education, and Welfare, DHEW Publication No (OS) 73-88; (Washington D.C.: Government Printing Office, 1973), p. 20. Referred to subsequently as *Medical Malpractice.*

2. Ibid., p. 105.

3. *Medical Economics* (January 11, 1965).

4. *Medical Economics* (December 5, 1960), pp. 38-60.

5. *Medical Malpractice,* p. 33.

6. Richard Carter, *The Doctor Business* (Garden City, N.Y.: Doubleday, 1958), pp. 240-41.

7. "Interview with Melvin Belli," *Playboy* (June 1965), pp. 87-88.

8. *Medical Malpractice,* Appendix, p. 522.

9. Ibid., p. 508.

10. *NBC Evening News,* January 7, 1975.

11. *Medical Malpractice, A Center Occasional Paper,* ed. by Donald McDonald, (Santa Barbara, Cal.: The Center for the Study of Democratic Institutions, 1971). Referred to subsequently as *Center Paper,* p. 5.

12. *Medical Malpractice,* p. 43.

13. Harry Nelson and John Goldman, "Medical Crisis: Doctors Finding Insurance Scarce," *Los Angeles Times,* January 7, 1975.

14. *Medical Malpractice,* p. 16.

15. "Interview with Belli," loc. cit., p. 87.

16. Carter, op. cit., pp. 238-39.

17. *Medical Malpractice,* pp. 6, 12.

18. Ibid., p. 24.

19. *Center Paper,* p. 4.

20. Ibid., p. 4.

21. *Medical Malpractice,* p. 35.

22. Ibid., pp. 10-11.

23. "She Dies Rich But Unaware," *Los Angeles Times,* May 12, 1972.

24. C. Joseph Stetler and Alan R. Moritz, *Doctor and Patient and the Law,* (St. Louis: C. V. Mosby, 1962), p. 380.

25. Louis Nizer, *My Life in Court* (New York: Pyramid Books, 1963), p. 400.

26. Ibid., p. 401.

27. *Center Paper*, p. 21.

28. Ibid., p. 21.

29. John L. Tovey, "The Most Inflated Malpractice Threat," *Medical Economics* (June 14, 1965), p. 142.

30. Stetler and Moritz, op. cit., p. 380.

31. Harry Nelson, "Malpractice Suits Here Called Deterrent to Full Health Care," *Los Angeles Times*, October 10, 1972.

32. *Medical Malpractice*, p. 18.

33. Ibid., p. 91.

34. "Inter-Professional Code for Physicians and Attorneys of the City and County of San Francisco," Adopted by the Bar Association of San Francisco, San Francisco County Medical Society, San Francisco Lawyers' Guild, April 1959.

35. *Medical Malpractice*, Appendix, pp. 424ff.

Chapter 8

1. Richard H. Blum, Unpublished report for an interim committee of the California Assembly Committee on Rules, 1961.

2. *Los Angeles Times*, August 28, 1965.

3. *Medical World News* (July 30, 1965), p. 60.

4. *Statistical Abstract of the United States, 1972* (Washington, D.C.: Government Printing Office, 1972), p. 72.

5. Ibid., p. 66.

6. Petition to the Cost of Living Council by Gary G. Grindler, A. Ernest Fitzgerald, and the Health Research Group, February 22, 1973.

7. "Financing for the Reorganization of Medical Care Services and Their Delivery," *Medical Cure and Medical Care*, ed. by Spyros Andreopoulos, Proceedings of the Sun Valley Forum on National Health, Inc., June 25–July 1, 1972, *The Milbank Memorial Fund Quarterly* (October 1972), Part 2, p. 204.

8. D. P. Rice and B. S. Cooper, "National Health Expenditures 1929-71," *Social Security Bulletin*, 35, 3-18 (January 1972); and B. S. Cooper and N. L. Worthington, "Medical Care Spending for Three Age Groups," *Social Security Bulletin*, 35, 3-16 (May 1972).

9. D. P. Rice and M. F. McGee, "Projections of National Health Expenditures, 1975 and 1980," *Research and Statistics Note*, No. 18, (October 30, 1970).

10. Edward M. Kennedy, *In Critical Condition, The Crisis in America's Health Care* (New York: Pocket Books, 1973), pp. 9-12.

11. Ibid., pp. 36-38.

12. Ibid., p. 15.

13. Godfrey Hodgson, "The Politics of American Health Care," Atlantic (October 1973), p. 52.

14. "2 Days in Hospital, 2 Operations Cost $10,000; Bill Is Rejected," *Los Angeles Times*, November 26, 1974.

15. Seymour E. Harris, *The Economics of American Medicine* (New York: The Macmillan Company, 1964), p. 214.

16. *Problems Associated with Reimbursements to Hospitals for Services Furnished Under Medicare*, Report to Congress by the Comptroller General of the United States, August 3, 1972 (Washington, D.C.: General Accounting Office, 1972), p. 2.

17. *Congressional Record* (August 2, 1973), S 15532.

18. Kennedy, op. cit., p. 62.

19. Ibid., p. 51.

20. Eric Sharp, "No One Notices They Die—Homeless, Penniless, and Sick," *Los Angeles Times*, October 2, 1973.

21. Jan de Hartog, *The Hospital* (New York: Athencum, 1964), p. 72.

22. William C. Selover, *The Christian Science Monitor*, January 31, 1966.

23. *Violence in the City—An End or a Beginning?* Report by the Governor's Commission, State of California, Sacramento, 1965.

24. Harry Nelson, "State Cities Doubt, Shelves Bid for Watts Hospital Funds," *Los Angeles Times*, December 20, 1965.

25. "Witnesses Cite Continued Discrimination by Hospitals Against Medicare Recipients," *The Nation's Health* (October 1973), p. 1.

26. Michael M. Davis, *Medical Care for Tomorrow* (New York: Harper & Brothers, 1955), p. 111.

27. Henry E. Sigerest, *On the Sociology of Medicine*, ed. by Milton I. Roemer (New York: Oxford University Press, 1951), pp. 321-25.

28. Mary Risley, *House of Healing* (Garden City, N.Y.: Doubleday, 1961), p. 215.

29. Richard Warren Lewis, "The Unsinkable Debbie Reynolds," *The Saturday Evening Post* (August 22-29, 1964), p. 79.

30. Sinclair Lewis, *Arrowsmith* (New York: The New American Library, 1961), pp. 281-83.

31. Seymour Kern, "Hospitals for Profit," *Frontier* (October 1960), p. 5.

32. Blum, op. cit., p. 46.

33. Victor Cohn, "There's Money in Hospitals," *Washington Post*, November 8, 1973.

34. *Medicare and Medicaid: Problems, Issues, and Alternatives*, Report of the Staff to the Committee on Finance, United States Senate, February 9, 1970 (Washington, D.C.: Government Printing Office, 1970), pp. 139-40.

35. Ibid., pp. 140-41.

36. "Surplus Hospital Beds Tied to Deaths," *Los Angeles Times*, May 8, 1975.

37. "Big Cut Possible in Hospital Patients," *Los Angeles Herald-Examiner*, February 24, 1970.

38. Narda Z. Trout and Jerry Belcher, "Alcoholics Illegally Held in 11 Hospitals, Suit Charges," *Los Angeles Times*, January 23, 1975.

39. *Medicare and Medicaid: Problems, Issues, and Alternatives*, p. 106.

40. Ibid., p. 107.

41. *Shopper's Guide to Surgery: Fourteen Rules on How to Avoid Unnecessary Surgery* (Washington, D.C.: Consumer Insurance, 813 National Press Building, Washington, D.C. 20004; $1.00 per copy.).

42. *Meeting the Challenge of Health Care Today*, Teamsters Joint Coun-

cil and Management Hospitalization Trust Fund (265 West 14th Street, New York, N.Y. 10011), pp. 15-16.

43. Ibid., p. 11.

44. Harry Nelson, "Cancer Care, All Facilities Aren't the Same," *Los Angeles Times,* November 2, 1973.

45. *U.S. News & World Report* (March 15, 1965), p. 55.

46. Ibid., p. 51.

47. *Study of Health Facilities Construction Costs:* Report to the Congress by the Comptroller General of the United States (Washington, D.C.: General Accounting Office, 1972), p. 95.

48. Donald C. Brodie, *Drug Utilization and Drug Utilization Review and Control* (Rockville, Md.: DHEW Publication (HSM) 72-3002, 1970), pp. 1-2.

49. *Medical Malpractice, Report of the Secretary's Commission on Medical Malpractice* (Washington, D.C.: Government Printing Office, 1973), p. 33.

50. *Medical Cure and Medical Care,* pp. 46-47. (see note 7)

51. *Study of Health Facilities Construction Costs,* p. 98.

52. *New York Times,* January 4, 1972.

53. "U.S. Revises Plan to Police Medicare," *Los Angeles Times,* November 29, 1974.

Chapter 9

1. *Health Care Services for the Aged,* Final Report to the Subcommittee on Institutions of the California State Legislature, Submitted to the Assembly on April 2, 1965, pp. 31-33. (Mimeo)

2. Ruth and Edward Brecher, "Nursing Homes," *Consumer Reports* (January 1964), p. 31. (The comprehensive series of articles ran in the January, February, March, and April issues.)

3. Statement of William Thomas of Columbia University School of Public Health and Administrative Medicine, *Conditions and Problems in the Nation's Nursing Homes,* Hearings before the Subcommittee on Long-Term Care of the Special Committee on Aging, U.S. Senate, Eighty-Ninth Congress (first session), (Washington, D.C.: Government Printing Office, 1965), Part 5, pp. 556-61. (In subsequent references identified as Moss Hearings.)

4. *Consumer Reports* (January 1964), p. 32.

5. *Health Care Services for the Aged,* p. 41.

6. Moss Hearings, Part 1, p. 32.

7. Ibid., Part 2, pp. 238-64.

8. Ibid.

9. Ibid.

10. *California Senior Citizens Sentinel* (August 1964), p. 1.

11. *Consumer Reports* (February 1964), p. 32.

12. *Moss Hearings,* Part 2, p. 106.

13. Ibid., p. 125.

14. *Medical World News* (August 27, 1965), p. 31.

15. *Consumer Reports* (January 1964), p. 32.

16. Ibid.

17. "Joint Commission to Accredit Nursing Homes," *Medical World News* (August 27, 1965), pp. 30-31.

18. *Medicare and Medicaid, Problems, Issues, and Alternatives: Report of the Staff to the Committee on Finance of the U.S. Senate, February 9, 1970* (Washington, D.C.: Government Printing Office, 1970), pp. 93-95.

19. Ibid., pp. 34-36.

20. David H. Pryor, "Where We Put the Aged," *New Republic* (April 25, 1970), p. 16.

21. Ibid., p. 17.

22. D. P. Rice and S. B. Cooper, "National Health Expenditures," *Social Security Bulletin 35*, 3018, January 1972.

23. "Gold in Geriatrics," *Time* (June 6, 1969), p. 103.

24. "Golden-Age Fraud," *Time* (January 1, 1973), p. 55.

25. "Nursing Firm That Got Loan from Ohio Files as Bankrupt," *Los Angeles Times,* June 27, 1970.

26. "Gold in Geriatrics," *Time* (June 6, 1969), p. 103.

27. Comptroller General of the United States, *Report to the Congress: Problems in Approving and Paying for Nursing Home Care Under the Medicaid Program in California* (Washington, D.C.: Government Printing Office, 1970), p. 1.

28. Ibid., pp. 17-19.

29. Charles A. O'Brien, Deputy Attorney General, *Report on MediCal by the California Department of Justice* (November 6, 1968), p. 11. (Mimeo)

30. Ibid., p. 16.

31. Ibid., pp. 24-26.

32. Ibid., p. 28.

33. Ibid., p. 10.

34. "The High Cost of Health," *Newsweek* (July 14, 1969), p. 61.

35. *Medicare and Medicaid, Problems, Issues, and Alternatives*, pp. 136-37.

36. *New York Times* News Service, "A Yacht on Medicaid," *Los Angeles Herald-Examiner*, September 6, 1974.

37. *Congressional Record* (February 24, 1970), pp. H 1213-21.

38. *Consumer Newsweek* (October 28, 1970), p. 1.

39. John A. Williams, "Surprise Inspection of Nursing Homes," *Los Angeles Times*, May 12, 1973.

40. Doug Shuit, "Three Indicted in Medical Fraud; Alleged Scheme Could Hit Total of $3 Million," *Los Angeles Times*, July 22, 1971.

41. Narda Trout, "State Examiners Investigating Charges Against Nursing Homes," *Los Angeles Times*, October 24, 1973.

42. *Nursing Home Care in the U.S.: Failure in Public Policy*, Report of the Subcommittee on Long-Term Care of the Special Committee on Aging, U.S. Senate (Washington, D.C.: Government Printing Office, 1974).

43. "Nursing Homes Under Fire," *Time* (February 3, 1975), p. 61.

44. Frank Del Olmo, "Beating of Patients at Rest Home Alleged," *Los Angeles Times*, April 22, 1975.

45. "Poor Nursing-Home Care Laid to Doctors," *Los Angeles Times,* March 3, 1975.

46. Ibid.

Chapter 10

1. Abraham B. Bergman and R. J. Werner, "Failure of Children to Receive Penicillin by Mouth," *New England Journal of Medicine* (June 13, 1963), pp. 1334-38.

2. Senator Gaylord Nelson, Statement, June 11, 1973, p. 1. (Mimeo)

3. For brief accounts of the hearings conducted by the Senate Subcommittee on Antitrust and Monopoly see Estes Kefauver and Irene Till, *In a Few Hands* (New York: Pantheon Books, 1965), and Richard Harris, *The Real Voice* (New York: Macmillan, 1963).

4. Tom Mahoney, *The Merchants of Life* (New York: Harper and Brothers, 1959), p. 4.

5. *Administered Prices, Drugs,* Hearings Before the Subcommittee on Antitrust and Monopoly of the Committee on the Judiciary, Eighty-Sixth Congress (second session), (Washington, D.C.: Government Printing Office, 1960), Part 1, pp. 48-55.

6. Robert Rosenblatt, *Los Angeles Times*, July 27, 1970.

7. Standard & Poor's figures, *U.S. News & World Reports* (May 7, 1973), p. 75.

8. Kefauver and Till, op. cit., p. 47.

9. Sinclair Lewis, *Arrowsmith* (New York: The New American Library, 1961), p. 132.

10. Mahoney, op. cit., p. 4.

11. Detailed histories of the beginnings of pharmacy are presented by Henry E. Sigerist, *A History of Medicine*, Vol. 1 (New York: Oxford University Press, 1951), and Kenneth Walker, *The Story of Medicine* (New York: Oxford University Press, 1955).

12. Ritchie Calder, *Medicine and Man* (New York: The New American Library, 1958), p. 19.

13. Donald G. Cooley, *The Science Book of Modern Medicine* (New York: Franklin Watts, 1963), p. 15.

14. Walker, op. cit., p. 135.

15. Ritchie Calder, op. cit., p. 211.

16. Ibid., p. 213.

17. Ibid., p. 187.

18. Mahoney, op. cit., p. 136.

19. *Los Angeles Times*, December 15, 1967.

20. *Competitive Problems in the Drug Industry: Present Status of Competition in the Pharmaceutical Industry*, Hearings Before the Subcommittee on Monopoly, Select Committee on Small Business of the United States Senate (Ninety-First Congress), (Washington, D.C.: Government Printing Office, 1968), Part 5, pp. 1819-20.

21. Ibid., p. 1824.

22. John Foster, "Drug Companies Broaden Their Base," *The Exchange* (May 1970), pp. 3-5.

23. *Competitive Problems in the Drug Industry*, Part 5, p. 1869.

24. Irma Hunt, "The Great American Medicine Show," *Modern Matur-*

ity (August-September 1973), pp. 58-59.

25. *Medical World News* (June 18, 1965), p. 66.

26. Richard Harris, op. cit., p. 79.

27. *Congressional Record* (May 17, 1965), pp. 10343-46.

28. J. W. Baxter, *World Patent Laws and Practice* (New York: Matthew Bender, 1970).

29. Seymour Harris, *The Economics of American Medicine* (New York: Macmillan, 1964), p. 77.

30. Richard Harris, op. cit., pp. 76-77.

31. Kefauver and Till, op. cit., p. 26.

32. *Administered Prices, Drugs*, p. 91.

33. Kefauver and Till, op. cit., p. 29.

34. Laurence Stern, "The Wonderful World of Wonder Drugs," *The Progressive* (November 1963), pp. 31-33.

35. "Two Companies Accused of Drug Patent Frauds," *Los Angeles Times*, June 16, 1969.

36. *Con$sumer New$week* (October 9, 1972), p. 3.

37. Morton Mintz, "Dual Drug Price System Hit," *Washington Post* April 1, 1973.

38. *Con$umer New$week* (March 20, 1972), p. 3.

39. "Bills Would Require Posting of Drug Prices," *Los Angeles Times*, January 27, 1972.

40. *Con$umer New$week* (March 20, 1972), p. 3.

41. "Disease: Anti-Competitive Practices in the Retail Drug Industry," *Consumer Federation of America News* (May 1974), p. 2.

42. Senator Gaylord Nelson, Statement (June 11, 1973), p. 1. (Mimeo)

43. Richard Harris, op. cit., p. 125.

44. *Journal of the American Medical Association* (November 9, 1964), p. 542.

45. A. Dale Console and Gaylord Nelson, "The Strange Story of the Marketing of Medicine," *The Progressive* (August 1969), p. 14.

46. Ibid.

47. Statement presented to the Senate Subcommittee on Monopoly, Washington, D.C. (February 6, 1973), p. 7.

48. HR 5734 (The Prescription Drug Freshness Act), HR 5735 (The Prescripton Drug Labeling Act), and HR 5736 (The Prescription Drug Information Act).

Chapter 11

1. Herman M. and Anne R. Somers, *Doctors, Patients, and Health Insurance* (Washington, D.C.: The Brookings Institution, 1961), pp. 103-4.

2. For brief accounts, see Estes Kefauver and Irene Till, *In a Few Hands* (New York: Pantheon Books, 1965), and Richard Harris, *The Real Voice* (New York: Macmillan, 1963).

3. Donald C. Brodie, *Drug Utilization and Drug Utilization Review and Control* (Rockville, Md.: DHEW Publication No. (HSM) 72-3002, 1970), pp. 1-2.

4. Milton Silverman and Philip R. Lee, *Pills, Profits, and Politics*

(Berkeley: University of California Press, 1974), p. 266.

5. Harry Nelson, "Prescription Drug Abuse Kills 100,000 Yearly, Two Claim," *Los Angeles Times*, June 10, 1974.

6. *Drug Utilization and Drug Utilization Review and Control*, pp. 24-25.

7. B. C. Hoddinott, et al., "Drug Reactions and Errors in Administration on a Medical Ward," *Canadian Medical Association Journal*, 97 (1967), p. 1001.

8. *Drug Utilization and Drug Utilization Review and Control*, p. 25.

9. "Antibiotics: Curative Drugs," ed. by Samuel Proger, *The Medicated Society* (New York: Macmillan, 1968), pp. 85-89.

10. "Deaths Laid to Needless Use of Antibiotics," *Los Angeles Times*, December 8, 1972.

11. *Competitive Problems in the Drug Industry: Present Status of Competition in the Pharmaceutical Industry*, Hearings Before the Subcommittee on Monopoly, Select Committee on Small Business, Ninetieth Congress (Washington, D.C.: Government Printing Office, 1967), Part 3, p. 1039.

12. Eleanor McBean, Statement, September 20 1973. (Typewritten)

13. *Con$umer New$week* (November 1, 1971), p. 4.

14. *Congressional Record* (October 15, 1971), pp. S16293-99.

15. *Con$umer New$week* (November 1, 1971), p. 4.

16. Kefauver and Till, op. cit., p. 60.

17. *San Francisco Examiner*, June 8, 1965.

18. *JAMA* (June 25, 1960).

19. Kefauver and Till, op. cit., p. 63.

20. Hubert H. Humphrey, "Myths About Federal Drug Policies," *New Republic* (May 16, 1964), p. 17.

21. "Diseases Due to Drug Treatment," *The Medicated Society*, pp. 165-79.

22. Ibid., p. 179.

23. ". . . *Particularly Chloromycetin*," Report by the California Senate Factfinding Committee on Public Health and Safety, January 1963.

24. Ibid., p. 10.

25. Bob Diebold, "Physician Urges Caution with Prescribed Drugs," *Los Angeles Times*, March 7, 1968.

26. "The Peculiar Success of Chloromycetin," *Consumer Reports* (October 1970), p. 617.

27. ". . . *Particularly Chloromycetin*," pp. 65-66.

28. "The Peculiar Success of Chloromycetin," *Consumer Reports* (October 1970), p. 618.

29. "$400,000 Award Against Drug Firm Upheld," *Los Angeles Times*, March 15, 1973.

30. *Advertising of Proprietary Medicines*, Hearings Before the Subcommittee on Monopoly of the Select Committee on Small Business, United States Senate, Ninety-Second Congress (Washington, D.C.: Government Printing Office, 1973), Part 3, p. 1142.

31. "At Wit's End to Stop Misuse of Potent Antibiotic—Goddard," *Los Angeles Times*, March 1, 1968.

32. "U.S. Admits Vietnam Gets Perilous Drug," *Los Angeles Times*, November 18, 1970.

33. "The Peculiar Success of Chloromycetin," p. 618.

34. Jeffrey Bishop, "Drug Evaluation Programs of the AMA, 1905-1966," *JAMA* (May 9, 1966), pp. 496-98.

35. Richard Harris, op. cit., p. 126.

36. "The Peculiar Success of Chloromycetin," p. 618.

37. *JAMA* (January 24, 1972).

38. *JAMA* (June 26, 1972).

39. *Advertising of Proprietary Medicines*, Part 2, p. 541.

40. *Competitive Problems in the Drug Industry,* Part 14, p. 5727.

41. Ibid., p. 5775.

42. Ibid., pp. 5509-10.

43. Ibid., Part 8, p. 3506.

44. Ibid., p. 3508.

45. Copies of the statements presented to the Nelson Senate subcommittee were provided me by Dr. Adriani, including the statement of February 6, 1973. In an accompanying letter, he described his grave concern about the "paid bureaucracy" in charge of AMA affairs and his desire to prevent the "further deterioration" of the organization.

46. *Drug Utilization and Drug Utilization Review and Control*, p. 29.

Chapter 12

1. *A Ship Called Hope* (New York: Dutton, 1964), p. 120.

2. Ibid., p. 148.

3. Speech delivered to the House Ways and Means Committee, July 28, 1961.

4. *Medical Malpractice: Report of the Secretary's Commission on Medical Malpractice* (Washington, D.C.: Government Printing Office, 1973), p. 15. (A note stated that the commission had learned of a malpractice suit filed in Hawaii in which the Hawaii Good Samaritan Statute was pleaded as a complete defense by the doctor who had been sued—the first suit officially recorded.)

5. Ibid., p. 16.

6. Robert J. Donovan, "Many Parents You Wouldn't Expect to Beat Up Their Children Are Doing It," *Los Angeles Times*, May 29, 1970.

7. Ibid.

8. Monrad G. Paulsen, "Legal Protections Against Child Abuse," *Children* (March-April 1966), p. 23.

9. Richard Carter, *The Gentle Legions* (Garden City, N.Y.: Doubleday, c. 1961), p. 71.

10. Ibid., p. 73.

11. Ibid., p. 172.

12. Ibid., p. 205.

13. Richard Carter, *Breakthrough* (New York: Pocket Books, 1967), pp. 259-63.

14. *New York Times*, April 17, 1956.

15. Leonard Engel, "The Salk Vaccine: What Caused the Mess," *Harper's* (August 1955), pp. 27-33.

16. Richard Carter, *The Doctor Business* (Garden City, N.Y.: Doubleday, 1958), pp. 42-43.

17. Ibid., p. 45.

18. "Salk vs. Sabin," *Consumer Reports* (February 1962), pp. 94-97.

19. James Burrow, *AMA: Voice of American Medicine* (Baltimore, Md.: Johns Hopkins Press, 1963), p. 160.

20. *Doctors, People, and Government* (Boston: Atlantic–Little Brown, 1953), p. 20.

21. *American Legion Magazine* (January 1954), p. 31.

22. Ibid., p. 34.

23. Ibid., p. 34.

24. (Arthur J. Connell), Ibid., p. 39.

25. Ibid., August 1954, pp. 18-19.

26. *Congressional Record* (March 6, 1973), pp. S4032-37.

27. August Gribbin, "Blood That Kills," *The National Observer*, January 29, 1972.

28. Ibid.

29. Richard Titmuss, *The Gift Relationship* (New York, Vintage Books, 1972), p. 146.

30. *H. R. 11828*, November 17, 1971.

31. Narda Z. Trout, "Medical Association Stand on Blood Banks Hit," *Los Angeles Times*, November 6, 1973

Chapter 13

1. *Smoking and Health: Report of the Advisory Committee to the Surgeon General of the Public Health Service, Department of Health, Education, and Welfare.* (Washington, D.C.: Government Printing Office, 1964).

2. *Los Angeles Times*, March 18, 1964.

3. Ibid., January 20, 1964.

4. Ibid., March 17, 1964.

5. *Congressional Quarterly* (1964), p. 250.

6. *Frontier* (June 1964), p. 25.

7. *Los Angeles Times*, March 18, 1964.

8. Ibid., March 25, 1964.

9. William Shannon, *The Progressive* (August 1964), p. 6.

10. Ruth and Edward Brecher, "Smoking and Lung Cancer," *Consumer Reports* (June 1963). Also *Smoking and the Public Interest* (Mt. Vernon, N.Y.: Consumers Union, 1965), pp. 25-26.

11. Elizabeth Drew, "The Quiet Victory of the Cigarette Lobby: How It Found the Best Filter Yet—Congress," *The Atlantic* (September 1965), p. 78. Also, *Consumer Reports* (October 1965), p. 490.

12. *Los Angeles Times*, June 24, 1964.

13. Ibid., June 25, 1964.

14. David Finn, "The Businessman and His Critics," *Saturday Review* (September 12, 1964), p. 59.

15. Weldon J. Walker, "Government-Subsidized Death and Disability," *JAMA* (Dec. 16, 1974), pp. 1529-30.

16. "Kennedy's Chief Science Adviser Warns on Danger of Pesticides," *New York Times*, May 17, 1963.

17. R. A. M. Case, "Toxic Effects of DDT in Man," *British Medical Journal* (December 15, 1945), pp. 842-45.

18. V. D. Wigglesworth, "A Case of DDT Poisoning in Man," *British*

Medical Journal (April 14, 1945), p. 517.

19. *Chemicals in Foods and Cosmetics*, Hearings Before the House Select Committee to Investigate the Use of Chemicals in Foods and Cosmetics, House of Representatives, Eighty-Second Congress, (Washington, D.C.: Government Printing Office, 1952-53), Part 2, pp. 948-63.

20. *Medical World News*, March 14, 1969; also, Laura Tallian, *The Pesticide Jungle* (privately printed, 1966), p. 25.

21. Robert Risebrough, *Chemical Fallout: Current Research on Persistent Pesticides*, ed. Morton W. Miller and George G. Berg (Springfield, Ill.: Charles C. Thomas, 1969), p. 21.

22. Karl Lutz, "FDA Discovers DDT Dangers—20 Years Late," *Prevention* (November 1969), pp. 74-77.

23. *Interagency Coordination in Environmental Hazards*, Hearings Before the Subcommittee on Reorganization of the Committee on Government Operations, U.S. Senate, Eighty-Eighth Congress (Washington, D.C.: Government Printing Office, 1963), Part 2, pp. 484-97.

24. Jerome B. Gordon, Statement before Senator Walter F. Mondale's Subcommittee, August 1, 1969.

25. *El Malcriado* (November 15-30, 1969), pp. 3, 7.

26. S. Gershon and F. H. Saw, *The Lancet* (June 1961), pp. 1371-74.

27. *Chemical Fallout: Current Research on Persistent Pesticides*, pp. 307-9.

28. "Chemical Hazards in the Human Environment," paper delivered at the 11th Science Writers Seminar of the American Cancer Society, March 28-April 2, 1969, pp. 3-4.

Chapter 14

1. "Mail-Order Health Insurance," *Consumer Reports* (May 1973), pp. 305-8.

2. *Consumers Health Protection Act*, introduced by State Senate Majority Leader George R. Moscone, California Legislature, March 14, 1972, p. 6.

3. Edward M. Kennedy, *In Critical Condition, The Crisis in America's Health Care* (New York: Pocket Books, 1973), pp. 33-36.

4. *Congressional Quarterly Almanac* (1972), pp. 578-79.

5. Kennedy, op. cit., p. 28.

6. Ibid., p. 30.

7. "Mail-Order Insurance," *Consumer Reports*, p. 306.

8. Ibid., p. 307.

9. Ibid., p. 307.

10. *Deceptive or Misleading Methods in Health Insurance Sales*, Hearing Before the Subcommittee on Frauds and Misrepresentations Affecting the Elderly of the Special Committee on Aging of the United States Senate, May 4, 1964 (Washington, D.C.: Government Printing Office), pp. 24-71.

11. Ibid., p. 135.

12. Anonymous, M.D., *The Healers* (New York: G. P. Putnam's Sons, 1967), p. 75.

13. Sidney Margolius, *A Consumer's Guide to Health Insurance Plans* (Public Affairs Pamphlet #325), pp. 5-9.

14. William Faulkner, *The Wild Palms* (New York: Signet Edition,

1959), p. 73.

15. Herman M. and Anne R. Somers, *Doctors, Patients, and Health Insurance* (Washington, D.C.: The Brookings Institution, 1961) p. 312.

16. "New Forms of Medical Practice: Hospital Insurance Schemes," *JAMA* (January 21, 1933), pp. 192-94.

17. James Burrow, *AMA: Voice of American Medicine* (Baltimore: The Johns Hopkins Press, 1963), p. 215.

18. Ibid., p. 243.

19. Somers, op. cit., pp. 319-23.

20. Seymour Harris, *The Economics of American Medicine* (New York: The Macmillan Company, 1964), p. 319.

21. *Evergreen Cooperative Newspaper*, December 1965, p. 4.

22. *Barriers to Health Care for Older Americans*, Hearings Before the Subcommittee on Health of the Elderly of the Special Committee on Aging, United States Senate, Ninety-Third Congress (Washington, D.C.: Government Printing Office, 1973), p. 15.

23. Godfrey Hodgson, "The Politics of American Health Care," *Atlantic* (October 1973), p. 50.

24. Ray E. Brown, "The Purchase of Health Care—Payments, Controls, and Quality," *Report of the National Conference on Medical Costs* (Washington, D.C.: Government Printing Office, 1967), pp. 280-85.

25. Hodgson, op. cit., pp. 53-54.

26. Alexander Auerbach, "Health Insurance by Mail—Does It Justify the Cost," *Los Angeles Times*, May 18, 1972.

27. Brown, op. cit., p. 282.

28. *Con$umer New$week* (May 15, 1972), p. 4.

29. Milton I. Roemer and William Shonick, "HMO Performance: The Recent Evidence," *Health and Society* (Summer 1973), p. 294.

30. Brown, op. cit., p. 282.

31. "Insurers Fight Increase in Health Policy Frauds," *Los Angeles Times*, August 22, 1973.

32. Howard and Martha Lewis, *The Medical Offenders* (New York: Simon and Schuster, 1970), pp. 127-28.

33. Herbert S. Denenberg, "Dr. Strangelove Joins Alice-in-Wonderland in Quest of a National Health Plan," *The Progressive* (May 1973), p. 20.

34. Ibid., p. 20.

35. "Commercial Health Insurance Industry Should be Eliminated, Says Regulator," *Con$umer New$week* (May 15, 1972), p. 1.

36. *More Needs to Be Done to Assure That Physicians' Services—Paid for by Medicare and Medicaid—Are Necessary*, Report to the Congress by the Comptroller General of the United States (Washington, D.C.: U.S. General Accounting Office, 1972), p. 20.

37. Ibid., p. 33.

38. Hodgson, op. cit., pp. 49-50.

39. Kennedy, op. cit., pp. 166-67.

Chapter 15

1. Michael A. Shadid, *Crusading Doctor* (Boston: Meador Publishing Co., 1956), p. 125.

2. Ibid., p. 39.

3. Michael A. Shadid, *Doctors of Today and Tomorrow* (New York and Chicago: Cooperative League of the USA, 1947), p. 140.

4. James Howard Means, *Doctors, People, and Government* (Boston: Atlantic–Little, Brown, 1953), p. 175.

5. *Crusading Doctor*, p. 147.

6. Ibid., pp. 168-69.

7. Ibid., pp. 154-55.

8. Ibid., p. 190.

9. Ibid., p. 262.

10. Means, op. cit., p. 176.

11. Helen Clapesattle, *The Doctors Mayo* (Minneapolis: The University of Minnesota Press, 1963), p. 411.

12. Ibid., p. 400.

13. Nathan Sinaid, Odin W. Anderson, and Melvin L. Dollar, *Health Insurance in the United States* (New York: The Commonwealth Fund, 1946), p. 13.

14. Means, op. cit., p. 142.

15. "Pioneer of Prepaid Medical Care," *Iowa Alumni Review* (April 1965), p. 7.

16. M. B. Rothfeld, "Sensible Surgery for Medical Costs," *Fortune* (April 1973), pp. 87-110.

17. Dan Wakefield, "Dr. Jekyll and the AMA," *Nation*, June 22, 1958; also, "The Miners and the AMA," *Commonweal*, September 19, 1958.

18. William A. MacColl, *Group Practice & Prepayment of Medical Care* (Washington, D.C.: Public Affairs Press, 1966), pp. 88-116.

19. Natalie Davis Spingarn, "A Successful Switch in the Economics of Medicine," *Los Angeles Times*, November 26, 1973.

20. Herman N. and Anne R. Somers, *Doctors, Patients, and Health Insurance* (Washington, D.C.: The Brookings Institution, 1961), p. 349.

21. Means, op. cit., pp. 174-75.

22. *Crusading Doctor*, pp. 290-91.

23. Means, op. cit., p. 174.

24. Ibid., p. 175.

25. *Crusading Doctor*, p. 295.

26. *Brief 31591*, Filed in the Supreme Court of the State of Washington by Houghton, Cluck, Coughlin & Henry and Mervyn F. Bell, pp. 242-43.

27. MacColl, op. cit., p. 142.

28. *Doctors of Today and Tomorrow*, p. 93.

29. MacColl, op. cit., pp. 132-33.

30. Robert Fairbanks, "New Gold Rush—Prepaid Medi-Cal Franchises Sought," *Los Angeles Times*, December 10, 1972.

31. Harry Nelson, "State Again OKs Health Plan Hit as Inadequate," *Los Angeles Times*, February 19, 1973.

32. "Prepaid Health Plan Practices Hit by Post," *Los Angeles Times*, November 16, 1973.

33. *America's Health Needs: The Government's Role* (AFL-CIO Publication No. 131, July 1963), p. 14.

34. Selig Greenberg, *The Troubled Calling* (New York: Macmillan, 1965), p. 171.

35. "The Quality of Prepaid Health Care," *Los Angeles Times*, January 29, 1973.

36. *Group Health and Welfare News*, November 1964, pp. 1-3.

37. *Doctors of Today and Tomorrow*, p. 98.

Chapter 16

1. *Life* (September 17, 1965), p. 105.

2. *JAMA* (March 30, 1946), p. 858.

3. Ibid. (November 9, 1946), p. 600.

4. "A Simple Error in Logic," *Fortune* (October 1961), pp. 122-23; *New York Daily News,* October 27, 1964.

5. William P. Keim, "What the AMA Really Fears," *The New Republic* (February 13, 1964), p. 11.

6. Roul Tunley, *The American Health Scandal* (New York: Harper and Row, 1966), p. 162.

7. *Los Angeles Herald-Examiner*, November 1, 1965.

8. Henry E. Sigerist, *On the Sociology of Medicine*, ed. by Milton I. Roemer (New York: M. D. Publications, 1960), p. 16.

9. *Health Services in Britain* (London: British Information Services, 1964), p. 1.

10. James Howard Means, *Doctors, People, and Government* (Boston: Atlantic–Little Brown, 1953), p. 94.

11. *Health Services in Britain*, pp. 10-16.

12. Sigerist, op. cit., pp. 113-38.

13. Tunley, op. cit., pp. 200-201.

14. Gunnar Biorck, *Trends in the Development of Medical Care in Sweden* (Stockholm: Swedish Institute, 1965), pp. 6-7.

15. Gillis Albinsson, *Public Health Services in Sweden* (Linköping: The Swedish Hospital Association, 1963), pp. 25-27.

16. Karl Evang, D. Stark Murray, and Walter J. Lear, *Medical Care and Family Security* (Englewood Cliffs, N.J.: Prentice-Hall, 1963), p. 80.

17. "The World's Most Socialized Medicine," *Life* (January 23, 1970), pp. 39-48.

18. "China's 'Politicized' Health Care Process; Three Views," *The Nation's Health* (May 1973), p. 5.

19. Ibid.

20. Ibid.

21. Janet Goldwasser, Stuart Dowty, and Maud Russell, "Dr. Norman Bethune: What This Canadian Comrade Means to the Chinese People," *Far East Reporter*, 1973.

22. George Roth, "Medical Care in North Viet Nam," *American Report* (December 18, 1972), p. 15.

23. John Champlin, "Poor Health Care in the South," *American Report* (February 12, 1973), p. 17.

24. "Grand Design for Europe's MDs," *Medical World News*, July 30, 1965, p. 46.

25. Pete Hamill, "Doctors Go on Strike," *Saturday Evening Post* (May 6, 1964), p. 82.

26. "Strike Prognosis," *The Observer* (July 18, 1965), editorial.

27. Milton I. Roemer, "Socialized Health Services in Saskatchewan," *Social Research* (Spring 1958), pp. 87-101.

28. *The Progressive* (April 1965), p. 8.

29. "2 and ½ Years Later: Canada's Doctor Strike," *Look* (March 23, 1965), pp. 101-5.

30. "Those Radical Canadians," *The Progressive* (August 1964).

31. H. Rocke Robertson, *Health Care in Canada: A Commentary* (Ottawa: Science Council of Canada, 1973).

32. Ibid., p. 71.

33. Ibid., p. 63.

34. Ibid., p. 51.

Chapter 17

1. *Group Health and Welfare News* (August 1973), p. 5.

2. *Study of Health Facilities Construction Costs*, Report to the Congress by the Comptroller General of the United States (Washington, D.C.: General Accounting Office, November 20, 1972), p. 95.

3. Caldwell B. Esselstyn, "Statement to the Ways and Means Committee of the House of Representatives in Support of H. R. 3920," November 20, 1963.

4. Bel Kaufman, *Up the Down Staircase* (Englewood Cliffs, N.J.: Prentice-Hall, 1965), p. 167.

5. John Schulman, Jr., and Carol Wood, "Experience of a Nurse Practitioner in a General Medical Clinic," *JAMA* (March 13, 1972), pp. 1453-61.

6. Doug Shuit, "Fire Bond Link to Paramedics Sought for 'Voter Salability,'" *Los Angeles Times*, December 16, 1974.

7. William A. MacColl, "Alternatives in Health Care," *Proceedings of a Seminar on Prepaid Group Practice Health Plans*, Conducted by the Center for Labor Education and Research, University of Colorado, March 20-21, ed. by Walter H. Uphoff, CLEAR Publication No. 2, pp. 63-64.

8. Robert Fairbanks, "Favoritism in Medi-Cal Spurs $50,000 Boon," *Los Angeles Times*, June 17, 1974.

9. "Consumers' Guide to Doctors Stirs Tempers," *Los Angeles Times,* October 23, 1974.

10. "Nursing 'Horror Tale' Being Probed Here," *Los Angeles Herald-Examiner*, January 24, 1975.

11. *Study of Health Facilities Construction Costs*, p. 98.

12. Ibid., pp. 109-10.

13. Ronald J. Ostrow, "Doctors, Professionals May Face Antitrust Action, Saxbe Says," *Los Angeles Times*, December 7, 1974.

14. John E. Deitrick, "Independence or Dependence," *Journal of Medical Education* (January 1964), p. 5.

15. *Planning for Medical Progress Through Education*, Association of American Medical Colleges, April 1965.

Index

H34
(010.573)